AF766575

FOOD SAFETY

FOOD SAFETY
Past, Present, and Predictions

DARIN S. DETWILER

ELSEVIER

ACADEMIC PRESS

An imprint of Elsevier

Academic Press is an imprint of Elsevier
125 London Wall, London EC2Y 5AS, United Kingdom
525 B Street, Suite 1650, San Diego, CA 92101, United States
50 Hampshire Street, 5th Floor, Cambridge, MA 02139, United States
The Boulevard, Langford Lane, Kidlington, Oxford OX5 1GB, United Kingdom

Library of Congress Cataloging-in-Publication Data
A catalog record for this book is available from the Library of Congress

British Library Cataloguing-in-Publication Data
A catalogue record for this book is available from the British Library

ISBN: 978-0-12-818219-2

For information on all Academic Press publications
visit our website at https://www.elsevier.com/books-and-journals

Publisher: Charlotte Cockle
Acquisitions Editor: Patricia M. Osborn
Editorial Project Manager: Emerald Li
Production Project Manager: Kamesh Ramajogi
Designer: Christian J. Bilbow

Typeset by Thomson Digital

I dedicate this work to the memory and legacy of my son.

Riley Edward Detwiler, 1991–1993

Riley Detwiler

Riley's death at the age of 18 months, due to *E. coli O157:H7* during the landmark 1993 Jack in the Box outbreak, "shook the nation."

When he was only a few months old, I justified being out to sea on a Navy submarine by telling myself that I was making the world a safer place for him, and I would spend the rest of my life making up lost time with him when he was older. I learned about the dangers of this deadly foodborne pathogen on his deathbed.

I have since spent more than half of my life having outlived Riley and trying one way or another to prevent other parents from looking at their family table with a chair forever empty due to preventable deaths from food safety failures.

Toddler's Death Shakes the Nation. (1993). *The Orlando Sentinel.* Available from: http://articles.orlandosentinel.com/1993-02-28/news/9302270333_1_detwiler-coli-infection-riley

Contents

Author biography

Dr. Darin Detwiler, LP.D., MA.Ed., is an internationally recognized and respected food policy expert with over 25 years' experience in shaping federal food policy, consulting with corporations, and contributing thought leadership to industry events and publications. He advises industry, NGOs, and government agencies, addressing food safety and authenticity issues in the United States and abroad. In 2018, Detwiler received the International Association for Food Protection (IAFP) Distinguished Service Award (Sponsored by *Food Safety Magazine*).

Since 1993, Detwiler has consulted with the USDA in strengthening food safety policies, particularly in the areas of consumer education, product labeling, and their pathogen reduction program. In addition to serving in various educational, editorial, and advisory capacities, his committee work includes appointments to two terms as a member of the National Advisory Committee on Meat and Poultry Inspection for USDA, where his work improved standards and policies related to risk-based sampling. As the senior policy coordinator for Stop Foodborne Illness, a national food safety organization, he evaluated pertinent regulatory issues for the USDA and the FDA as a consumer advocate in their stakeholder advisory group. His work supported the FDA's efforts for implementation of the Food Safety Modernization Act. He later served as a council member for the Conference for Food Protection, identifying and addressing emerging problems of food safety to influence model laws and regulations among all government agencies.

Detwiler is the Assistant Dean at Northeastern University's College of Professional Studies and the Lead Faculty of the Master of Science in Regulatory Affairs of Food and Food Industries. As a Professor of food regulatory policy, he has specialized in food safety, global economics of food and agriculture, Blockchain, and food authenticity.

Detwiler received his Doctor of Law and Policy from Northeastern University with a research focus on state implementation of federal food policies.

Foreword 1

Darin Detwiler and I met under the most dire of circumstances: the 1993 Jack in the Box *E. coli* O157:H7 outbreak in the Pacific Northwest. About 700 people became ill and, tragically, 4 children died, when contaminated hamburger patties were undercooked by grill operators in this restaurant chain. This event was a watershed event in the history of food safety. At the time of the outbreak, I was the Director of Microbiology for the United States Department of Agriculture, Food Safety and Inspection Service's Office of Science and Technology (the precursor of the Office of Public Health and Science). I was a member of the USDA leadership team investigating this outbreak and I led the laboratory investigations to identify the contaminated lots of meat and remove them from commerce. Darin's son Riley tragically lost his life due to a secondary infection in the outbreak.

The Jack in the Box outbreak was the catalyst for unprecedented food safety changes in US government regulations, the meat industry, and consumer practices in the 1990s. No other event had radically changed the meat industry since Upton Sinclair's book, *The Jungle*, exposed unsanitary practices of the meat industry and led to two new regulations: the Pure Food and Drug Act of 1906 and the Federal Meat Inspection Act of 1906. In the aftermath of this crisis, FSIS declared *E. coli* O157:H7 an adulterant in raw ground beef, published the Pathogen Reduction/Hazard Analysis and Critical Control Points Rule, added safe handling labels to raw meat and poultry products, and created the Office of Public Health and Science, among other initiatives. All were designed to improve the safety of meat and poultry products, especially raw ground beef.

Parents of the *E. coli* victims lobbied to change the government and industry practices to better protect the health of consumers and improve the safety of the US food supply. I believe these parents were the true heroes of the outbreak since they worked beside those of us in government seeking to enact regulatory and industry reform, often working despite their grieving. They were true partners to us in seeking regulatory change: testifying beside us in federal and state legislative hearings, participating in USDA hearings and briefings, and sharing their tragic stories with the media so other consumers could learn how to better protect their families from a similar fate. Darin personally worked with the USDA on their initiative to add safe handling instruction labels for consumers to packages of raw meat and poultry products.

After leaving USDA, Darin and I worked in the same food safety circles but did not have the chance to work together again as closely as we had during the outbreak and its aftermath. Our friendship was rekindled when we both spoke on a panel at the 2017 Food Safety Consortium in Schaumburg, IL. With a focus on looking back at the 1993 *E. coli* outbreak, we were joined by Bill Marler (noted attorney and expert on foodborne illness) and Mike Taylor (former FDA Deputy Commissioner for Foods). This was an emotional, yet powerful moment for all of us, and one that was 25 years or so in the making.

Darin and I also had breakfast together in Salt Lake City, UT, during the 2018 annual meeting of the International Association of Food Protection (IAFP). Darin was receiving IAFP's prestigious Distinguished Service Award, sponsored by *Food Safety Magazine*, and I was presenting the John H. Silliker lecture. As we reminisced about the past and our current interests, we learned that we shared a passion for advocating for complete adoption of the Food and Drug Administration's Food Code. This code is guidance material that describes current best practices for storing, preparing, and serving food in foodservice and retail establishments and is used as a model by local, state, federal, and tribal regulators to develop their own food safety policies. Content is developed by academicians, regulators, consumer advocates, and industry members of the Conference for Food Protection. However, since the code is guidance material and not law, regulators in the about 3000 state, local, territorial, and tribal jurisdictions may choose to adopt some, none, or all of the current code versions and recommendations.

The lack of complete adoption requires owners of establishments that cross-jurisdictional lines using various codes (or parts of codes) to have differing training programs for employees to be in compliance for health inspections. Lack of uniform national standards also results in health inspections that are not consistent in content across all states and jurisdictions leading to incomplete data for trending and analysis and differences in inspection criteria and grading. Most importantly, the lack of complete adoption of the current version of the food code means that state and local regulators are not using the most up-to-date scientific recommendations for storing, preparing, and serving safe food. Indeed, one state is currently using a version of the code that is 24 years old! United in the cause of campaigning for complete adoption of the food code by regulatory agencies, Darin and I collaborate and speak about this issue in various industry symposia. We urge you to join in this cause.

Darin has been in the forefront of food safety reform since the tragic events of the Jack in the Box outbreak. This book is a compelling look at the history and future of food safety and regulatory policy written from the perspective of a person who is not only an academic, but also a parent who turned the loss of a son during an outbreak into a mission to support the industry and government, as well as a respected food safety professional who has long been involved in the issues. It should be read by every food safety professional. I highly recommend it.

Dr Ann Marie McNamara

About the Foreword 1 Author

Dr. Ann Marie McNamara is the former Director of Microbiology, USDA, Food Safety and Inspection Service, Office of Public Health and Science during the Jack in the Box outbreak. She has worked in all areas of food safety: in the government, in manufacturing as Vice President of Food Safety and Technology at Sara Lee Corporation, in research/consulting as Vice President of Food Safety and Scientific Affairs at Silliker, Inc., in foodservice as Vice President of Food Safety and Regulatory Affairs at Jack in the Box, Inc., in retail as Vice President of Food and Essentials Safety and Quality Assurance at Target Corp., and in foodservice and manufacturing as Vice President of Food Safety and Quality Assurance at US Foods. For her work in investigating the Jack in the Box outbreak, Dr. McNamara and her team won a Superior Service Award from the Secretary of Agriculture. Among her honors and awards, she was the recipient of five USDA Superior Service awards including recognition as a coauthor of the USDA Pathogen Reduction/HACCP regulation, and most recently accepted the Food Marketing Institute's Food Safety Innovation Award on behalf of Target for the development and implementation of a health inspection management program supported by Hazel Analytics automated analysis platform.

Foreword 2

I never met Riley. However, I have a vivid memory 27 years later of his tiny white casket flashing across the front page of Seattle papers and evening news. I remember the picture of Riley that Darin carries a smiling toddler, planning mischief.

Riley's life was cut short by a deadly pathogen that had been long ignored by government and industry and was virtually unknown to consumers. In 1993 we all thought hamburgers were the all-American meal - not a recipe for death.

Riley and my daughter, Morgan, would have graduated from high school in 2010 and would be 28 this year. For Darin, instead of 28 years of memories and a future with his grown son, he has photos and videos of a forever young Riley and faded clippings of the public's view of Riley's agonizing death and the pain on his parents' faces.

It is an honor to be a part of Riley's story but it's with anguish I recognize that the beginning of my life's work is forever linked to Riley's death and the deaths of Lauren Rudolph, Michael Nole and Celina Shribbs, and the devastating life-long illnesses of so many others caused by *E. coli* O157:H7, including Brianne Kiner, who was hospitalized for several months after Riley died a few hospital rooms away.

In the intervening years, there have been too many stories like Riley's and Brianne's. I have done what I could to help those families impacted by *E. coli*, *Salmonella*, *Listeria*, and other foodborne pathogens. I have done what I could to change government and industry behavior by using the levers of the legal system. However, regardless of how passionate I might be at times to be "put out of business," it pales to what Darin Detwiler has done in the memory of his son.

As a lawyer, I have seen what can happen to a parent of a child that dies or has life-long complications caused by a pathogen like *E. coli*. Understandably, many never recover or simply cope by ignoring the pain. Few, like Darin, stare directly at the pain, embrace it, learn from it and teach us from it. Every word of this book written by Riley's father carries a bit of Riley in every sentence, page, and chapter. This book is important. Thank you, Darin, for writing it and thank you, Riley, for inspiring it.

William "Bill" Marler

About the Foreword 2 Author

William "Bill" Marler has become the most prominent foodborne illness lawyer in America and a major force in food policy in the U.S. and around the world. He is the managing partner of Marler Clark, a Seattle, Washington, based law firm that specializes in foodborne illness cases. He began litigating foodborne illness cases in 1993, during the landmark Jack in the Box *E. coli* O157:H7 outbreak. For over 25 years, he has represented thousands of individuals in claims against food companies whose contaminated products have caused life altering injury and even death. Marler's advocacy for a safer food supply includes petitioning the USDA to better regulate pathogenic *E. coli*, working with nonprofit food safety and foodborne illness victims' organizations, and helping spur the passage of the 2010 FDA Food Safety Modernization Act. His work has led to invitations to address local, national, and international gatherings on food safety, including testimony before the U.S. House of Representatives Committee on Energy and Commerce. He is the publisher of the online news site, *Food Safety News* and in 2016 the American Bar Association listed his award-winning blog, www.marlerblog.com as one of the top 100 legal blogs. Marler's numerous awards include the 2010 NSF Food Safety Leadership Award for Education. Marler contributes to Food Safety News and the Food Poison Journal.

Marler's latest efforts include petitioning (along with some victims and activist groups) the USDA's Food Safety Inspection Service to ban dozens of *Salmonella* strains from meat and poultry (Kindy, 2020).

Reference

Kindy, K. (2020). He helped make burgers safe. Now he's fighting food poisoning again. The Washington Post. Available from: https://www.washingtonpost.com/national/he-helped-make-burgers-safer-now-hes-fighting-food-poisoning-again/2020/01/18/5b979cf8-38ad-11ea-9541-9107303481a4_story.html..

Preface

Certain newspaper headlines are frozen in our minds. The ones that seem to rise to the top of the lists for conversations—especially for those "Where were you when ...?" scenarios—most often pertain to tragedy.

I remember vividly the 1979 headlines about the Three Mile Island incident involving a nuclear power electricity-generating station in Pennsylvania, on the other side of the country from where I was living at the time. Sure, we only had a few TV network stations at that time, but it seemed like we were bombarded by 24-hour coverage of the partial meltdown of a nuclear reactor and radioactive releases with potential public health effects. I also remember the leadership shown by President Jimmy Carter as he walked through the plant's control room only a few days after the incident began. Even though I was only 11 years old at that time, it created in me an awareness of an invisible threat: something from which we cannot necessarily hide.

I also remember, not too many years later, the 1986 Space Shuttle Challenger explosion. What started out as live TV coverage of American astronauts launching into space ended shortly after the shuttle broke apart only seconds into its flight, killing all seven crew members, including one who would have been the first teacher in space. For me, again, the idea frozen in my mind is that as great as we are as a nation in terms of scientific development and technological advancement, we are all still vulnerable. There are always opportunities for flaws and for something perceived as insignificant to cause catastrophic failure.

In 1993, a third headline captured my attention, this one regarding an *E. coli* outbreak at Jack in the Box fast-food restaurants in the Pacific Northwest. At the time the news was breaking, I had finished serving in the Navy, where I worked in the engineering plant of a nuclear submarine. I thought I was reasonably intelligent, yet I had never heard of *E. coli*. My wife and I, along with our 9-year-old and 16-month-old sons lived about 90 miles north of Seattle. Our first thoughts were that we would be safe if avoided eating in Seattle. As the news revealed more information, my precautions grew to include my family avoiding hamburgers. Finally, we learned that we should avoid eating hamburgers from a specific restaurant. If I were afraid for any one of us, it was for my stepson, thinking that he was vulnerable. But I soon became aware of the fact that some of those assumptions would fall short of protecting my family.

We all learned an important lesson. There are different ways in which people get sick from contaminated food. In 1993, my youngest son Riley was the child I thought we would not have to worry about because at his very young age he had never even eaten a hamburger and would not any time soon. That did not matter, however, as he became ill with *E. coli* not from directly eating food contaminated with a foodborne pathogen, but because of *person-to-person* contamination—from another child in his day care who was sick with *E. coli*.

Even while sitting by my son's bedside for weeks, I assumed that this was going to be a long, difficult recovery from a horrible illness and that my son was going to survive. I clipped newspaper articles about the outbreak, articles that mentioned his name, and articles about the investigators. Friends and family sent clippings along with "get well" cards. I planned to create an album to use when he was old enough to explain how brave he was and how he overcame incredible medical challenges.

I still have many of those old newspaper clippings. And, aside from family photos and video of a young boy being loved and learning how to walk, I have four immortal images burned into my memory from 1993.

One image is a look in my son's eyes as he sat on my lap while I held him in his hospital bed the day he was first admitted. At only 16 months of age, he could not understand how his IV bag, hanging at the bedside, was not a bottle that he could hold and drink.

The second image comes from something I saw on the TV news, as I had been prevented from getting close enough to be there in person. I saw the immediately recognizable characteristics of my son's face, peeking out from under the blankets and the sides of a basket that was being loaded into a helicopter, as he was about to be airlifted to Seattle Children's Hospital almost 90 miles away.

The third is from that hospital's pediatric intensive care unit, where I saw barely visible portions of my son's face and body surrounded by medical equipment while in a medically induced coma for weeks.

The final image comes from when I watched two men carrying my young son in a white coffin on a cold February morning. That coffin was far smaller than a coffin should ever be.

I remember how I long held on to a belief—based on what I recognized as the enormous reaction of the government, the overwhelming coverage from the media, and the outpouring of support from people around the country—that somehow science or policy or industry would find a way to prevent these failures from happening again. In the years that followed, I helped leaders at the USDA make changes in safe handling labels, in federal food safety policies, and in inspection criteria. My goal at the time was that my son's death from *E. coli* might, at least, play a role in preventing other parents from going through my experience.

Unfortunately, I am not alone in carrying the burden of memories like these stemming from failures in food safety. All these years later, we are still bombarded on a weekly basis with the coverage of outbreaks and recalls, of victims, and of other families who bury little children due to *E. coli*, *Salmonella*, or some other foodborne pathogen. While those most often hospitalized or killed are young children, no age group is immune to foodborne pathogens.

No large corporation is immune to failures that happen before, during, or after their involvement with a product. Since 1993, we have seen the seemingly uninterrupted cycle of crisis-and-reform through headline after headline of multistate outbreaks and huge recalls involving major labels and national retail or restaurant chains. The early food safety focus on meat and poultry soon included recalls and outbreaks tied to cantaloupe, leafy greens, sprouts, caramel apples, ice cream, peanut butter, and other produce. Ready-to-eat and commercially packaged goods such as cereals and salads also found their way onto lists of contaminated products.

Many times, even the efforts of those companies and leaders who did everything they could to protect their consumers would be thwarted by improper handling, inadequate cooking, or some other action down the line. However, news coverage and even documentaries have highlighted investigation after investigation and lawsuit after lawsuit. We have even watched executives discuss their companies' stock values fall and, often, rise again.

I often hear the voices of other victims and their families who have also shared the true burden of disease with industry, policymakers, and consumer advocates who also served on committees and boards involved in improving food safety for others. Today, the FDA Food Safety Modernization Act stands as an example of one of the most significant pieces of food safety legislation made law only because of the hard work of young survivors, parents, experts, victims' lawyers, and advocacy groups.

A few years ago, I met with an official in Washington, DC, who stated that we only needed to be concerned with young children who ate contaminated food. His assessment was far from complete. My message to him was that foodborne pathogens affect people of *all* ages, but certain "vulnerable populations," such as very young children, pregnant women, the elderly, and people with a compromised immune system, are more likely to develop severe symptoms or even die. Further, I pointed out that foodborne illnesses could be transmitted through contaminated food, contaminated water/air, person-to-person contact, or through contact with animals.

The Centers for Disease Control and Prevention (CDC) estimates that each year, 48 million Americans become ill from foodborne pathogens, 128,000 are hospitalized, and 3,000 die (CDC, 2018). Since Riley's death in the landmark 1993 *E. coli* outbreak, the math shows that over 75,000 American consumers have died from foodborne illnesses, a large portion of which could have been prevented (Mead et al., 1999). However, I often hear federal food regulators and industry executives make statements that the American food supply is "the safest in the world." Many experts have criticized these misleading statements as they portray a lesser sense of risk to policymakers and to consumers (Krebs, 2004). The frequency and quantity of meat recalls, along with the number of outbreaks, illnesses, and deaths tied to foodborne pathogens indicate that problems still exist somewhere between the farm and the table.

Even with government regulations, science-based inspections, and audit systems in place, America's "safest in the world" food supply is far from perfect. The investigation and reporting of foodborne illnesses by state and county health departments are critical in the prevention of foodborne disease in the United States. The past, present, and future of food safety involves reform across the full spectrum of economic, geographic, legal, political, and social systems.

Invisible threats are not always thousands of miles away from us, brought to our attention solely through a news story. Catastrophic failures are not exclusive to undertakings far from those of normal daily activities. And inevitably, no matter how hard we try to avoid being at risk, families are often vulnerable to outside threats great and small.

There will never be an end to pathogens in our food, but we can change the culture around the future of food safety. To do so will require a Herculean effort: an enormous amount of work, strength, and courage.

The first-hand accounts in this book are included with the goal of benefiting industry and consumers such that the future of food safety will result in few chairs forever empty at family tables.

References

Centers for Disease Control and Prevention (2018). Estimates of Foodborne Illness in the United States. Available from: http://www.cdc.gov/foodborneburden/index.html.

Krebs, A. (2004). Debunking the myth that the U.S. "Has the Safest Food in the World. The Agribusiness Examiner. Available from: http://www.organicconsumers.org/foodsafety/foodmyth040504.cfm.

Mead, P., Slutsker, L., Dietz, V., McCaig, L., Bresee, J., Shapiro, C., et al. (1999). Food-related illness and death in the United States. Centers for Disease Control and Prevention. Available from: http://wwwnc.cdc.gov/eid/article/5/5/99-0502.

Acknowledgments

Had I been asked 25 years ago if there would be a need to tell these stories, to connect with other families, and to share the true burden of disease with policymakers today, I would have responded with the assumption that the problem of foodborne pathogen outbreaks would be solved by now.

I wish to acknowledge the support from my family and friends and all those who have been touched by Riley's death and my message over these years.

This book would not have been possible if not for the contributions of many people who allowed me to share their firsthand knowledge. Many fine leaders and consumer advocates in organizations, such as Stop Foodborne Illness, The Center for Science in the Public Interest, The Consumer Federation of America, and The Pew Charitable Trusts, inspired me to dig deeper into my work with consumer advocacy and policy. Key figures at the USDA and the FDA, including Mike Taylor, Dr. Stephen Ostroff, and Jill Hollingsworth have been instrumental and extremely supportive of my collaboration with regulators. Tanya Roberts has been someone whose economics of food safety work I have read for years. Meeting with her in person and interviewing her for this book was a gift. I also can say the same about Dr. John Kobayashi, whose work in epidemiology played a key role over the decades, and about Caroline Smith DeWaal, whose leadership through the decades greatly inspired me. I am forever thankful to Bill Marler for his direct and indirect impacts on my knowledge and my actions.

Additional voices in this book come from many dedicated and respected experts in their respective fields. I wish to also acknowledge the following for their time and their willingness to share their perspectives: JoNel Aleccia, Jeff Almer, Mitzi Baum, Alan Baumfalk, Doug Beach, Ali Berlow, Dennis Bounds, Linda Byron, Joseph Corby, Christine Haughney Dare-Bryan, Sandra Eskin, Adam Friedlander, Thomas Gremillion, Rylee Gustafson, Jorge Hernandez, Michael Hicks, Anna Jesus, Nathan Libbey, Lisa Lupo, Valerie Madamba, Gina McCarthy, Brad McNamara, Sean O'Leary, Kevin Otto, Patrick Quade, Joseph Robertson, Brian Ronholm, Robin Strombler, Dr. Barbara VanRenterghem, and Jeremy Zenlea.

Writing a book like this is personal and professional. The many interviews became opportunities for reconnection as well as validation. I found moments of new connections amid moments of reflection and healing.

For me, the work behind this book drew support and inspiration from some who are not part of this topic, but who became part of my process, including Dr. Keenan Davis, Anne Elliott, Dr. Dustin Harp, Dr. Jonathan Kramer, Dr. Kristin Lee, and Shane Zimmer.

Dr. Neenah Estrella-Luna provided incredible guidance through my doctoral research into food safety policy. Dr. Ann Marie McNamara worked generously with me and with my graduate students at Northeastern University to explore new directions in FDA Food Code adoption for states. Anna Jesus also collaborated with my graduate students and played a significant role in my comfort with collaborating with industry. As someone who placed one foot in academia and the other in food policy for many years, I wish to thank the leadership at Northeastern University's College of Professional Studies for supporting my academic work for graduate students in the food industry. I also wish to acknowledge my teaching peers in Washington State (Leah Smith and David Roderick to name just a few) who supported my work in and out of the classroom.

Finally, I wish to acknowledge my best friend and wife, Gennette. She saw in me the capability and the significance of which I had lost sight long ago. She pushed me when I was stubborn, pulled me when I was weak, cared for me when I was sick, and always greeted me with excitement when I returned after my many trips to spread the word about food safety. I would never have accomplished this if it were not for her love and support.

CHAPTER 1

2018: past and present collide

"What's evolved is an understanding that the interests of consumers are aligned with the industry's interests."
Mike Taylor, FDA Deputy Commissioner for Foods, 2010–16

"Continuous improvement is still needed."
Dr. Stephen Ostroff, FDA Deputy Commissioner for Foods, 2016–18

Although 1993 is referred to frequently as a pivotal year for the current state of food safety, many years before and since have seen failures and successes resulting in improvements to science, policy, and culture around protecting consumers. A broad look at the many significant food safety-related events of 2018, however, affords a useful opportunity to examine the past, present, and future predictions for food safety.

On January 4, 2018, the Trump administration's Food and Drug Administration (FDA) published *Guidance for Industry: Policy Regarding Certain Entities Subject to the Current Good Manufacturing Practice and Preventive Controls, Produce Safety, and/or Foreign Supplier Verification Programs* in which the administration stated:

> *"The purpose of this document is to state the intent of the Food and Drug Administration (FDA, we, or the Agency) not to enforce certain regulatory requirements as they currently apply to certain entities and/or activities .... we intend to exercise enforcement discretion with regard to the preventive controls requirements."*
> ***(FDA, 2018a)***

Thus, the FDA, previously sued by the Center for Food Safety and the Center for Environmental Health in 2012 for failure to implement provisions of the 2010 FDA Food Safety Modernization Act (FSMA) in a timely manner, now stated that they may not "exercise enforcement" as previously outlined in their rules. Specifically, that 2012 lawsuit asserted that the FDA failed to meet several mandated enforcement action deadlines related to Section 204 of FSMA related to the goal of "rapidly and effectively" preventing or mitigating foodborne illness (Bottemiller, 2012). Just as delaying enforcement deadlines caused concern, this new idea of "enforcement discretion" on the part of the FDA did not sit well with many.

Food Safety
http://dx.doi.org/10.1016/B978-0-12-818219-2.00001-6

As pointed out by Dr. Peter G. Lurie, President of the Center for Science in the Public Interest, "The announcement is a rotten anniversary present," given that President Barack Obama signed FSMA into law on this very day 7 long years ago (January 2011) (Lurie, 2018). This announcement also took place just as investigators and health officials were dealing with a multistate/multinational outbreak (17 cases across 13 states and 17 cases across 5 eastern provinces in Canada) tied to lettuce (Scutti, 2018). Only a few months later, multistate outbreaks of *Escherichia coli* tied to romaine lettuce sickened 210 consumers across 36 states, sending 96 to the hospital and identified as the cause of 5 deaths (CDC, 2018).

These legislative actions and *E. coli* outbreaks all coincided with the 25th anniversary of the landmark, 1993 "Jack in the Box" *E. coli* outbreak that shocked the nation. That outbreak, tied to ground beef sold in fast-food restaurants, resulted in a shock to public health. State public health departments in Washington, Idaho, Nevada, and California reported laboratory-confirmed infections of 723 people, hospitalization of 171 people (45 were children under the age of 10), and the deaths of 4 toddlers (Heiman, Mody, Johnson, Griffin, & Gould, 2015). Today, food safety experts still refer to the 1993 outbreak as the "9/11 of the food industry" (Childers, 2015).

A panel discussion of that seminal outbreak took place at the December 2017, Food Safety Consortium, in Schaumburg, IL. The timing of this panel sat in stark contrast to what some attendees reported about a handful of major companies. They talked about how some chains who rarely attend such industry events still prioritize that their company's well-being over consumers' complaints (about food-related illnesses or metal objects found in products) should be viewed with suspicion.

The panel of leading food scientists and authorities included Michael Taylor, former FDA deputy commissioner and FSIS administrator, Seattle attorney William Marler (noted for his representation of foodborne illness plaintiffs over the last 25 years), Ann Marie McNamara, who succeeded Dr. David Theno at Jack in the Box when he retired, and myself—Dr. Darin Detwiler, an Assistant Dean and Professor of Food Regulatory Compliance at Northeastern University's College of Professional Studies. My son, Riley, became ill from pathogenic *E. coli* O157:H7 and died from hemolytic uremic syndrome (HUS) during that 1993 outbreak.

Panelists credited the late Dr. David Theno with demonstrating the effectiveness of biological sampling and a HACCP-based approach in restaurants to contaminant control. His work changed the tradition of face-value acceptance of supplier assurances. Hired by the corporate offices at Jack in the Box immediately after the 1993 outbreak, Theno pioneered customer inspections of production facilities, an unusual practice in the early 1990s. His work also paved the way for the independent, third-party food safety audits, now standard practice throughout the industry.

Panelists also reminded industry leaders in the audience of what was normal before the 1993 outbreak: companies "passing-the-buck" and distancing themselves from taking responsibility for deaths and illnesses from adulterated meat, companies blaming the US Department of Agriculture (USDA) inspectors and even blaming consumers who failed to adequately cook ground beef.

One important message about then, versus now, was that gathering critical public health information in 1993 was nowhere near as easy as it is now. Ann Marie McNamara shared how the 4- to 5-day wait for lab confirmation of *E. coli* infection "was a big frustration during the outbreak when every hour mattered for children in intensive care units" (Beach, 2017).

William Marler reflected on the aftermath of the 1993 event, describing the USDA's war on *E. coli* O157:H7 as "a huge success story," in that the cost of recalls and multimillion-dollar settlements forced beef processors to change their business model and invest heavily in preventive actions (Higgins, 2018).

Earlier in the consortium, William Shaw, the USDA Food Safety Inspection Service (FSIS)'s food safety risk manager, shared a sign that these actions have made an impact. Sampling of raw ground beef for *E. coli* O157:H7 by FSIS in 2018 is producing positive results 0.09% of the time, down significantly from 0.87% back in 2001 (Higgins, 2018).

Mike Taylor reminded the audience for context that the recalls and hearings over melamine (an industrial chemical compound used in the production of laminates, glues, and flame retardants) in pet food, milk powder, and infant formula and the *E. coli*-related recalls of ground beef were seemingly daily headlines. He also discussed the crisis of confidence in the safety of processed foods that emerged during high-profile recalls that reached a head with Peanut Corporation of America (PCA)'s *Salmonella* outbreak of 2008–9 (more about PCA in Chapter 6). Taylor stated that, "What's evolved is an understanding that the interests of consumers are aligned with the industry's interests" (Higgins, 2018).

I took the stage after Taylor to share the true burden of disease with details of my son's death. I showed photos from Riley's brief life: a few before he became sick, then ones of him in my arms as I held him in a hospital bed early after being admitted, being airlifted to Children's Hospital, after being placed in a coma, and being carried in a far-too-small white coffin. I also took the time to honor the other children who perished in the outbreak. The young lives of Lauren Rudolph, Michael James Nole, and Celina Shribbs were cut short earlier in that outbreak. Their families and I have seen the repeated stories of outbreaks and deaths play out again and again over the last 25 years. Outlining the impact that families have had, I then described my work—to prevent others from suffering like my son and family—with the government, with industry, and with consumers in the 25 years since my loss. I also stated that my work with organizations and industry groups has placed me in a position to observe that "There are some in the food industry that do not take food safety as seriously as others" (Higgins, 2018).

Finally, I shared how I see hope for social media's role in shrinking the size of outbreaks and larger preventive efforts by the food industry. Social media has shown time after time the power to gather information. One such example is IWasPoisoned.com—a crowdsourcing website that gives consumers the ability to report their food-poisoning experiences as they occur. This website has already helped health officials identify and shorten outbreak investigations, such as the 2015 Chipotle Mexican Grill outbreaks. Facebook has also helped to convey information and shape an awareness of food safety. I also highlighted the role of consumers in driving some change through these kinds of sites.

Dr. Stephen Ostroff, who was at the time serving as the FDA's Deputy Commissioner for Foods and Veterinary Medicine, discussed how *Campylobacter* and *Salmonella* cases had not seen much improvement since the 1990s. FDA-regulated food companies continue to lag behind, he said. Better diagnostics and surveillance systems mask progress in processor performance, and, as Ostroff suggested, "Continuous improvement is still needed" (Higgins, 2018).

Ostroff also addressed concerns about food safety priorities under the Trump administration. At the time the White House had not yet requested any relaxation in enforcement, and Ostroff's (then) boss, FDA Commissioner, Scott Gottlieb, had signaled his commitment to food safety (Gottlieb, 2018), Dr. Ostroff went on to add that while we have an administration "focused on reducing regulatory burdens … 'What are the implications' for FSMA's [the 2010 FDA Food Safety Modernization Act] preventive-control rules?" (Higgins, 2018).

The year 2018 would find a series of challenges to food safety become rather visible to the public as glaring warnings that threats to the family meal could not be simply solved with our current actions and policies.

First, the romaine lettuce outbreak in early 2018 was followed by another romaine lettuce outbreak in late November sickening 62 consumers across 16 states (along with illnesses reported in Canada) with 25 hospitalizations and no reported deaths. The outbreak investigation from multiple stakeholders traced the romaine lettuce to harvest areas of the central coastal growing regions of Northern and Central California (CDC, 2019). This was the second one in 2018 and the third in just 1 year, as a December 2017 outbreak tied to romaine lettuce sickening 25 consumers across 15 states (and in Canada) with nine hospitalizations and one reported death (CDC, 2018).

Food safety experts were not alone in their criticism of the industry not having learned any lessons in prevention and in traceability through these three outbreaks, as well as having had the opportunity to learn from the 2006 outbreak tied to romaine lettuce. This criticism was met with opposition to the CDC's call to stop eating romaine lettuce until more information was available. In his November 30, 2018, guest op-ed published in the *Wall Street Journal*, Jim Prevor wrote "Lettuce Try Not to Panic," declaring that the CDC overreacted by advising consumers not to eat romaine lettuce from the Northern and Central California growing regions or if they do not know where it was grown (Prevor, 2018). Founder and publisher of Produce Business magazine and known as the "Perishable Pundit," Prevor justified his position using incomplete reported data from an ongoing outbreak and completely ignored data from previous outbreaks tied to the same product.

This served as an eye opener in terms of food safety and how some may be reacting to the current state of "fake news" or "alternative facts" and the shift away from a reliance on science and data. Stephen Ostroff, MD, the FDA's Deputy Commissioner of Foods and Veterinary Medicine at the time, is still not too shy to state how he views the science on this issue. "… there's just something inherently problematic about things like leafy greens. Even with all of the research trying to figure out how you can make them safer, there's still going be a risk associated with those types of products" (Stephen Ostroff, Personal Communication, 2019).

Second, only 1 week before Thanksgiving, the USDA recalled over 250,000 pounds of four Jennie-O Turkey products linked to a *Salmonella* outbreak which sickened 216 consumers across 38 states (and in Canada), hospitalizing 84 people and resulting in 1 death (CDC, 2018). This holiday warning of ongoing outbreaks and recalls tied to romaine lettuce, cake mixes (FDA, 2018b), and ground beef (USDA, 2018) came at a time at odds with a holiday season known for cooking. *Fortune Magazine* characterized these recalls as "Cramping Thanksgiving Dinner Menus This Year" (Laursen, 2018).

As for the ground-beef recall, most who work in the food safety arena are frustrated to still see this news, frustrated but not surprised. Attorney William Marler openly points out that, from the 1993 *E. coli* outbreak through the 2002 ConAgra *E. coli* outbreak, "at least 95% of Marler Clark [his law firm] revenue was *E. coli* cases linked to hamburger" (Marler, 2019). He further clarifies, however, that "there is still much the industry can do .... *E. coli* will always be an issue .... The industry cannot let up. Even with the success there still have been isolated tragedies ..." (Marler, 2019).

Last, but perhaps most concerning is the impact of the Trump administration's long government shutdown that started on December 22, 2018, and ultimately lasted until January 25, 2019 (Schaul & Uhrmacher, 2019). In the end, this went down in the record books as the longest federal government shutdown in US history (Foran, 2019).

Although some reported 800,000 federal employees were prevented from doing their jobs and from receiving their paychecks (Rein & Whoriskey, 2019), consumer advocacy organizations, experts, food safety advocates, and many within the food safety community expressed significant concerns regarding the shutdown's reduction of food safety efforts for American consumers (Goldschmidt & Scutti, 2019).

Barbara VanRenterghem, PhD, the Editorial Director for Food Safety Magazine, recalls how consumers did benefit from the television news coverage of this event:

> *"I noticed during the government shutdown, there were a lot of broadcast news reporting on this and how it was affecting food safety. And I thought, 'Oh, I should watch this'—but they said nothing. It was click bait for broadcast television. They had a headline that sounded really good and people should pay attention and see how that affects their safety. But they really didn't say anything substantive. I think that the media really missed an opportunity to educate."*
>
> ***(Barbara VanRenterghem, Personal Communication, 2019)***

The USDA Food Safety and Inspection Service plays a lead role in regulating meat, poultry, and egg products (including dried, liquid, or frozen eggs, and excluding shell eggs, which fall under the FDA's jurisdiction). According to the USDA's FY 2019 contingency plan, about 11% of FSIS staff were placed on furlough during this time (USDA, 2019).

The US FDA regulates foods, including: dietary supplements, bottled water, food additives, infant formulas, and most (some 85%) other food products not regulated by the USDA. The FDA placed about 41% of their staff on furlough during the shutdown, according to an HHS 2019 contingency plan (HHS, 2018).

In summary, as a result of this shutdown, 85% of Americans' food lost over 40% of the people working to keep America's tables safe.

According to a Senior Advisor at the FDA, who asked not to be identified: "What folks don't realize is that the 41% number for FDA translates to much higher number for the foods program, including CFSAN and field food inspectors in ORA" (Personal Communication).

According to Thomas Gremillion, the Director of Food Policy at the Consumer Federation of America, Americans should be concerned that these agencies' food safety functions are not happening during the shutdown. "The inspection activity, the regulatory activity that helps to prevent people getting sick, has been suspended or dramatically diminished" (Firth, 2019).

Ali Berlow, Publisher of Edible Vineyard Magazine and author of *The Food Activist Handbook: Big & Small Things You Can Do to Help Provide Fresh, Healthy Food for Your Community* (2015), believes that "this government shutdown will have long-term effects. We have to look closer to the source of our food and regulate for that there, because clearly the federal government … may not always be there for us in terms of food safety" (Ali Berlow, Personal Communication, 2019).

The Center for Food Safety and Applied Nutrition (CFSAN) carries out the mission of the FDA by providing services to consumers, domestic and foreign industry, and other outside groups regarding field programs. The Office of Regulatory Affairs (ORA) is the lead office for *all* agency field activities. ORA inspects regulated products and manufacturers, conducts sample analyses of regulated products, and reviews imported products offered for entry into the United States. In pursuit of the FDA's mission, ORA also works with its state, local, tribal, territorial, and foreign counterparts. According to (then) FDA Commissioner Scott Gottlieb, foods categorized by the agency as "high risk" are continuing to be inspected. At the same time, many USDA food inspectors will continue to work, but without pay (Mulero, 2019).

Some industry experts have predicted that the relaxation of food safety policies would be seen under the Trump administration, especially as his first year in office had seen the reversal of, or at least the attempt to reverse anything accomplished under the Obama administration. Previous administrations have demonstrated a completely different appreciation for the need to take action to protect consumers from failures in our food safety systems.

Regardless of the political party that holds the Executive Office or the majority in Congress, historical data regarding foodborne illness cannot be reversed. No consumers should have to fear the safety of the food they buy or suffer the consequences of lapses in food safety protections. Unfortunately, however, this happens far too often. To understand how our food safety infrastructure has come to be what it is, it may be useful to review its past developments in the following chapter.

References

Beach, C. (2017). Time after time, food safety comes down to information. Food Safety News. Available from: https://www.foodsafetynews.com/2017/11/time-after-time-food-safety-comes-down-to-information/.

Bottemiller, H. (2012). Obama administration sued for delay of FSMA implementation. Food Safety News. Available from: https://www.foodsafetynews.com/2012/08/obama-administration-sued-for-delay-on-fsma-implementation/.

Centers for Disease Control and Prevention (CDC). (2018). Multistate outbreak of shiga toxin-producing *Escherichia coli* O157:H7 infections linked to leafy greens (final update). Available from: https://www.cdc.gov/ecoli/2017/o157h7-12-17/index.html.

Centers for Disease Control and Prevention (CDC). (2018). Multistate outbreak of *E. coli* O157:H7 infections linked to romaine lettuce. Available from: https://www.cdc.gov/ecoli/2018/o157h7-04-18/index.html.

Centers for Disease Control and Prevention (CDC). (2018). CDC investigation notice update: salmonella outbreak linked to raw turkey products. Available from: https://www.cdc.gov/media/releases/2018/s1221-raw-turkey-update.html.

Centers for Disease Control and Prevention (CDC). (2019). Outbreak of *E. coli* infections linked to romaine lettuce: Final Update. Available from: https://www.cdc.gov/ecoli/2018/o157h7-11-18/index.html.

Childers, E. (2015). Fast food restaurants that have had *E. coli* outbreaks. Rebel Circus. Available from: https://www.rebelcircus.com/blog/fast-food-restaurants-that-have-had-e-coli-outbreaks/2/.

Firth, S. (2019). Shutdown impact: food inspections get spottier. MedPage Today. Available from: https://www.medpagetoday.com/publichealthpolicy/fdageneral/77376.

Foran, C. (2019). Current shutdown breaks record for longest government shutdown in US history. CNN. Available from: https://www.cnn.com/2019/01/12/politics/government-shutdown-breaks-record-longest-ever/index.html.

Goldschmidt, D., & Scutti, S. (2019). Are there foods you should avoid during the government shutdown? It depends who you ask. CNN. Available from: https://www.cnn.com/2019/01/15/health/shutdown-fda-food-inspections-risk/index.html.

Gottlieb, S. (2018). Statement from FDA Commissioner Scott Gottlieb, M.D., on FDA's commitment to modernizing food and nutrition programs. FDA. [Press Statement].

Available from: https://www.fda.gov/news-events/press-announcements/statement-fda-commissioner-scott-gottlieb-md-fdas-commitment-modernizing-food-and-nutrition-programs.

Heiman, K., Mody, R., Johnson, S., Griffin, P., & Gould, L. (2015). Synopsis: *Escherichia coli* O157 outbreaks in the United States, 2003-2012. *Emerging Infectious Diseases*, *21*(8), 1285–1496 Available from: http://wwwnc.cdc.gov/eid/pdfs/vol21no8_pdf-version.pdf.

Higgins, K. (2018). Why Jack in the box still matters: by ushering in audits, microbiological testing and HACCP, the Chain's *E. coli* O157:H7 poisonings continue to impact the industry. Food Processing. Available from: https://www.foodprocessing.com/articles/2018/why-jack-in-the-box-still-matters/.

Laursen, L. (2018). How recalled foods are cramping thanksgiving dinner menus this year. Fortune Magazine. Available from: http://fortune.com/2018/11/21/turkey-recall-romaine-lettuce-thanksgiving-2018/.

Lurie, P. (2018). Trump administration indefinitely delays key food safety protections. Center for Science in the Public Interest. Available from: http://mailchi.mp/cspinet/trump-administration-indefinitely-delays-key-food-safety-protections.

Marler, B. (2019). Beef Industry, Seriously, I thought you were putting me out of Business? Marler Blog Lawyer Op-Ed. Available from: https://www.marlerblog.com/lawyer-oped/beef-industry-seriously-i-thought-you-were-putting-me-out-of-business/.

Mulero, A. (2019). Gottlieb: Government Shutdown is 'Not Business as Usual'. Regulatory Focus (Regulatory Affairs Professionals Society). Available from: https://www.raps.org/news-and-articles/news-articles/2019/1/gottlieb-government-shutdown-is-not-business-as.

Prevor, J. (2018). Lettuce try not to panic. Wall Street Journal. Available from: https://www.wsj.com/articles/lettuce-try-not-to-panic-1543534658.

Rein, L., & Whoriskey, P. (2019). While federal workers go without pay, senior trump administration officials are poised to get $10,000 raises. The Washington Post. Available from: https://www.washingtonpost.com/business/2019/01/04/while-federal-workers-go-without-pay-senior-trump-administration-officials-are-poised-get-raises/?utm_term=.b40e929ca299.

Schaul, K., & Uhrmacher, K. (2019). This shutdown was the longest ever—by a lot. The Washington Post. Available from: https://www.washingtonpost.com/graphics/2019/politics/longest-shutdowns-history/?noredirect=on&utm_term=.b0ff323fba47.

Scutti, S. (2018). Lettuce suspected in deadly US *E. coli* outbreak. CNN. Available from: http://www.cnn.com/2018/01/04/health/e-coli-outbreak-leafy-greens-suspected-cdc/index.html.

US Department of Agriculture (USDA). (2018). Swift Beef Company recalls ground beef products due to possible *E. coli* O157:H7 contamination. FSIS News Release. Available from: https://www.fsis.usda.gov/wps/portal/fsis/topics/recalls-and-public-health-alerts/recall-case-archive/archive/2018/recall-114-2018-release.

US Department of Agriculture (USDA). (2019). United States Department of Agriculture FY19: summary of activities to be continued in the event of a government shutdown. Available from: https://www.usda.gov/sites/default/files/documents/usda-shutdown-plan-summary-3.pdf.

US Department of Health and Human Services (HHS). (2018). Department of Health and Human Services Fiscal Year 2019 contingency staffing plan for operations in the absence of enacted annual agriculture and interior appropriations. Available from: https://www.hhs.gov/sites/default/files/fy-2019-hhs-lapse-contingency-plan-narrative-december-ag-interior.pdf.

US Food and Drug Administration (FDA). (2018). Guidance for industry: policy regarding certain entities subject to the current good manufacturing practice and preventive controls, produce safety, and/or foreign supplier verification programs. Available from: https://www.fda.gov/Food/GuidanceRegulation/GuidanceDocumentsRegulatoryInformation/ucm590646.htm?utm_campaign=CFSANCU_01042018_EnforcementPolicy&utm_medium=email&utm_source=Eloqua&elqTrackId=2fad7dba9a814f1b94fe481acd43de8b&elq=dc4bc02b5de94e8588965575cea10307&elqaid=1971&elqat=1&elqCampaignId=1336.

US Food and Drug Administration (FDA). (2018). Duncan Hines classic white, classic butter golden, signature confetti and classic yellow cake mixes recalled due to potential presence of salmonella. Available from: https://www.fda.gov/Safety/Recalls/ucm625144.htm.

CHAPTER 2

"Modernization" started over a century ago

"The things described by Mr. Sinclair happened yesterday, are happening today, and will happen tomorrow and the next day, until some Hercules comes to cleanse the filthy stable."
From literature Review of* The Jungle *in* The London Times, *1906

"You wouldn't know the industry as we know it today."
Ann Marie McNamara
Silliker Lecture, 2018

In terms of food safety concerns (including quality, defense, security, and authenticity), experts are quick to point out that though the industry is virtually an ocean of good behaviors, bad behaviors continue to exist and muddy the waters with serious impacts. Such bad behaviors include failures in following food industry best practices or health codes, economically motivated adulteration, and unethical practices impacting the environment and/or workers.

With increased processing and global sourcing, our food has become dramatically more vulnerable, raising concerns that are more than theoretical and come with interesting historical precedents. Early published articles in Europe hint at food safety's past even some 200 years ago.

Early concerns in Europe

An article in an 1819 edition of *Philosophical Magazine* recounts how a woman, concerned by the unusual appearance in green tea she had purchased, "took a sample of the suspected tea leaves to Mr. Accum [a German chemist], who analyzed it and pronounced it to contain copper" (Accum, 1819). The article goes on to explain the science of how Accum validated the adulteration. A year later, Accum published his 1820 *A Treatise on Adulteration of Food and Culinary Poisons*, exposing and criticizing

Food Safety
http://dx.doi.org/10.1016/B978-0-12-818219-2.00002-8

"normal" practices—especially the use of chemical additives—within the food processing industry (Accum, 1819). This groundbreaking work marked the start of Accum's noted crusade for national adulteration legislation. It also marked the beginning of public awareness of the need for food safety oversight. In his 1934 book *History of Food Adulteration*, Frederick Filby credits Accum's work for having "finally brought the storm over adulteration in 1820 .... From that time onward, adulteration has come more and more before public attention" (Filby, 1934).

In the early 1850s *The Lancet*, a British medical journal published a series of devastating reports on food adulteration, relying on commissioned analyses of food samples (Wilson, 2005). Dr. Arthur Hassall, a British physician and chemist, exposed, among other practices, how pickled vegetables were dyed with lead- and copper-based colors. Hassall used *The Lancet* as a platform to "name and shame" individual shops for the fraudulent products they sold. His work led directly to the passage of the 1860 Food Adulteration Act and later British legislation against these practices (Coley, 2005).

After the 1860 Adulterated Food Act, changes in British laws came in the form of the 1872 Adulteration Act, describing how adulteration causes a "great hurt" to Her Majesty's subjects and endangers their lives (The Adulteration of Food Act, 1872, 1874).

England's Sale of Food and Drugs Act of 1875, only 2 years later, not only set out to repeal the 1872 Adulteration of Food Act and replace it with stronger legislation, but went further to define the term "food," require consumer-driven standards, and set strict liability for food-related offences (Sale of Food and Drugs Act, 1875). Changes later put forth in the 1879 Sale of Food and Drugs Amendment Act aimed to solve conflicts in court interpretations and decisions from England and Scotland courts (Howman, 1901).

Start of regulations in the United States

Around that time, significant food regulatory changes began in the United States. On May 15, 1862—during the US Civil War—President Lincoln signed an Act to establish a US Department of Agriculture (An Act, 1862) with a focus mostly on research and discovery. Domestically, this newly-established USDA hired botanists trained to search for new plants and varieties that would launch new agriculture in the United States. At the same time, the USDA financed agricultural exploration in foreign lands. Not until

40 years later, however, was the USDA granted authority to regulate and inspect meat.

In 1883 Harvey W. Wiley, MD, was appointed chief chemist at the USDA (US Department of Agriculture, 2018). Wiley had already made a name for himself while serving an appointment as Indiana's state chemist, having protested against the practice of adulteration in fertilizers and in food. After taking his new position at the USDA, 21 years into the life of the department, he focused his attention and government funding toward the investigation of food adulteration (Harvey Washington Wiley, 2018).

Wiley published by 1887, at the direction of the Commissioner of Agriculture, a series of Technical Bulletins on Foods and Food Adulterants (US Department of Agriculture, 1887). By the end of the decade, the USDA issued Bulletin 25: "A Popular Treatise on the Extent and Character of Food Adulterations," clearly advocating for national legislation on food adulteration (Wedderburn, 1890).

In a number of unsuccessful attempts between 1897 and 1901, Wiley worked with various organizations to propose various versions of pure-food legislations to Congress (Harvey Washington Wiley, 2018). Wiley would also go on to experiment with live volunteers, referred to as his "Poison Squad," to determine the effects of preservatives on the human body.

The first significant public call-to-action for "just" food in America came through the landmark reform-oriented work of investigative journalists, often referred to as "Progressives" or "Muckrakers," These investigative journalists emerged after the era of "Yellow journalism."

Yellow journalism was characterized by newspapers that used sensationalism to increase sales and shape public opinion, often through exaggerated headlines and biased stories. Newspapers sometimes used misleading images in the form of drawings and political cartoons, which appealed to immigrants who read little or no English. Around the turn of the century, in their attempt to drive up circulation, some newspapers, such as Joseph Pulitzer's *New York World* and William Hearst's *New York Journal*, would sensationalize stories or publish highly subjective stories as if they were purely objective. The height of Yellow journalism came during the Spanish–American War. Both of the New York newspapers ran extensive, exaggerated front-page coverage of the war.

Investigative journalism, however, is a practice in which reporters go to great lengths to investigate a single topic of interest. These topics often involved crime, political corruption, or corporate wrongdoing. An investigative journalist may spend months or sometimes years researching and even going undercover to prepare a report, article, book, or "exposé."

The most prominent journalist to become known as the ultimate Muckraker was Upton Sinclair because of his investigative journalism that lead to his landmark 1906 book, *The Jungle*. In 1904 Upton Sinclair spent seven weeks working undercover in Chicago's meatpacking plants. A year later, he wrote a series of articles for a socialist political newspaper called *Appeal to Reason*. The articles exposed how unsanitary working conditions were in the plants, and how the meat industry was putting consumers at risk for disease.

His original intentions were not so much about shining a light on the food industry as much as they were to look at the "slave-like" working conditions of immigrants and to support socialism in America.

Unlike similar journalists of that time, who turned their newspaper exposés into nonfiction books, Sinclair made the brilliant decision to publish his exposé in the form of a novel. Because readers had become sensitized and more experienced judging the exaggerated and fake stories written during the era of Yellow journalism, perhaps Sinclair wanted his readers to ask if he is accurate, yet horrific descriptions of meat processing in his novel could be true.

Enter *The Jungle*

The world first took significant notice of the unseen dangers on their dinner plates with the publishing of Upton Sinclair's 1906 novel *The Jungle*. Even though Sinclair's intended message was support for socialism, readers paid a great deal of attention to the two chapters in which he described in detail the conditions under which meat was prepared. The impact of Sinclair's novel on readers can be seen in an excerpt from *The London Times* Literary Supplement review of the book in 1906 (*The London Times*, 1906) (Fig. 2.1).

Because Sinclair published the book as fiction, his first-hand observations from inside a Chicago meatpacking house eluded censure, thus exposing his readers to the grotesque nature of the meat industry. The reviewer connected Sinclair's book to its real-world context and validated the reality of the novel's content. The 1906 *London Times* review reinforced *The Jungle* as a factual warning and accurately predicted the concerns Americans would continue to face 100 years later.

> *"The book is published as a novel, and it might claim to be reviewed, therefore, under the head of fiction. But the very first thing to be said about it is that, if it is a novel, a work of imagination and invention, the conduct of an author who invented and*

published in a form easily accessible to all readers, young and old, male or female, such disgusting, inflammatory matter as this would deserve the severest censure .... Unhappily we have good reason for believing it to be all fact, not fiction. The action of the President ... remove all doubt, and give the book very great importance ... it is with nothing less than horror that we learn it to be true. The things described by Mr. Sinclair happened yesterday, are happening today, and will happen tomorrow and the next day, until some Hercules comes to cleanse the filthy stable."

Source:* The London Times *(1906).

Readers' concerns soon became a political issue and escalated into a full-blown "meat scandal" in President Theodore Roosevelt's administration. Though initially referred to by Roosevelt as a "Muckraker" for his role as an investigative journalist who exposed a social/corporate ill, Sinclair would later engage directly with the president over the food conditions in Chicago. In one of many letters between Sinclair and President Roosevelt, the author described how the industry in Chicago took steps, after he published his novel, to prevent others from taking a look at what took place inside the processing facilities or, as Sinclair wrote: "The lid is on in Packingtown" (Sinclair, 1906). In response President Roosevelt sent his own team of commissioners to personally see if the conditions reported by Sinclair were authentic.

On June 8, 1906, the Franco-American Food Company in New Jersey purchased the majority of a whole newspaper page in the *New York Times* to publish an "Open Letter to President Roosevelt and the American Nation."

They described themselves as the "Packers of Honestly and Cleanly Made" products and then made a plea to the president:

"The report of your Commissioners on the packing industry of Chicago is being published and commented upon by the press of this country, also by the newspapers throughout the world. After reading that report, it stands to reason that a vast number of people at home and abroad, who are not well posted as to the difference between brands, will stop using, not only canned meats from Chicago, but canned goods of every description.

We regret that if you feel confident the report of your Commissioners is true, you did not make the investigation more thorough, so that the American public and the world at large might know that there are packers and packers and that if some are unworthy of public confidence, there are others whose methods are above board and whose goods are of such high quality as to be a credit to the American nation.

For twenty years we have manufactured canned soups and canned meats of the highest grade, both as to quality and purity. We have spared neither effort or expense to make them as good as possible. The cleanliness of our entire plant from cellar to roof is a matter of astonishment to our numerous visitors. By these methods we have established a unique reputation, our best customers being those who know how our goods are made.

> *But what about the millions who, owing to distance, lack of time or some other reason, are not able to visit us? How is the average consumer to know that the methods of all packers are not alike? ... What can we do to counteract the bad impression which is being created against our products? Advertise? Outside of the heavy expense that this will entail, no one will believe us after reading your report ...*
>
> ***(The Franco-American Food Company, 1906)***

By this time, however, the American public was already convinced of the deplorable conditions in the meatpacking industry and was not persuaded by the open letter or other attempts by leaders in the food industry to improve public relations. Consumers across the nation, as well as merchants in many other countries who lost sales due to the "scandal" with bad meat from Chicago, supported strong food safety legislation. This, along with the findings of Roosevelt's investigative commission, no doubt gave strength to the president's decision to sign into law two key piece of food safety legislation.

When adding Sinclair's novel to a list of books that shaped America, the Library of Congress describes his work as a "graphic exposé of the Chicago meat packing industry" that "lead directly to national legislation" (Lamolinara, 2012). President Roosevelt intended for two new pieces of legislation to end the meat industry scandal that impacted not only the American consumer at home, but also the industry's efforts to sell products abroad.

The Pure Food And Drug Act of 1906—described by the Acting Secretary of Agriculture in 1925 as "one of the most beneficent pieces of legislation ever passed by Congress" (Dunlap, 1925)—banned the manufacture, sale, or transportation of adulterated or misbranded or poisonous or deleterious foods, drugs, medicines, and liquors and established what would later become the US Food and Drug Administration (FDA).

The Federal Meat Inspection Act (FMIA) of 1906 established authority for federal meat inspection.

Sinclair's 1906 novel motivated more than significant changes in legislation, as it sparked consumers' perception of not only the food industry, but also of food safety in general. Changes in regulation at the time sufficiently addressed the problems in the nation's food supply. The Food, Drug, and Cosmetic Act of 1938, a subsequent law, repealed some of the 1906 FMIA while empowering the FDA to require food (other than that regulated by the USDA) to conform to three kinds of food standards:

1. standards (definitions) of identity,
2. standards of quality, and
3. standards regulating the fill of container.

No provisions were established, however, for federal inspection by the FDA related to food safety.

From public and government awareness of failures in our food system came new regulations and greater levels of regulatory control. These did not come without criticisms and opposition from some within the food industry. Experts, including Harvey Wiley, the USDA chief chemist 1883–1912, criticized the often-relaxed implementation of new food safety regulations.

In 1925 Wiley wrote a letter to President Calvin Coolidge in which he addressed "a 'shocking' neglect on the part of the United States Government to enforce the Food and Drugs Act, for which I labored incessently (sp) for twenty-five years" (Wiley, 1925). He did not technically send the letter to the President, as he published the letter in *Good Housekeeping Magazine*, then the director of the Bureau of Foods, Sanitation, and Health for the magazine. Wiley criticized the government for having often turned a blind eye on specific cases that appeared to violate the law, and he discussed how "failures to administer the law" by those superior to him were so "shocking" that he ultimately retired voluntarily. Wiley noted in his letter that "The proper enforcement of the Food and Drugs Act is intimately related to the public health," but offered his assessment in that "the health and efficiency of our citizens are continually threatened" (Wiley, 1925).

Though Wiley's criticisms may have been justified, food safety had come a long way since the turn of the century.

Taking a summary review, England's 1860 Adulteration Act and the 1906 Pure Food and Drug Act in the United States were two of the earliest pieces of legislation to provide generalized regulation of food and drugs on a national scale. In both the European and American events, political landscapes conducive to reform in protecting consumers and becoming modern regulatory states came about through the hard work of individuals who campaigned for legislation to prevent adulteration. Legislative changes came about after the hard work of investigative journalists who were enthusiastic to bring the evils of adulteration to the forefront of the public mind, and the ignited demands from consumers.

Over the next several decades, new sciences, new food production technologies, and new consumer trends, demands, and behaviors would collide to erode the level of food safety and reverse some of the progress that had been made. Frozen foods and improved means of transportation allowed for raw ingredients and prepared foods to last longer and travel farther. At the same time, mid-century Americans were gradually beginning consuming more meals outside the home and, along with Americans' passion for driving, fast food restaurants eventually grew in numbers and popularity, even securing their place as part of the "American culture."

Late 20th century

In order to understand the impact of the Jack in the Box outbreak (discussed in Chapter 3), Dr. Ann Marie McNamara, in her 2018 John H. Silliker Lecture at the conference of the International Association for Food Protection, took audiences back to the 1980s. McNamara served as the Director of Microbiology for the USDA's Food Safety and Inspection Service. She later led efforts for food safety at Jack in the Box corporate office and Target Stores' corporate office.

> *"This was the decade when the CDC was focused on AIDS and the USDA was focused on chemical contaminants in food. Soon, the USDA would focus mainly on preventing animal diseases in food, then change slowly to a focus on human illnesses carried by food. The FDA was battling an outbreak of O157 in apple cider."* Salmonella *was well known since the 1960s as pathogen, but much of the research work was focused on farms. Listeria was a new foodborne pathogen and in 1989 had just caused the first death of a cancer patient with complications listeriosis due to consumption of a hotdog. You wouldn't know the industry as we know it today. There were no pathogen or microbial testing requirements and if any intervention was used, it was used for shelf life extension" (McNamara, 2018).*

In the 1980s and leading up to the Jack in the Box outbreak, Oregon and Washington had active health departments related to epidemiology, surveillance, and outbreak investigation. Dr. John Kobayashi worked in Washington as the state's Epidemiologist for Communicable Diseases at the State Department of Health (DOH) from 1982 to 2001, after serving 2 years in Washington State as a CDC Epidemic Intelligence Service officer. He joined a well-regarded team.

> *"During the 80s, Washington State had a reputation for aggressive reporting of foodborne illness. The [state DOH] reported more foodborne outbreaks than any other state except New York, and more foodborne outbreaks than any other state by population than Hawaii .... The collaboration with the various people who work on things, like* E. coli *O157 or other infectious diseases ... had a good reputation. In Oregon, they had a long, long history of a stable epidemiology program and good people there" (John Kobayashi, personal communication, April 26, 2019).*

While a few foodborne pathogens, such as *Salmonella,* gained the popular attention of consumers in the second half of the 20th century, during those decades experts soon discovered threats from other pathogens.

The CDC identified *Escherichia coli* O157:H7 for the first time in 1975 (Marler, 2010) in a case involving a 50-year-old woman in California (Riley et al., 1983). In total 7 years later, in 1982, state and federal heath investigators first recognized *E. coli* O157:H7 as a pathogen tied to food. Area hospitals in Jackson County, Oregon, noted a cluster of 47 patients who were all displaying the same symptoms, though not responding to any treatment (Riley et al., 1983). Assumed to be an issue isolated to that area, officials called the outbreak "The Jackson County Syndrome" for months until noting similarities with a cluster of patients in Michigan (Terry, 2011).

With the common element from the public health investigation proving to be the consumption of hamburgers at McDonald's fast food restaurants, these were the first occurrences of O157 as a new human pathogen linked to beef products. However, health officials collected reports of illnesses at a time when this serotype was thought of as rare (Marler, n.d.). In fact, the outbreak resulted in no cases of hemolytic uremic syndrome (HUS) and no deaths, thus prompting Mike Doyle, PhD, Director of the Center for Food Safety at the University of Georgia, to note that this case was "almost viewed as a freak event" (Green, 2001).

Fortunately, the work investigating this outbreak resulted in ways to solve and control future outbreaks with greater speed and accuracy.

> *[The USDA's Food Safety Inspection Service] microbiologists developed new ways to isolate and identify this new pathogen. They published four papers in the Journal of Food Protection on new cultural media, enrichment broths, and screening methods to detect O157. These researchers were Anita Okrend, Bonnie Rose, Chuck Lattuada, and others. I have often wondered what would have happened if the Jack in the Box outbreak occurred and FSIS did not have a validated and peer-reviewed method for isolating and identifying O157 in beef products (McNamara, 2018).*

After the 1982 "Jackson County Syndrome," the USDA continued to regard the pathogen as an accepted or allowable element to be noted during inspections. Federal regulators established no critical limits or control protocols. It would take not only consumer outcry, but public tragedy before such changes were put in place.

In total, 2 years later, Oregon health officials were again challenged as followers of Bhagwan Shree Rajneesh, a mystic, guru, and spiritual teacher in India, carried out "the first and largest bioterrorism attack in the U.S., of Food Poisoning/Bioterrorism on American soil" (Powell, 2018). The "1984 Rajneeshee Incident" resulted in 751-recorded illnesses, 45 hospitalizations, (no deaths) of citizens in The Dalles, Oregon, from *Salmonella enterica* Typhimurium (Detwiler, 2016). A lengthy investigation found that the perpetrators spread liquid tainted with the *salmonella* pathogen on surfaces in the Wasco County Courthouse, and introduced it into the drinking water, salad bars, and salad dressing at 10 local restaurants. Their purpose was to incapacitate voters in order to influence the outcome of a local 1984 election in their favor, placing cult members, known as Rajneeshees, into office. This unprecedented act of terrorism would eventually force policy makers to focus on food defense in the form of "defining the illegality of ill-intended use, production, dissemination, or storage of biological agents" (Ryan & Glarum, 2008).

Bill Keene, a senior epidemiologist with the Oregon Public Health Authority in Portland, OR, began collecting mementos from outbreak investigations as early as the late 1970s. Today his museum, located in his small, former Portland office, exhibits hundreds of items, including some from the 1984 Rajneeshee Incident: buttons, signs, some tarot cards, and mugs bearing the image of cult leader Bhagwan Shree Rajneesh.

In April 1986 six children near Spokane, WA, became ill from *E. coli*, with one patient, a 2-year-old girl, dying from her illness. Health detectives never determined the source. Later that year, an outbreak of *E. coli* in Walla Walla, WA, sickened 37 people. A common factor for 27 of these victims was having eaten ground beef at a fast food Mexican restaurant. Two became ill with secondary infections—the mother and grandmother of infected children. Of the 37 victims, 17 were hospitalized, 1 patient (under 5 years of age) developed HUS, 2 had surgery, and 2 elderly women died (*Escherichia coli* O157:H7, 2012).

In 1987 the first year that Washington State mandated *E. coli* be reported to county health officials, 93 cases were reported from the state—most of which were of children under age 5. Researchers speculate the number of *E. coli* cases was actually much higher, as inadequate testing and reporting existed at that time. By 1993, however, health officials noted 150–200 state cases of *E. coli* infections are reported each year in Washington State (Gilmore, 1993).

Kobayashi was a friend of Bill Keene, a senior epidemiologist with the Oregon Public Health Authority, in Portland, OR. Keene often drove all across the state to collect samples from victims, his car easily identified by his personalized license plate that read O157:H7. In a *USA Today* article announcing his untimely death in 2013, Keene was described as being "responsible for saving countless lives because of his dogged investigations of food-borne illness outbreaks" (Weise, 2013). Kobayashi remembered him and his impact on later events in Washington State.

"[Keene] was a great guy and he was sort of like my cohort. In fact, we'd talk back and forth all the time. And that generated an atmosphere of cooperation and collegial work. I knew all about that [McDonald's] outbreak in 1982. That was one of the first outbreak investigations. The reason why we [Washington State] got on board with regards to [tracking incidents of] E.coli *O157 is that 1982 outbreak. After that, one of the folks that was in my office set up surveillance for* E.coli *O157 here in Washington state starting in 1984. And the reason we were able to do that is because we were working well with them. At that time there was a lab at group health and we cooperated with the CDC and so on. So there was this groundwork that got laid that went on for about 10 years before Jack in the Box. And like I say, Seattle and Washington State had a good reputation for foodborne investigations" (John Kobayashi, personal communication, 2019).*

These events in Washington and Oregon highlight significant firsts in food safety failures and in intentional adulteration. However, the Pacific Northwest was not alone in challenges to their consumers and to those who protect them.

In 1985 "the largest number of culture-confirmed cases ever associated with a single outbreak of salmonellosis in the United States" (Epidemiologic Notes and Reports Update: Milk-borne Salmonellosis—Illinois, 1985) in the form of an outbreak traced to two brands of pasteurized 2% milk produced by a single dairy plant. (Ryan et al., 1987; *The New York Times*, 1985). The incident resulted in over 16,000 culture-confirmed cases in five states, the vast majority of them in Illinois. Investigators at the time estimated that the true amount was actually closer to 10 times that number (Ryan et al., 1987). The culprit milk was produced in Illinois and distributed to supermarkets in that state, as well as in other adjacent states (Indiana, Iowa, Michigan, and Wisconsin) also affected by the outbreak. At least nine deaths were attributed to the outbreak (*The New York Times*, 1985).

These incidents through the 1980s served to strengthen the resolve of disease detectives and health officials at a time when another dark storm was on the horizon. A decade after the discovery of food as a vehicle for *E. coli* O157:H7, the landmark 1993 "Jack in the Box" *E. coli* O157:H7 outbreak, tied to ground beef sold in fast-food restaurants, would change how consumers, media, public health experts, doctors, lawyers, the food industry, and even policy makers looked at food safety (O'Hagan, 2011). According to Kobayashi:

"I don't have any doubt that if there had not been this groundwork that had been going on since the 1982 outbreak and this great relationship between Oregon and Washington and the collaboration and the active surveillance and the health departments, that the [1993] outbreak with Jack in the Box could have been much worse" (John Kobayashi, personal communication, 2019).

Nobody could predict just how bad the 1993 Jack in the Box *E. coli* outbreak would be, nor how significant to the future of food safety it would become.

References

Accum, F. (1819). *Philosophical Magazine 54*, 218. Reprinted in Cole, R. (1951). Friedrich Accum (1769-1838). A Biographical Study. *Annals of Science*, 7(2), 128–143, doi: 10.1080/00033795100202291. Available from: https://www.tandfonline.com/doi/pdf/10.1080/00033795100202291.

The Adulteration of Food Act, 1872. (1874). *The law magazine and review*. Available from: https://heinonline.org/HOL/LandingPage?handle=hein.journals/lmagb3&div=58&id=&page.

Coley, N. (2005). The fight against food adulteration. *Education in Chemistry, 52*(2). Available from: https://eic.rsc.org/feature/the-fight-against-food-adulteration/2020253.article.

Detwiler, D. (2016). Death should not be on the Menu. *EC Nutrition, 5*(3), 1148–1149. Available from: https://www.ecronicon.com/ecnu/pdf/ECNU-05-0000158.pdf.

Dunlap, R. W. (1925). Letter of USDA Acting Secretary R.W. Dunlap to President Calvin Coolidge. Archival Copy. Available from: https://6sd6hj41ya-flywheel.netdna-ssl.com/images/pdfs/109_Dunlapletter.pdf.

Escherichia coli O157:H7. (2012). *Bad Bug Book*. (2nd Ed.). U.S. Food and Drug Administration: Center for Food Safety and Applied Nutrition. Available from: https://www.fda.gov/media/83271/download.

Filby, F. A. (1934). *A history of food adulteration and analysis*. London: Allen & Unwin.

The Franco-American Food Company. (1906). An open letter to President Roosevelt and the American Nation. *The New York Times*. Microfilm Collection, Western Washington University.

Gilmore, S. (1993). Walla Walla cases prepared the state for this outbreak -- Washington became a pioneer in reporting, cooking standards. *The Seattle Times*. Available from: http://community.seattletimes.nwsource.com/archive/?date=19930131&slug=1682833.

Green, E. (2001). The bug that ate the burger. *The Los Angeles Times*. Available from: https://www.latimes.com/archives/la-xpm-2001-jun-06-fo-6863-story.html.

Harvey Washington Wiley. (2018). Science History Institute. Available from: https://www.sciencehistory.org/historical-profile/harvey-washington-wiley.

Howman, M. (1901). The Sale of Food and Drugs Acts, 1875 to 1899 with Notes: Decided Cases in England and Scotland, and Appendix Containing Forms, Etc. Edinburgh: William Green & Sons.

The London Times. (1906). Literary Supplement: *The Jungle*. Microfilm collection, Western Washington University.

Lamolinara, G. (2012). "Books that shaped America" Exhibition to Open June 25 list includes popular favorites, forgotten titles. Library of Congress. Available from: https://www.loc.gov/item/prn-12-123/. Marler, B. (n.d.). McDonald's Restaurant Hamburger 1982. Foodborne illness outbreak database. Available from: http://www.outbreakdatabase.com/details/mcdonalds-restaurant-hamburger-1982/.

Marler, B. (2010). *E. coli* outbreak litigation – $500,000,000 recovered in 18 years. Marler Blog. Available from: https://www.marlerblog.com/articles/e-coli-information/.

McNamara, A. (2018). John H. Silliker lecture: heroes: past and future. IAFP Journal for Food Protection. Available from: https://www.foodprotection.org/upl/downloads/meeting/archive/5c91137f3262435bd43ee.pdf.

O'Hagan, M. (2011). What You Eat Can Kill You if You Don't Watch Out. *The Seattle Times*: Pacific NW Magazine. Available from: http://seattletimes.com/html/pacific-nw/2016550578_pacificpsickfood30.html.

Powell, D. (2018). Your vomit and diarrhea is our bread and butter: Portland's outbreak museum. Barf Blog. Available from: https://www.barfblog.com/tags/bill-keene/.

Riley, et al. (1983). Hemorrhagic colitis associated with a rare *Escherichia coli* serotype. *New England Journal of Medicine, 308*(12), 681–685. Available from: https://www.marlerblog.com/uploads/image/nejm198303243081203.pdf.

Ryan, et al. (1987). Massive outbreak of antimicrobial-resistant salmonellosis traced to pasteurized milk. *JAMA, 258*(22), 3269–3274. Available from: https://www.ncbi.nlm.nih.gov/pubmed/3316720.

Ryan, J., & Glarum, J. (2008). *Biosecurity and bioterrorism: Containing and preventing biological threats*. Burlington, MA: Elsevier.

Sale of Food and Drugs Act (1875). Chapter 63. Available from: http://www.legislation.gov.uk/ukpga/1875/63/pdfs/ukpga_18750063_en.pdf.

The New York Times. (1985)Salmonella outbreak is traced. *The New York Times*. Available from: https://www.nytimes.com/1985/04/17/garden/salmonella-outbreak-is-traced.html.

Sinclair, U. (1906). Letter from Upton Sinclair to President Theodore Roosevelt, 03/10/1906 (National Archives Identifier: 301981); Letters Received, 1893-1906; Records of the Office of the Secretary of Agriculture, 1839-1981; Record Group 16; National Archives. Available from: https://www.archives.gov/historical-docs/todays-doc/?dod-date=310.

Terry, L. (2011). *E. coli* first linked to food poisoning in Oregon; 30 years later, deadly strain hits Europe. *The Oregonian*. Available from: https://www.oregonlive.com/environment/2011/06/ecoli_first_linked_to_food_poi.html.

US Department of Agriculture. (1887). Technical Bulletin 19330 – Number 13: Foods and Food Adulterants. Available from: https://archive.org/details/foodsfoodadulter13unit/page/n10.

US Department of Agriculture. (2018). FSIS History. Available from: https://www.fsis.usda.gov/wps/portal/informational/aboutfsis/history.

Wedderburn, A. (1890). US Department of Agriculture Technical Bulletin 25: A Popular Treatise on the Extent and Character of Food Adulterations. Available from: https://archive.org/details/populartreatiseo25wedd/page/n2.

Weise, E. (2013). Top Food-safety Sleuth Bill Keene, 56, dies. *USA Today*. Available from: https://www.usatoday.com/story/news/nation/2013/12/03/bill-keene-food-safety-obituary/3863283/.

Wiley, H. (1925). Letter to President Coolidge: enforcement of the food law. *Good Housekeeping Magazine*. Archived copy. Available from: https://6sd6hj41ya-flywheel.netdna-ssl.com/images/pdfs/53_Letters%20to%20President.pdf.

Wilson, B. (2005). Food scares are one of the great British traditions. *The Telegraph*. Available from: https://www.telegraph.co.uk/news/uknews/1484479/Food-scares-are-one-of-the-great-British-traditions.html.

CHAPTER 3

1993: the "9/11" of the food industry

"...I knew that, when Phil called me, that it was something serious . . ."
Dr. John Kobayashi, Washington State Epidemiologist, 1982–2001

"No product, no industry, no job is more important than a life—particularly a child's life."
Darin Detwiler, testimony before a Congressional panel, 1993

On January 12, 1993, Dr. Phil Tarr, then a pediatric gastroenterologist at the University of Washington and Seattle's Children's Hospital, filed a report with the Washington State Department of Health (DOH) about a perceived cluster of children with bloody diarrhea and hemolytic uremic syndrome (HUS) likely caused by *Escherichia coli* O157:H7 (McNamara, 2018). Complicating these findings at the time was the fact that, in 1993, hospitals did not routinely test for *E. coli*. He contacted Dr. John Kobayashi, the Washington State Epidemiologist, who started the epidemiological trace-back, linking these cases to undercooked hamburger patties. Dr. John Kobayashi remembers the call:

> *"The call I got was directly from Phil Tarr . . . . I knew that, when Phil called me, that it was something serious, because he had worked with us for well over 10 years on* E. coli *O157 and other things. And for him to say, 'this is something that I've never seen before,' that was a big red flag" (John Kobayashi, Personal Communication, 2019).*

Because these cases were in King County, WA, where Seattle sits, the Washington State DOH called Dr. Ross Alexander in the King County Health Department immediately to make sure his office was informed and would take action. The state DOH was not investigating the issue at the time, per protocol. A few days went by before the state DOH had any further activity. Later that week it became clear that there were cases located outside Seattle. When cases occur only within the city, that is Seattle's responsibility to investigate. Within a county, that is each respective county's responsibility. But when cases expand to more than one county in Washington State, the problem becomes the state's responsibility.

Food Safety
http://dx.doi.org/10.1016/B978-0-12-818219-2.00003-X

"Frankly speaking, I don't think there were any discussions with the people in the Department of Health in [the WA state capitol in] Olympia at that time. I may have told them that something was going on, but it was very common for outbreaks to be investigated for a few days without having any higher-level discussions" (John Kobayashi, Personal Communication, 2019).

By the end of that week, the DOH speculated that they had 11 cases of *E. coli* O157 or possibly cases of O157 with HUS, or maybe just people who had bloody diarrhea. They sent out a bulletin to all the emergency rooms and labs within King County by fax, telling them of these reports and requesting that if they had any further cases to report them to the DOH. Reporting increased rapidly to 40 cases by Friday of that week. Scientists at the CDC, including Patricia Griffin, Rob Tauxe, and Joy Wells, joined together as the outbreak investigation progressed. At an alarming rate, they saw a rapid increase of young victims admitted to local hospitals and being airlifted to Children's Hospital in Seattle.

At first, the DOH believed it was very suspicious that this problem was related to eating hamburgers but three quarters of the cases had a history of consuming a hamburger. Unfortunately, as these cases were not simply from any one restaurant or one particular event, this created a greater challenge during the investigation: they ate hamburgers at fast-food chains scattered around Seattle. And the difficult part (because a lot of people eat hamburgers) was confirming whether the hamburger connection was simply being reported because a lot of people eat hamburgers or because there was something specific going on related to hamburgers.

Within a few days after this initial alert, the Washington State DOH had enough suspicion to alert Robert Nugent, president of Jack in the Box, that the *E. coli* outbreak was being investigated as being at least partly attributed to hamburgers purchased at his restaurants. Upon receiving this alert, Jack in the Box executives dispatched a research team to Seattle (Sellnow & Ulmer, 1995).

By that first weekend, the major focus of the DOH was to identify and confirm cases, and then confirm the contaminant source. Even by that Saturday night the DOH staff were still rather suspicious of Jack in the Box as a potential source, but they were not 100% certain. Dr. Kobayashi characterized Jack in the Box as "a big organization" with "a lot of outlets all over the place" (John Kobayashi, Personal Communication, 2019). It was, at the time, the fifth largest fast-food chain in the United States (Sellnow & Ulmer, 1995). The DOH decided to meet the next day with the Jack in the Box team to go over what they had found and what information they might have to help solve the problem.

Meanwhile, Dr. Kobayashi and the DOH were calling neighboring jurisdictions: California, Oregon, British Columbia (Canada), and the CDC in Atlanta. The Washington DOH reported this to Atlanta at a time when literally nobody else was reporting anything unusual with regard to O157, as not very many states were reporting O157 at that time. As a result, no information of note was coming in through the CDC.

That first Saturday night and into Sunday, the DOH focused on doing a case control study by getting interviews from parents of children who were not sick but who were of the same age as the children who were ill. Most of these control study cases were of children who lived in the same neighborhood as the ill children. They found out that Jack in the Box was not like McDonald's, where virtually every neighborhood in Seattle had a McDonald's restaurant. Jack in the Box was located only in certain neighborhoods. The DOH thought it important that to establish accurate conclusions the controls be matched with people who lived in the same areas where these cases were coming from, resulting in a complicated and time-consuming procedure.

On Sunday, January 17, 1993, the DOH met with the Jack in the Box team. Dr. Kobayashi describes the event as "a very long meeting" with people from Environmental Health, King County Health Department, the DOH, the lab people, Jack in the Box management, and epidemiology specialists. First and foremost was to sort out what could be a possible explanation for the outbreak. They looked at details right down the temperature level of the cooking. Kobayashi wanted to know where Jack in the Box got their meat from and how it was handled. One of the important details officials learned at the very beginning of this meeting was that the meat passed through a central distribution system. All the meat was produced in southern California and driven by truck up to a warehouse in Tukwila, WA, just south of Seattle. From there the products were distributed to about 66 restaurants around the state and in Idaho. Of those 66, the DOH had identified 13 potential cases of O157 infected people who had eaten a hamburger at one of the Jack in the Box restaurants.

This raised a key question for Dr. Kobayashi:

> *"Why were only 13 of them named? We knew that 66 of the restaurants got the same hamburger meat through this distribution center. The DOH asked the Jack in the Box management new questions: Was there anything unique or unusual about these 13 restaurants that were being named at that time? Was there any particular truck distribution system that went there? Were there any common employees who worked in more than one of those restaurants? Was there any problem with refrigeration failure or some sort of problem in handling of the meat for those particular restaurants? We also asked about other items because sometimes things like hamburger meat can be a 'red herring' in an outbreak, that it's not the hamburger, but it ends up being the lettuce, the tomatoes, the bread, or the milk, etc" (John Kobayashi, Personal Communication, 2019).*

By the end of that meeting, unfortunately, they were not able to identify any other explanation for why the 13 restaurants were named.

One key piece of the puzzle that the DOH did learn at that meeting, however, was that about 10 of the 13 Jack in the Box restaurants were inspected by the King County Environmental Health staff. They were checking on how well the hamburgers were cooked and how other food-handling procedures were performed. The main finding the inspectors noted was that employees were not cooking hamburger patties to the temperature of 155 degrees Fahrenheit required by Washington State. In early 1992, the Washington State Board of Health mandated that all restaurants should cook ground beef to the internal cook temperature of 155 degrees Fahrenheit, having earlier identified O157 as a problem in the state and proper cooking temperature as a solution. Experts had also found that hamburger was frequently the source of an infection for the people who got sick. Thus, Washington State had a more stringent requirement than the national level at that time. This state-mandated minimum temperature was actually higher than the national mandate of 140 degrees Fahrenheit—the Federal Food Code temperature at that time (Marler, 2018).

Washington State health officials reached out to all restaurants in the state with the new standards. Although Jack in the Box leaders executives claimed that they knew nothing of state's change to the 155 degrees Fahrenheit mandate (and perhaps they did not directly), the new standards were found filed away at their corporate headquarters in San Diego (Marler, 2013).

On June 18, 1992—3 months after the state-mandated minimum cooking temperature and 7 months before the contaminated patties would cause the 1993 *E. coli* outbreak—a shift leader at a Arlington, WA, Jack in the Box restaurant faxed a suggestion to an inbox at the Jack in the Box corporate headquarters in San Diego, CA: "I think regular patties should cook longer. They don't get done and we have customer complaints" (Marler, 2013).

After receiving notification of the corporate office receipt of the message, and a pen/highlighter combination as a token of appreciation, the shift leader later was notified by the corporate office that increasing the cooking time made burgers "tough" (Marler, 2013).

This state-mandated minimum cooking temperature is not a meaningless bureaucratic hoop: it is imperative for ground beef to reach the proper minimum cooking temperature as the critical "kill step" to prevent consumers from eating contaminated meat. According to Bert Bartleson, the Washington State DOH's Food Program technical expert who investigated the outbreak, "Had Jack in the Box followed state regulations ... the [1993] epidemic would have been prevented." He also pointed out that "Either

[Jack in the Box] didn't believe in science, or they didn't read the literature. If they followed the standards ... no one would have gotten sick" (Porterfield & Berliant Mcclatchy, 1995).

The DOH learned another, more critical piece of information: some of the cooking temperatures taken in the inspected Jack in the Box outlets did not even reach the federal-level mandate minimum of 140 degrees Fahrenheit.

> *"Food workers would take a frozen hamburger patty out of the freezer when somebody ordered a hamburger. They would put it on the grill on one side for one minute and another side for another minute. They had little timers that they would use to make sure that the time of cooking was the same. And then the hamburger was ready to eat. Workers didn't look at the inside of the hamburger or anything like that. They were just following procedures. So there was, to our knowledge, a pretty uniform procedure that was going on throughout all of these Jack in the Box restaurants" (John Kobayashi, Personal Communication, 2019).*

Thus, there were problems with how well the hamburgers were being cooked. With this information, Dr. Kobayashi stated to the management from Jack in the Box that "while we cannot confirm that you guys are the source of the outbreak, we are very suspicious that you are" (John Kobayashi, Personal Communication, 2019). He went on to point out that they knew the restaurants were not cooking the hamburgers according to Washington State law.

Finally, Dr. Kobayashi gave the representatives from Jack in the Box an ultimatum: "Unless you can change this now, we will go public with this even though we don't have confirmation epidemiologically" [of Jack in the Box as the source of the outbreak] (John Kobayashi, Personal Communication, 2019). Jack in the Box immediately sent out an electronic communication to all their facilities instructing them to cook their hamburgers longer.

The DOH continued to gather information about the controls all during that Sunday, January 17, 1993. By the end of that day, the DOH still had not gathered enough controls to make a definitive conclusion regarding Jack in the Box.

> *"We were working during this time. And so that's when we actually went public with this, saying that we had an outbreak of* E. coli *O156:H7, and that a frequent cause of this type of pathogen was hamburger and everybody should be careful about cooking their hamburger properly. But we weren't naming Jack in the Box that Sunday night. I was bombarded with questions from the media about what we knew, and I said we're working on it as fast as we can. The pressure was enormous to provide information about where we thought this outbreak was coming from" (John Kobayashi, Personal Communication, 2019).*

But by the next morning, they did have enough. Having interviewed 16 controls, which were matched with 16 of the 30 cases, the DOH determined their evidence was conclusive. On Monday, January 18, 1993, DOH officials went public with an announcement about the source of the O157 outbreak. This news conference took place during the Martin Luther King holiday weekend at the state lab. After that press conference, Jack in the Box agreed to stop serving hamburgers and quarantine the meat.

But that's only part of the story.

Only two days after the DOH officials made the announcement, and on the day of President Bill Clinton's inauguration, a powerful storm swept through the Puget Sound area, which includes Seattle and King County, WA. The storm ravaged the Puget Sound area, knocking out the power for hundreds of thousands of residents across three counties, some living in the dark for 5 days. Worse, the deaths of six people were attributed to the storm.

> *"I remember the lights went out because of the storm. We looked outside and the wind was blowing things all over the place. Fortunately the state lab, where we were working with the epidemiology people, was well prepared. That building was built with the foresight to have emergency generators. And so, even though things looked gloomy, we had power in every single office in one hour. I think if the disaster preparedness had not been adequate for the state lab, then that would have been a real, real problem for us" (John Kobayashi, Personal Communication, 2019).*

Coming so soon after the public announcement made for difficult circumstances. Some health officials talked to Jack in the Box executives over the phone from their homes, often in the dark without power in their homes. They also talked with executives at other restaurants and food retails establishments in the region about their fears when the power came back on.

"Restaurants wanted to open up and go back to cooking right away. But you had to make sure that things were refrigerated properly and, and the stove you have to temperature" (John Kobayashi, Personal Communication, 2019). Many doctors and health officials were tracking how many people were sick in an effort to determine if the outbreak was getting worse or had it reached its peak. Data would later show that the peak took place between the dates of the DOH announcement of the source of the outbreak and the middle of the storm.

> *"The amount of conversations with the federal level at the federal level at that time was enormous. It was very clear that we were not just dealing with a regional outbreak, that we were dealing with a national problem. And when things change from a regional outbreak to a national outbreak, it makes life a lot more complicated. But you also had the complication of the person to person infections. And that, that was a big concern."(John Kobayashi, Personal Communication, 2019)*

The power outage would impact proper cooking temperatures, proper refrigeration temperatures, and even proper handwashing—all critical factors in preventing foodborne illnesses.

Additionally, Dr. Kobayashi and the DOH were concerned about the secondary transmission of *E. coli* O157:H7 and how it can be passed from person to person as easily as it can from food to person. "We knew that there were over 60 kids who had been in daycare centers who had *E. coli* O157:H7 And the risk was very great that children might spread that disease to other children and to family members" (John Kobayashi, Personal Communication, 2019).

The news of these cases found their place in the headlines and in the evening news, stories of the 45 infected children who required hospitalization, 38 of whom suffered serious kidney problems and 21 required dialysis (Huemer & Challem, 1997).

Only days after taking the oath of office, President Bill Clinton discussed the ongoing food safety situation on a live, televised "Town Meeting," talking directly to live audiences in Detroit, Miami, and Seattle. The Seattle ABC affiliate invited me, as the father of 16-month-old Riley Detwiler, and Riley's mother to attend the Town Meeting and tell the president about our son, listed in critical condition—sick with *E. coli*—in Seattle Children's Hospital. In his response, President Clinton stated that "We can do more (meat) inspections in a more effective way, hire more inspectors, and do a better job. We can empower the inspectors to do more things" (Schaefer, 1993).

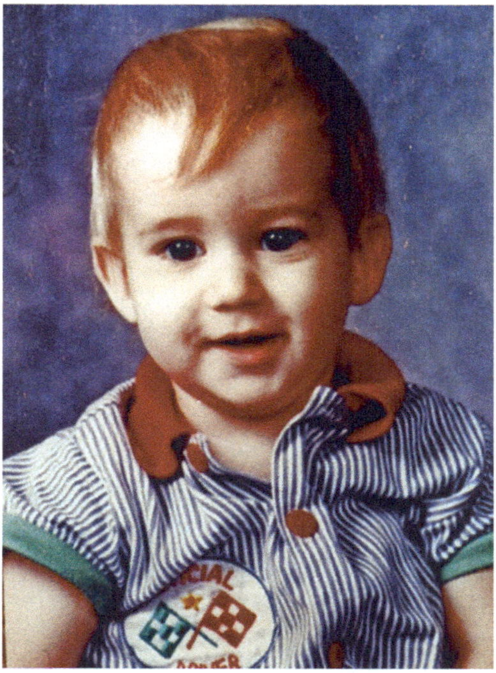

***Riley Detwiler** Photo, taken in 1992, from Author*

Riley Detwiler: Loss and Legacy

Reports on the outbreak in newspapers and on television through January 1993 informed consumers that investigators had tied the outbreak to beef in hamburger sold at Jack in the Box restaurants. I believed that to keep our family safe, we only needed to avoid eating at that fast-food chain or any restaurant in Seattle. And with Riley being just 16 months old, I thought he was out of harm's way. After all, Riley had never eaten a hamburger and certainly was not going to start now. But I soon became alarmed.

Even though the outbreak's focal point was 90 miles south of where we lived, I picked Riley up from his day-care center one day and found a health department notice asking parents to watch for signs of foodborne illness in their children. Whatcom County health officials were concerned about a sick, 18-month-old child named Tristan at the day-care center.

Tristan's father was a shift supervisor at the local Jack in the Box restaurant, the only location in Bellingham, WA. Tristan's mother was an assistant manager at the same restaurant. She regularly cooked burgers for herself and her son, which she would bring home after work. One night, after eating hamburgers from work, Tristan and his mother became ill. She suspected they had *E. coli* poisoning.

Immediately, Tristan's mother rushed her son to the hospital for testing. Back then, that meant a 48-hour wait time for results. The next morning she took her son to day care, but did not say a word to the staff about his illness for fear he would be sent home. It was not until the following day, after she again dropped her son off at day care and went to work, that day-care staff got concerned about Tristan, who was suffering with diarrhea.

Tristan's parents left him in a day-care center, interacting with many children, for 2 days before the lab returned their son's test results for what could have been a life-threatening, communicable foodborne disease.

Unfortunately, the results came back positive for the exact strain of *E. coli* O157:H7 identified in the Jack in the Box outbreak.

In short order, health officials warned all parents of children attending the day-care center that Tristan could have infected other children through direct, person-to-person contact or through contaminated surfaces/items. This meant Riley, too.

Late that evening, Riley began showing symptoms. He was not his normal, active toddler self and started to suffer bloody diarrhea. Early the next morning, he was in really bad shape, so we rushed him to the hospital. I soon learned from Riley's medical team that he was indeed one of over 600 patients known to be sickened in the *E. coli* outbreak now known to have spread across Washington, Oregon, California, and Nevada.

After spending several days in a smaller hospital, doctors airlifted Riley to Seattle's Children's Hospital. He went from being "under observation" to having IV and monitors to being transferred to the Pediatric ICU. As I tried to sit close and hold him on his bed, the look of fear in his eyes grew painfully deeper with every hour. Riley wanted to go home. He wanted comfort from his bottle, but he could not have one. With only a few words at his disposal, he kept reaching for the hanging bag of IV fluids and saying "Ba Ba" for bottle. These were the last words I heard Riley said.

Through the night and into the morning, Riley fell in and out of consciousness.

The next day, doctors performed exploratory surgery and removed a large portion of his colon. When the staff brought Riley back to his hospital room, the doctors could not look us in the eyes as they related how bad things were and that they had placed him in a medically induced coma. I painfully remember Riley's eyes, coated with an ointment, remained closed. His little arms and legs arranged to serve as a bridge between his small body and the web of wires and towering machines surrounding his bed. The little blonde boy, who had hardly been able to walk and talk just a week earlier, now remained medically paralyzed and breathing on a respirator. Over the next few weeks, Riley's little body, dwarfed by wires, tubes, and devices, developed renal failure, heart problems, and respiratory distress.

Meanwhile, a flurry of local and national news coverage led to brief national attention of the *E. coli* problem. Many in media and government initially treated *E. coli* as a regional problem, of no concern to the rest of the country, but that soon changed. Executives in the meat and restaurant industries, and government officials, announced that the outbreak was "over." But, the opposite was true. Cases of children infected from secondary (or person-to-person) transmissions were increasing rapidly. Doctors predicted that a second wave of victims of mostly children could well outnumber those who actually ate the tainted meat. The hospital arranged for special dialysis machines designed for toddlers to be flown in from other states to handle the expected patients.

During that time, President Clinton told the nation during the televised town hall that his administration, including his new USDA Secretary Mike Espy, would "look into this *E. coli* situation and put forth changes in policies and regulations as needed" (C-SPAN, 1993). A week later, President Clinton flew to Seattle and had planned to meet with me and with my son Riley in Children's Hospital, but his plan would prove untimely.

On February 20, 1993, only 23 days after he became ill, Riley died from a massive brain hemorrhage and organ failure. Along with the news of Riley's death, investigators confirmed that he had not eaten any of the contaminated product but became ill through person-to-person transmission from another child who had eaten the contaminated meat (*The New York Times*, 1993a; Andrews, 2013).

The day after Riley's death, President Clinton called me from a phone on Air Force One. Echoing JFK's famous "Ask Not" statement, President Clinton asked what his administration could do to help parents in this situation. I suggested that perhaps the best course of action would be to let parents like myself help the government make food safer.

Media coverage

"The 1993 outbreak changed everything. It was the pivotal event in food safety," according to Lynda Byron, an award-winning investigative journalist at the NBC affiliate KING 5 News in Seattle, WA, who covered the Jack in the Box outbreak and many others after. "This is the one that really struck at people's hearts and opened up their minds. It ultimately created the new level of vigilance. Food safety became a much more high profile area of discussion and people started to care about it in different ways because their eyes were opened" (Lynda Byron, Personal Communication, 2019).

Byron's recollection of her awareness of food safety concerns before the 1993 outbreak related to how she and her classmates read Upton Sinclair's 1906 novel "The Jungle" in journalism school. She was outraged at how food-packing plants were described as being so filthy and unhealthy a century earlier. "I thought we had moved way ahead of that, and that really, food safety, especially fatalities from consuming food, were an event of the past" (Lynda Byron, Personal Communication, 2019).

For over 25 years, Byron worked with Dennis Bounds, a television news anchor for KING-TV. Bounds also started his presence 2 years before the outbreak. He recalls how the "devastating" news of children in hospitals and of deaths captured the attention of his peers.

Bounds argues that the press coverage of this outbreak was important for many reasons, chiefly for accountability. "What does the company do to make it right?" "How do they atone for this problem?" Another major question was "Why was this happening?"

Dr. Kobayashi, serving as the main DOH information source for the press, was extremely busy dealing with the media during that week after the major announcement was made. He told the DOH public affairs person, Dean Owen, that he thought they had done everything they could possibly do in terms of intervention and maybe he could get some rest from the media this weekend. Owen's advice to Dr. Kobayashi:

> *"Don't stop talking to the media ... this story has become a national event. Once a story starts going like this, you have to keep feeding information to the media into the public and not stop. And he said that the public and the media is sort of like a big animal that needs to be fed. And if you don't provide information, people will start looking around for other people to get information from and that those who may not have as accurate of information as you have" (John Kobayashi, Personal Communication, 2019).*

The news coverage served to give viewers a sense of the idea that behind the news are people and families affected and have stories to tell.

> *"This was a huge story, one of the worst stories to cover, because it was about sick kids. Beyond simply being newsworthy, we featured compelling stories, told by families affected by* E. coli, *and each family's experience ran the gambit. Yes, families lost children, but there were also those youngsters who survived and we revisited over the years" (Linda Byron, Personal Communication, 2019).*

Bounds points out that, when covering a tragedy or death, especially of a child, it becomes a challenge of doing the story justice. "If the family would look at that coverage, they would not be offended" (Dennis Bounds, Personal Communication, 2019).

Viewers were not the only ones to learn about *E. coli* and foodborne pathogens in general. "I can't recall covering any kind of outbreak before 1993," admits Bounds. "I followed with interest as my own nine-year-old was in the same grade in school as Brianne Kiner, a young girl who barely survived only to live with so many health problems" (Dennis Bounds, Personal Communication, 2019).

"As journalists, we look for what I call motivators, the reasons that people would care about a story," describes Byron. "These stories hit several key motivators. The first one being safety, but others include health, family, community, and this kind of hidden threat" (Linda Byron, Personal Communication, 2019).

As a result, the unfolding story of this outbreak of a rather unheard-of pathogen appealed to viewers and readers. At the same time, reporters felt the personal impact of these stories.

> *"The idea that the sort of thing that all Americans do—taking your family out for a burger could end up sickening hundreds of people and killing people—that seemed way above the threats that I had been aware of and that I think most of us*

in the media had been aware of. We were witnessing something happening that could affect my family, my community, my safety, the health of people I love and help ... even those people I don't even know" (Linda Byron, Personal Communication, 2019).

The local story also drew national coverage, with Riley's funeral being covered on national news. Riley's mother and I appeared on CNN and television shows such as ABC's Turning Point, The Phil Donahue show, and twice on Good Morning America. Local TV station shows and news programs featured us even more.

"It was a story that was really important on a local level, because there's a strong local connection," explains Byron. "As it affected so many people, however, it became a national story and a certain momentum can build in these kinds of stories. And I think that happened with the Jack in the box and the *E. coli* outbreak—that there was a sense of outrage and then it snowballed and that reinforced the outrage. When you have children dying, that strikes at our collective sense of wrong and of caring" (Linda Byron, Personal Communication, 2019).

The news of these illnesses and deaths "shook the nation" and grabbed national headlines (*The Los Angeles Times*, 1993; *The New York Times*, 1993b; *The Orlando Sentinel*, 1993). Images of toddlers in hospitals and of tiny caskets made for compelling footage for the new 24-hour news cycle.

According to Byron, "As journalists, we look for what I call motivators—the reasons that people would care about a story. These stories hit several key motivators. The first one being safety, but others include health, family, community, and this kind of hidden threat" (Linda Byron, Personal Communication, 2019).

The unfolding story of this outbreak—of a rather unheard-of pathogen at the time—captured the attention of viewers and readers. Victims and their families gained the attention of the media and policymakers at the state and federal levels. Parents of the victims became consistent fixtures on the nightly news. Consumers and advocacy groups demanded safer meat policies and increased inspections.

They sent warnings to families about the hidden danger in the foods parents fed to their children. Simply avoiding fast-food hamburgers was not enough to guarantee any kind of immunity from *E. coli*, as public health investigators found cases of illness tied to ground beef cooked at home (King, 1993; Penhale, 1993).

During the outbreak, USDA Secretary Espy, along with other key leaders of his staff, made trips out to the Seattle area to visit with patients and parents, talk with investigators and industry, and face the press. Jill Hollingsworth, DVM, was the USDA's Food Safety Inspection Service (FSIS) Assistant Deputy Administrator at the time, traveled in that group. Hollingsworth describes the scene:

> *"That was one of the most difficult things I have ever done in my life. There were a lot of the parents there and I remember one of the mothers just started really yelling at us. And I remember thinking that if I were in her shoes, I'd probably be yelling at someone too. I just remember telling [H. Russell Cross, FSIS Administrator at the time],* 'I just don't know how much longer I can do this ... this is just taking a real toll on me.' *And he was so nice. He said,* 'No, you don't understand. That's why you do need to be here'" *(Jill Hollingsworth, Personal Communication, 2019).*

The 1993 "Jack in the Box" *E. coli* O157:H7 outbreak resulted in the restaurant chain's parent company losing nearly $140 million in profit, a drop in stock value by over 30%, and over 20,000 pounds of meat being destroyed (American Association for Justice, 2015). More important to remember, however, is the human toll of this landmark event. By the end of February 1993, four children had died, including:

- Six-year-old Lauren Beth Rudolph of southern California, who died on December 28, 1992 (Sylvester, 1995);
- Two-year-old Michael Nole of Tacoma, WA, who died on January 22, 1993 (*The New York Times*, 1993b);
- Two-year-old Celina Shribbs of Mountlake Terrace, WA, who died less than a week later on January 28, 1993 (Kelley, 1996); and
- Eighteen-month-old Riley Detwiler of Bellingham, WA, who died on February 20, 1993.

Of Riley's legacy, Warren King of *The Seattle Times* wrote: "A week before he became ill with the *E. coli* infection that eventually killed him, 16-month-old Riley Detwiler took his first five steps alone. That little-boy distance—from the playpen to the television—was huge in his life and perhaps symbolic of what he was to become in an epidemic that sickened 500 people and killed three children" (King, 1993).

While Riley's death "shook the nation," its impact is evident to this today. *The Seattle Times* acknowledged that Riley and other victims created a huge national awareness, "Of a relatively little-known foodborne illness. Of the simple hand-washing that can prevent its spread from person to person. Of inadequate government meat-inspection requirements" (King, 1993).

When he was only a few months old, I justified being out to sea on a Navy submarine by telling myself that I was making the world a safer place for him, and I would spend the rest of my life making up lost time with him when he was older. I learned about the dangers of this deadly foodborne pathogen on his deathbed.

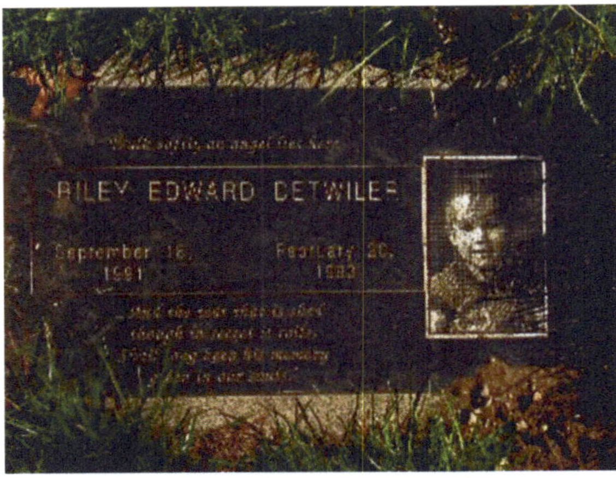

Photo from Author of gravestone for Riley Detwiler.

Making "*E. coli*" and "foodborne outbreak" commonplace phrases in popular vocabulary and impacting new legislation, the 1993 Jack in the Box *E. coli* outbreak became a seminal event in building the future of food safety in America (King, 1993).

References

American Association for Justice. (2015). Food safety and the civil justice system. Available from: https://www.justice.org/sites/default/files/FoodSafety.pdf.

Andrews, J. (2013). Jack in the Box *E. coli* Outbreak: Riley Detwiler's Story. *Food Safety News*. Available from: http://www.bigy.com/FoodSafety/CurrentNews/eColiRiley.

C-SPAN. (1993). Clip of presidential town meeting. Available from: https://www.c-span.org/video/?c4506516/clinton-town-meeting.

Huemer, R. P., & Challem, J. (1997). The natural health guide to beating supergerms. New York: Pocket Books, p. 8.

Kelley, T. (1996). Chronology of *E. coli* outbreak. The Seattle Times. Available from: http://community.seattletimes.nwsource.com/archive/?date=19960707&slug=233804.

King, W. (1993). *E. coli* victim leaves legacy of awareness. The Seattle Times. Available from: http://community.seattletimes.nwsource.com/archive/?date=19930225&slug=1687443.

Marler, B. (2013). Publisher's platform: lessons learned the hard way. Food Safety News. Available from: https://www.foodsafetynews.com/2013/01/publishers-platform-lessons-learned-the-hard-way/.

Marler, B. (2018). 25 Years Ago—Jack in the Box—Lessons Learned the Hard Way. Marler Blog. Available from: https://www.marlerblog.com/legal-cases/25-years-ago-jack-in-the-box-lessons-learned-the-hard-way/.

McNamara, A. (2018). John H. Silliker lecture: heroes: past and future. IAFP Journal for Food Protection. Available from: https://www.foodprotection.org/upl/downloads/meeting/archive/5c91137f3262435bd43ee.pdf.

Penhale, E. (1993). A cry for better meat safety. The Seattle Post-Intelligencer (Washington, DC).

Porterfield, E., & Berliant Mcclatchy, A. (1995). Jack in the box ignored food safety regulations, court documents say. The Spokesman (WA) Review. Available from: http://www.spokesman.com/stories/1995/jun/17/jack-in-the-box-ignored-food-safety-regulations/.

Schaefer, D. (1993). A prime time for the President—Clinton pledges to work on *E. coli*, Boeing's woes. The Seattle Times. Available from: http://community.seattletimes.nwsource.com/archive/?date=19930211&slug=1684984.

Sellnow, T.L., & Ulmer, R.R. (1995). Ambiguous argument as advocacy in organizational crisis communication. Argumentation and Advocacy, 31, 138–150. Available from: https://www.researchgate.net/publication/292267039_Ambiguous_Argument_as_Advocacy_in_Organizational_Crisis_Communication.

Sylvester, R. (1995). Children risk death from burger bug. The Sunday Telegraph (London), p. 9.

The Los Angeles Times. (1993). Child dies from bacteria; parents had voiced an appeal to Clinton. The Los Angeles Times. Available from: https://www.articles.latimes.com/1993-02-21/news/mn-825_1_town-meeting.

The New York Times. (1993). 17-month-old is 3rd child to die of illness linked to tainted meat. The New York Times. Available from: http://www.nytimes.com/1993/02/22/us/17-month-old-is-3d-child-to-die-of-illness-linked-to-tainted-meat.html.

The New York Times. (1993). Jack in the box's worst nightmare. The New York Times. Available from: https://www.nytimes.com/1993/02/06/business/company-news-jack-in-the-box-s-worst-nightmare.html.

The Orlando Sentinel. (1993). Toddler's death shakes the nation. The Orlando Sentinel. Available from: http://articles.orlandosentinel.com/1993-02-28/news/9302270333_1_detwiler-coli-infection-riley.

CHAPTER 4

Changes brought about after the 1993 outbreak

"Hard-working American parents deserve the peace of mind that comes from knowing that the meal they set before their children is safe"
President Bill Clinton, January 27, 1997, radio address.

February 23, 1993, the American Meat Institute (AMI) sponsored an industry briefing in Chicago to discuss the *Escherichia coli* 0157:H7 outbreak tied to contaminated hamburgers sold at Jack in the Box. Starting off the meeting, Jim Marsden, AMI's Vice President for scientific and technical affairs, informed the group that "Riley Detwiler, the 17-month old son of the parents who you just saw featured at the town meeting with President Clinton, died last Saturday" (Best, 1993). After a long list of regulators, scientists, and industry experts presented their thoughts, Marsden returned to the podium to offer a positive note, stating that "a year from now, *E. coli* will probably no longer be a problem for the meat industry" (Best, 1993). This prediction would prove to be overly optimistic.

At the time of the 1993 outbreak, inspectors from the USDA's Food Safety Inspection Service would engage in sensory-based "organoleptic inspections," which involved approving or rejecting meat by using sight, taste, smell, and touch to detect signs of disease or contamination on each carcass as it moved through the slaughterhouses. This meat inspection procedure of "poke and sniff" had been used since the passage of the 1906 Federal Meat Inspection Act. Within a year after the 1993 outbreak, however, the USDA initiated research into new inspection policies and proposed a "pathogen reduction program" in federally inspected meat processing facilities. These specific policy changes would require a radical change in how the USDA viewed pathogens.

As time was required to complete these changes, USDA Secretary Mike Espy proclaimed that, in the absence of a way to detect or prevent the presence of *E. coli* bacteria, the USDA must do "everything [it] can do to help inform consumers about proper preparation and storage of not-ready-to-eat meat and poultry" (Detwiler, 2014a). To this end, the USDA added to

Food Safety
http://dx.doi.org/10.1016/B978-0-12-818219-2.00004-1

the program a consumer awareness portion, described as a "bold action" that will educate the general public.

The USDA postcard

Secretary Espy invited me, Riley's mother, and other consumer advocates to join in discussions with USDA administrators about building public awareness. I expressed frustration over the forces within the industry that thwarted consumer education. Many within the department also expressed a level of frustration toward the many setbacks. Some in the meat industry objected to the postcard idea because it would emphasize educating consumers specifically about the dangers of undercooked ground beef.

After debates on wording and the specific message, the USDA decided that the postcard would be addressed to parents from USDA Secretary Mike Espy, and it would feature images and language advocating the "Recipe for a Safe and Delicious Hamburger." The postcard mentioned "ground meat" and "raw meat" but never actually included the word "beef." On May 3, 1994, the USDA began distributing (but not mailing) more than 5 million of these postcards to consumers (Fig. 4.1).

The postcard included a short message from Secretary Espy identified himself as the secretary of agriculture and wrote how the hamburger is "truly an American tradition," but also warned that "hamburgers and other meat products could contain bacteria that is (sic) harmful if not cooked or handled properly." His message reiterated four key points, which would appear on safety labels scheduled for mandatory placement after May 27, 1994, on all raw meat and poultry products. Though the safety labels advised only to "cook thoroughly," the postcards elaborated on methods consumers can follow to make sure hamburger patties are cooked properly, and at the correct temperature.

Beyond the actual message, the way the postcard was distributed also played an important role in its effectiveness. The USDA sent out more than 5 million of these cards across the nation, distributing them through the School Nurses Association of America, which in turn sent the cards home with elementary school students as a message from the school nurse. The idea was that parents would pay attention to a message from a school nurse and feel motivated to reconsider and change their perception of meat hazards, leading to safer cooking habits (Detwiler, 2014a).

The school children were also exposed to this information as school nurses discussed food safety issues with them in their classrooms. In talking

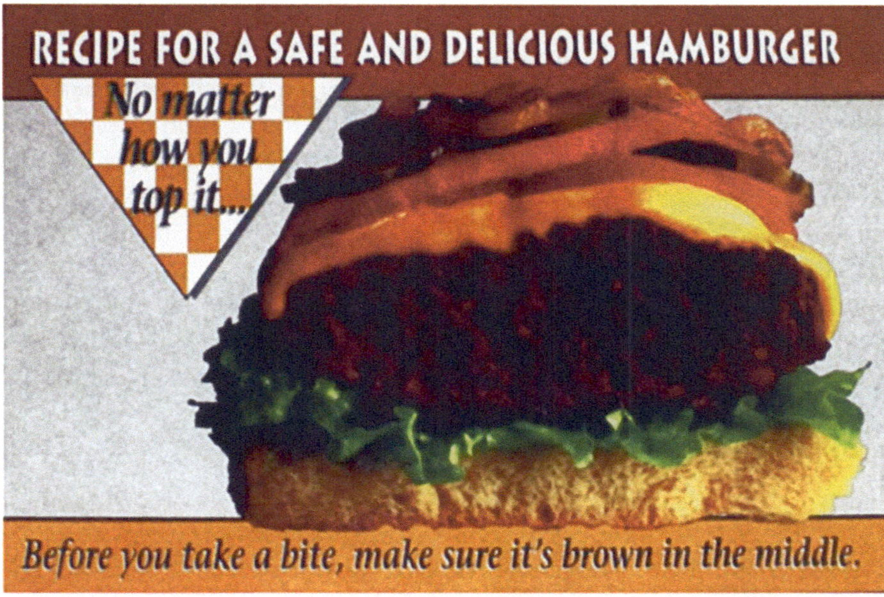
RECIPE FOR A SAFE AND DELICIOUS HAMBURGER
No matter how you top it...
Before you take a bite, make sure it's brown in the middle.

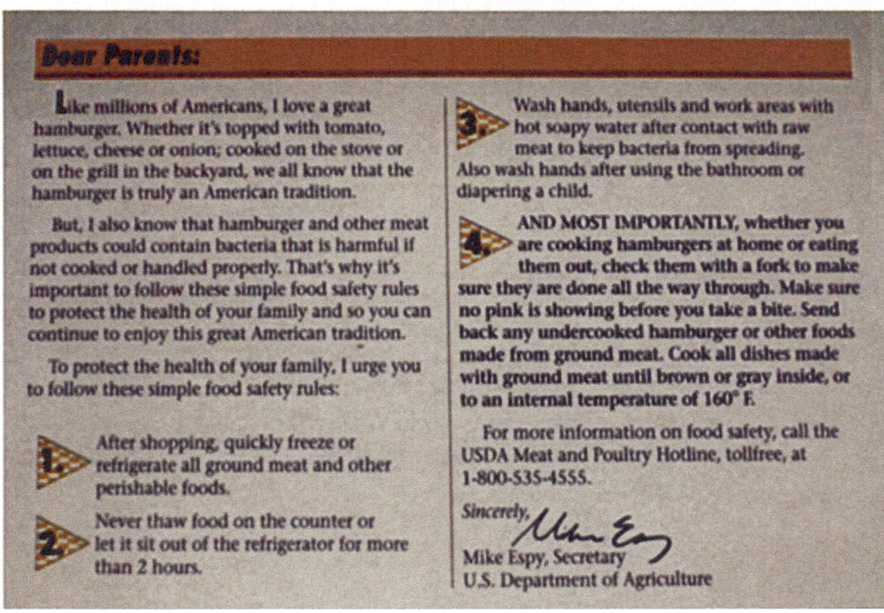

Dear Parents:

Like millions of Americans, I love a great hamburger. Whether it's topped with tomato, lettuce, cheese or onion; cooked on the stove or on the grill in the backyard, we all know that the hamburger is truly an American tradition.

But, I also know that hamburger and other meat products could contain bacteria that is harmful if not cooked or handled properly. That's why it's important to follow these simple food safety rules to protect the health of your family and so you can continue to enjoy this great American tradition.

To protect the health of your family, I urge you to follow these simple food safety rules:

1. After shopping, quickly freeze or refrigerate all ground meat and other perishable foods.
2. Never thaw food on the counter or let it sit out of the refrigerator for more than 2 hours.
3. Wash hands, utensils and work areas with hot soapy water after contact with raw meat to keep bacteria from spreading. Also wash hands after using the bathroom or diapering a child.
4. AND MOST IMPORTANTLY, whether you are cooking hamburgers at home or eating them out, check them with a fork to make sure they are done all the way through. Make sure no pink is showing before you take a bite. Send back any undercooked hamburger or other foods made from ground meat. Cook all dishes made with ground meat until brown or gray inside, or to an internal temperature of 160° F.

For more information on food safety, call the USDA Meat and Poultry Hotline, tollfree, at 1-800-535-4555.

Sincerely,

Mike Espy, Secretary
U.S. Department of Agriculture

Figure 4.1 ***USDA 1994 "Recipe For A Safe And Delicious Hamburger" Postcard front and back.*** *Image from Detwiler, 2014a*

with many of the school nurses and teachers involved, I learned of the almost complete lack of discussions around food safety in classrooms at the time. Many classroom talks after the distribution of the USDA postcards, however, lead to additional education in related topics, such as personal hygiene. Exposure to food safety issues at a young age, with continued exposure through the years (as students become adult consumers, parents, perhaps even food workers) could be powerfully effective in preventing outbreaks of *E. coli* and other food-borne illnesses.

The postcards represented a step toward more educated consumers, but the message was still vague as to the true threat to food safety. The postcard also indirectly supported the beef industry. Several months after the postcards were mailed, the USDA sent a stronger message directly to the beef industry.

A stunning announcement

On September 28, 1994, Michael R. Taylor, then the USDA's Food Safety Inspection Service Administrator, stunned the audience in a speech before the AMI when he said:

> *"To clarify an important legal point, we [the USDA] consider raw ground beef that is contaminated with* E. coli *O157:H7 to be adulterated within the meaning of the Federal Meat Inspection Act. We are prepared to use the Act's enforcement tools, as necessary, to exclude adulterated product from commerce. We plan to conduct targeted sampling and testing of raw ground beef at plants and in the marketplace for possible contamination. We know that the ultimate solution to the [*E.coli *] O157:H7 problem lies not in comprehensive end-product testing but rather in the development and implementation of science-based preventive controls, with product testing to verify process control" (Taylor, 1994).*

In other words, the USDA was declaring *E. coli* O157:H7 an illegal adulterant in meat and poultry under the USDA's regulatory authority and initiating a "zero tolerance" policy for the pathogen, implying potential legal ramifications for meat manufacturers.

The "safe handling" label

The USDA took another controversial step by requiring meat manufacturers to affix all packages of not-ready-to-eat meat and poultry at retail a label outlining safe-handling instructions. The goal was to ensure that the public understood not only how to handle raw meat and poultry products safely, but also how to properly cook it.

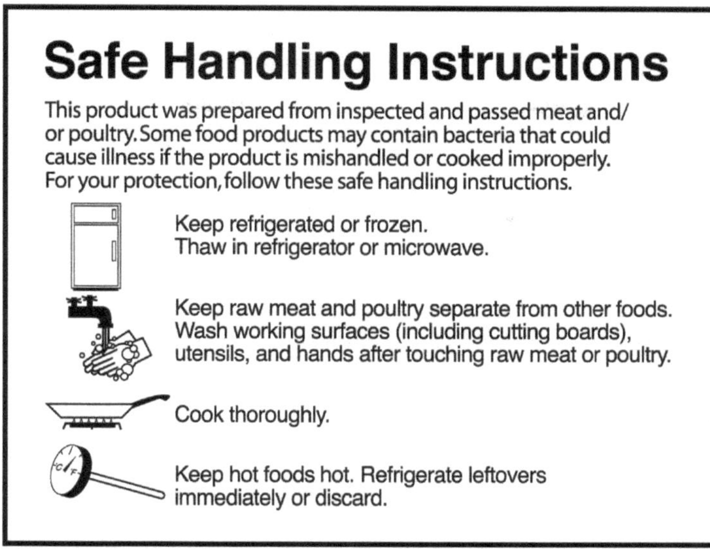

Image of USDA "Safe Handling Instructions" Label *US Department of Agriculture, 2015*

Agriculture Secretary Espy proclaimed that, in the absence of a way to detect or prevent the presence of the bacteria, the USDA must do "everything [it] can do to help inform consumers about proper preparation and storage of not-ready-to-eat meat and poultry" (Detwiler, 2014b). In the wake of the outbreak, the USDA's new pathogen reduction program included a consumer awareness portion described as a "bold action" to educate the general public. The program included the mandated use of food safe handling labels affixed to packages of raw meat and poultry. This effort was a complete reversal of the USDA's position on such labeling held some 20 years earlier.

In the early 1970s the USDA supported the interests of the meat industry over public health organizations when it came to warning or educational labels. The American Public Health Association (APHA) opposed the USDA's position, arguing that the USDA's "stamp-of-approval" misleads the public into thinking falsely the meat was free of pathogens. In 1971 the APHA sued the USDA in an attempt to force the agency to require a warning label with cooking instructions on all packages of raw meat and poultry. Among other things, the APHA argued that the USDA "stamp-of-approval" misled the public into thinking that the meat was free of pathogens, like Salmonella, when, in fact, it was not. In this case, the USDA sided with the meat industry in opposing the warning labels.

Since 1994 when the USDA reversed its policy on labeling, the warning label has been the most visible device the USDA has employed to educate consumers about food safety. The label does constitute progress, but many consumer advocates, including myself, believe the information on these labels was incomplete from the start.

In a 1993 discussion with Espy, I specifically asked why the cooking information was vague. He responded that because meat and poultry have different cooking temperatures, having those different temperatures listed may lead to confusion on the part of the consumer. He also stated that if there were different labels to be applied to different kinds of meat, mislabeling could occur at the plant or grocery store.

The USDA had, only a few years earlier, issued their 1990 Food Safety Inspection Service fact bulletin (not widely released to consumers, especially in a time before the internet) in which the USDA simply stated:

> *"Cook meat and poultry thoroughly—meat to at least 160 degrees Fahrenheit, and poultry to at least 180 degrees Fahrenheit. Using a meat thermometer is the best way to ensure that large cuts of meat are done. Greyish color and clear juices show when patties and individual pieces are done."*

In 1993 the USDA's intention for mandating their food safe handling instruction labels on all packages of raw meat, and poultry products was to inform consumers how to protect themselves. The meat industry took a position against this mandate as the labels may result in shoppers' knowledge that problems may exist. This warning indicated that more detailed information can be put out in a simple, precise way that would not require different labels for many products.

Though many newspapers across reported that the USDA's decision for issuing new consumer information was in part motivated by the 1993 *E. coli* outbreak, there was one other significant motivating factor for their decision: legal pressure.

This same fear that consumers may not know about their meat's safety was evident some 20 years earlier when, in 1971 the APHA sued the USDA on the grounds that their mark of inspection was misleading in APHA vs. Butz, 511 F.2d 331, 334 (1974). Claiming that consumers were not aware that the USDA's stamp of approval on a piece of mead did not actually mean that they tested it for bacteria that posed a risk to public health, the APHA argued that the USDA should require that meat carry a warning label with handling and cooking instructions to protect the consumer from foodborne pathogens. The court decided in favor of the USDA and denied a rehearing in 1975.

In May of 1993 the government agreed to require the food safe handling labels as part of its settlement of a lawsuit filed in Washington, DC's US District Court by Jeremy Rifkin from the consumer coalition "Beyond Beef." Rifkin criticized the USDA on how the information on the labels was insufficient, thus creating a weak message. His group even demanded that "cook thoroughly" be replaced with more explicit instructions.

USDA Secretary Espy requested that Riley's mother and I join the USDA in Washington, DC to help finalize efforts on launching the labels and other means of educating consumers about food safety. On August 11, 1993, we shared the stage with the USDA as they held a press conference to announce the food safe handling labels campaign and to show what the label would look like to deliver this message before the cameras and before the public.

Prior to the safe food handling label mandate taking effect, The USDA also reached out to consumers through "emotional" public-service advertisements for broadcast over 5500 radio stations to "help educate Americans about the importance of preparing meat and poultry safely" (Webb, 1993). The first USDA radio ad features my voice along with that of Riley's mother (from comments recorded at the August event in DC) to help educate Americans about the importance of preparing meat and poultry safely. The second one features solely a message from USDA Secretary Mike Espy.

ANNOUNCER: *A public service of the United States Department of Agriculture.*

ANNOUNCER: *January, 1993, A food poisoning outbreak in the Northwest takes the lives or several small children.*

RILEY'S PARENTS: *We went through the most torturous experience any parents could.*

RILEY'S PARENTS: *There is a great lack of knowledge nationally about issues of food safety and E. coli.*

ANNOUNCER: *[The Detwilers] lost their child to a deadly strain of E. coli bacteria. E. coli can be found in undercooked meat. But proper handling and thorough cooking of meat and poultry can keep your family safe. The US Department of Agriculture now requires safe handling labels on all uncooked meat and poultry products. These labels will tell you how to safely handle, prepare and store meats, and reduce your risk of food poisoning. Read the new safe handling labels on all raw meat and poultry ...*

RILEY'S PARENTS: *Because the torture of losing your child is enough, the torture of seeing it continue with nothing being done about it is worse.*

ANNOUNCER: *A public service of the United States Department of Agriculture.*
USDA SECRETARY MIKE ESPY: *In America, we have the safest food supply in the world. But we never stop learning how to make it safer. I'm Mike Espy—Secretary of Agriculture. Today, we know we must improve our meat inspection system—and we know we must keep—you—the consumer informed. That is why we want to send you an important message about proper handling of meat and poultry. It's important because some animal products may contain bacteria that could cause an illness. That's why the USDA is beginning to require safe handling labels on raw meat and poultry products. The labels will tell us how to safely store meat and poultry. They will tell us to thaw meats in the refrigerator or microwave. They will tell us to keep raw meats away from other foods—and to wash all working surfaces and hands after touching raw meat or poultry. They also will tell us to cook meats thoroughly. Look for these labels. Read them. Follow the instructions. And keep your food and your family safe.*

(Top) Script from USDA public service radio ad #1. (Bottom) Script from USDA public service radio ad #2.
Source: US Department of Agriculture, 1993

While consumer advocacy groups applauded the USDA's unprecedented and rather pro-consumer stand, various groups in the meat industry did not approve of the first, emotional appeal approach. Alisa Harrison of the National Cattlemen's Association called the radio ad a "scare-tactic approach" that placed a "skull-and-crossbones on American food." Furthermore, she complained of the use of grieving parents because "To make it so emotional is not going to give people the real information they need to avoid what happened to the Detwilers" (Webb, 1993). Industry groups voiced a preference for the second, less emotional USDA ad.

On October 14, 1993, one day before the initial rule of the labeling was to take effect, the National American Wholesale Grocers Association convinced a Texas federal judge to issue an injunction to delay the labeling because "unlabeled meat was not a significant health threat, and that the tainted meat outbreak in January was isolated to the Pacific Northwest." Ironically, though sad, only two weeks later, the Texas State Department of Health issued a statewide warning similar to the one contained in the USDA's intended food safe handling labels because of the deaths of two 3-year-old Texas boys from *E. coli* (Egan, 1993).

Though some stores voluntarily labeled their meat packages, the labeling requirement did not start until May 27, 1994—and even then, only ground meat products required labeling. All other meat and poultry products required labeling as of July 6, 1994 (a delay of three months from the USDA's initially intended date.) According to the pathogen reduction program's description of consumer awareness in the Federal Register, the food safety and inspection service (FSIS) will "inform consumers of the risks associated with unsafe food handling." However, in order to get the federal judge to release the injunction, the labels had to be designed in such a way that they would state proper handling techniques, but not any health hazards.

> *"This product was inspected for your safety. Some animal products may contain bacteria that could cause illness if the product is mishandled or cooked improperly."*

This message does not warn consumers of the possible dangers associated with meats in general. Instead, the issue is now discussed in terms of a public health, not an industry or USDA problem.

Neither *E. coli*, nor any other foodborne pathogen is named on the labels. The labels do not explain how bacteria contaminates get into the meat in the first place. What angered consumer advocates the most was that the labels do not describe the severity or the consequences of the problem to consumers. While words such as "may" and "could" make the problem sound insignificant, not every package of meat will be contaminated. Parents, such as myself, knew far too well that there is a great difference between something that "could cause illness" and something that could cause toddlers to suffer and in too many cases, die.

Progress by the USDA, relating to educating consumers, was thwarted by the efforts of the meat industry and the dual responsibilities of the USDA. Some of the department's administrators and assistants expressed concern over the pressures associated with the labels and with public awareness in general from within the industry, as some meat groups feared that an educated public would stop buying their product. Even the USDA was apprehensive of giving the consumer too much information as the consumer may not only be motivated to stop old behaviors associated with the products but be motivated to discontinue purchasing the product as well. This highlights an inherent conflict of interest for the USDA, for its charge is not only to regulate the quality of meat, but also to promote the sale and use of food products.

According to Janet Riley, a spokesperson for the AMI, "Warning labels really frighten the public, if consumers follow safe handling procedures, there's no need to scare people about what is really a very wholesome and nutritious product" (Egan, 1993). This description of the clean product may be very easy for the general public to believe, but what if a product is contaminated? In its 1990 FSIS fact bulletin, the USDA described contaminated meat and poultry as causing "thousands of individual cases, hundreds of outbreaks, and several deaths each year." The USDA went on to report

"6.5–8.1 million Americans may actually suffer [foodborne illness] symptoms each year" (Detwiler, 2014b). Mind you, this statement was made in 1990—four years before the USDA declared *E. coli* as an adulterant and well before reporting of illnesses from many food sources, let alone the systems to report, record, and monitor were in place.

Perhaps by placing a weak message on the labels, the USDA was at least able to mandate that some form of food safe handling instructions ought to be placed on every package of meat and poultry sold in the United States. But requiring labels and enforcing their use are two different things. I have visited plenty of grocery stores with their own butcher and packaging stations in which labels were not used on the products.

The USDA was able to get this label mandated in spite of backlash from the industry that delayed the labels and resulted in criticism not only over USDA radio ads promoting food safety but also criticism over the USDA's conflict of interest in regulating the safety of the products that the agency also protects in terms of commercial interest (Blake, 1994; Oleck, 1993; Webb, 1993). Ultimately, retailers across the nation began affixing or incorporating into packaging the safe handling instruction labels, a public education campaign that has been in effect for over 20 years, though new studies are questioning their effectiveness (Adu-Nyako, Kunda, & Ralston, 2003).

The 1993 outbreak prompted many improvements in food safety. In 1993 *E. coli* O157 infection was reportable in only 12 states. By October of 1993, the USDA had ordered safe-handling labels on all packages of raw meat and poultry products, temporarily shut down 30 meatpacking plants, hired more inspectors, and began developing a more sophisticated inspection system. By the end of 1994, 33 states had made it reportable, and by the end of 1996, it was reportable in 44 states. Several other federal changes stemmed from the 1993 outbreak as well.

Positive, systemic changes, but challenges ahead

In total, 6 years after the 1993 outbreak, the *Journal of Epidemiology & Infection* published a report on the event identifying two areas of change within the US Centers for Disease Control and Prevention (CDC) (Tuttle et al., 1999). First, in 1995, the CDC initiated the Foodborne Diseases Active Surveillance Network (FoodNet), an active, laboratory-based surveillance system that monitors trends in foodborne diseases across 10 surveillance areas around the United States. The system captures detailed data from about

15,000 laboratory-diagnosed cases each year, such as patient demographics, comorbidities, hospital stay details, and laboratory results, and then conducts special studies to identify their sources. This innovation allows federal entities to have access and share information from the states.

The second change at the CDC was the creation of the "PulseNet," a centralized national data collection system where multistate outbreaks could be detected. This system compares DNA fingerprints of microorganisms before analyzing to standardize comparisons. The CDC introduced the first major use of a DNA typing in foodborne outbreak epidemiology during the Jack in the Box outbreak. This DNA typing technique is used to identify the relatedness of bacterial isolates from victims from different states whose illness could be tied to food distributed through interstate commerce, as is common for large retail and fast food chains. The CDC trained and funded state health departments to test samples, which the states could now report to PulseNet.

Nevertheless, even with these two systems in place, the problem of food safety has continued to be a challenge and a danger in many ways (Tuttle et al., 1999).

The CDC's analysis of data collected over the past 20 years shows that between 48 and 76 million Americans get sick from foodborne diseases annually, 128,000 to 350,000 are hospitalized, and 3,000 to 5,000 die each year (CDC, 2014). Furthermore, experts attribute recent illnesses and recalls to numerous strains of pathogens including *Salmonella, Campylobacter, Listeria, E. coli,* and others in domestic and imported meat, poultry, produce, dairy goods, and spices. Soon, another outbreak would add more complexity to how people understood sources of outbreaks.

In October, 1996, the Seattle-King County (WA) Department of Public Health reported over a dozen cases of *E. coli* illness. Public health investigators isolated a genetically indistinguishable strain of *E. coli* O157:H7 from case patients. They soon found the same "fingerprint" pattern in O157:H7 isolates cultured from a previously unopened container of unpasteurized apple juice. With these cultures from a product proven to be indistinguishable from case-related isolates, investigators clinically tied the outbreak to its source.

On October 30, 1996, the Seattle-King County Department of Public Health and the Washington State Department of Health reported that the group of *E. coli* infections had been epidemiologically associated with drinking unpasteurized apple juice or juice mixtures containing apple juice produced by Odwalla Inc. of Half Moon Bay, CA (CDC, 1996).

On October 31, 1996, the Food and Drug Administration (FDA) announced Odwalla Inc.'s voluntary recall of juice products containing unpasteurized apple juice.

Additional, similar cases in from California, Colorado, and from British Columbia, Canada, through November. Meanwhile, the FDA began to inspect Odwalla's manufacturing plant in California. Although unable to pinpoint the exact source of the *E. coli* bacteria at the location, FDA investigators found numerous violations of health and safety codes: lack of proper sanitizing procedures, poor employee hygiene, and decayed fruit accepted from suppliers.

Ultimately, this outbreak resulted in 65 individuals reported and confirmed infected with the *E. coli* in the western United States and British Columbia. Many cases go unreported or undiagnosed in such outbreaks. Of this outbreak's reported cases, more than a dozen victims developed HUS, and of those, one 16-month-old Denver girl died from complications arising from her *E. coli* O157:H7 infection. At least one patient with *E. coli* O157:H7 infection acquired illness by secondary transmission from a patient with juice-associated infection (CDC, 1996).

In 1998 Odwalla was indicted and held criminally liable for the 1996 *E. coli* outbreak. The company pleaded guilty to 16 federal criminal charges plead guilty to 16 counts of shipping an adulterated food product and agreed to pay a $1.5 million fine—the largest such fine at that time in a food-poisoning case (Odwalla Pleads Guilty, 1998; Flynn, 2009). No individuals received jail time for their role in this outbreak.

The Odwalla outbreak was, in 1996, perhaps the first major *E. coli* outbreak tied to a major brand since the landmark outbreak tied to Jack in the Box in 1993. For me, the news of another 16-month-old child's death from complications arising from an *E. coli* O157:H7 infection hit far too close to home. For others, the fact that this outbreak was not tied to ground beef was a shock. Even journalists noted how odd it was that this was being investigated by the FDA and not the USDA.

As a direct result of the outbreak, Odwalla began pasteurizing its juices. The outbreak also spurred a response by the federal government, as they now require warning labels to be placed on all unpasteurized fruit and vegetable juice containers.

Some 20 years later, the fact that this incident caused illnesses, hospitalizations, long-term health implications, and a death still haunted Odwalla's founder, Greg Steltenpohl. In an interview in *the New York Times*, Steltenpohl recalled with tears in his eyes them moment when the King County department of health called in 1996 to inform him of the common element in many people's *E. coli* poisoning being his apple juice (Strom, 2016).

In his January 27, 1997, radio address, President Clinton addressed the 1996 *E. coli* outbreak tied to unpasteurized apple juice from Odwalla. The president announced a goal to prevent future outbreaks through a new food safety initiative.

> *"Nothing is more important to meeting this goal than seeing to it that Americans live in a world with clean air, safe food, and pure water. Hard-working American parents deserve the peace of mind that comes from knowing that the meal they set before their children is safe" (Clinton, 1997).*

By May of 1997, the Department of Health and Human Services (DHHS), Environmental Protection Agency (EPA), and USDA published "Food Safety from Farm to Table: A National Food-Safety Initiative – A Report to the President" identifying produce as a source of concern for foodborne pathogens (EPA, DHHS, and USDA, 1997). In total 5 months later, President Clinton announced a plan to protect American families from foodborne pathogens tied to nonmeat foods. He also issued Executive Order 13100 creating the President's Council on Food Safety (Exec. Order No. 13100, 3 C.F.R. 45661, 1998), and the "Initiative to Ensure the Safety of Domestic and Imported Fruits and Vegetables," wherein he directed appropriate executive branch food agencies to issue guidance through good agricultural practices and good manufacturing practices for produce (Clinton, 1998).

The USDA's Food Safety Inspection Service "Beef Products Contaminated with *E.coli* O157:H7" (FSIS, 1999) stated in 1999, "Given the low infectious dose of *E.coli* associated with foodborne disease outbreaks and the very severe consequences of an infection," the USDA would use the FMIA rules to require "adequate assurance that subsequent handling of the product will result in food that is not contaminated when consumed." This policy definition acknowledged the severity of the pathogen and introduced required activity beyond slaughter and packaging of the raw product.

Changes in industry went unchecked by regulators until significant public health issues not only arose but also persisted, encompassing many pathogens and sources of contaminated foods. Advances in technology, both scientific and computer, improved data collection and analysis for outbreak investigation. In the late 1990s the CDC and other agencies began using Pulse Field Gel Electrophoresis as a new means of identifying bacterial strains (DNA isolates from product and patient samples), thus allowing labs to compare their patterns to deduce if the strains are the same or different. This allows public officials to connect otherwise seemingly random and unconnected illnesses, hence identifying outbreaks and often identifying the source. This data allows regulators to inform the public, work with industry to stop the source of an outbreak, and to initiate recalls. Through the use of this technology, the CDC notes the incidences of illnesses have decreased, but the number of outbreaks identified has increased. The reason for this change is that increase in the early detection of pathogens in nonmeat foods allowed for outbreak sources to be identified and stopped sooner (Liang, 2016).

In keeping with the goals and mission of President Clinton's Food Safety Initiative, the FDA took steps in 1996 to improve its retail food protection program. Meeting with personnel from the FDA's Center for Food Safety and Nutrition, state and local regulatory officials from the six FDA regions, the Association of Food and Drug Officials, the Conference for Food Protection, and industry representatives, the FDA established a goal of "providing national leadership, being equal partners, being responsive, providing communication, and promoting uniformity" (FDA, 2015).

The collaboration of the many stakeholders produced the "Voluntary National Retail Food Regulatory Program Standards." After pilot testing in each of the FDA regions in 1999, pilot participants reported the results at the 2000 biennial meeting of the Conference for Food Protection, which endorsed improvements and refinements to these voluntary standards 2 years later.

In 1999 the USDA's Food Safety Inspection Service "Beef Products Contaminated with *E. coli* O157:H7" (FSIS, 1999) stated, "[g]iven the low infectious dose of *E. coli* associated with foodborne disease outbreaks and the very severe consequences of an infection," the USDA would use the FMIA rules to require "adequate assurance that subsequent handling of the product will result in food that is not contaminated when consumed" (FSIS, 1999). This policy definition acknowledged the severity of the pathogen and introduced required activity beyond slaughter and packaging of the raw product. The policy change did not, however, specify any one protocol for managing food safety in meat production. A few years later, the FSIS published a similarly titled policy change "*E. coli* O157:H7 Contamination of Beef Products," (FSIS, 2002), stating that the agency viewed the prevalence of O157:H7 on cattle brought to slaughter as being "higher than expected."

As a result, the USDA now required all manufacturers of beef products are required to reassess their Hazard Analysis and Critical Control Point

(HACCP) plans relating to *E. coli* O157:H7. The FSIS also issued compliance guidance for establishments on controlling *E. coli* O157:H7. In 2011 FSIS published "Shiga Toxin-Producing *E. coli* (STEC) in certain raw beef products" that revised policies relating to verification procedures, including sampling and testing manufacturing trim and other raw ground beef product components, to ensure the control of *E. coli* O157:H7 and six other serogroups of STEC—O26, O45, O103, O111, O121, and O145 (FSIS, 2011).

These compliance guidelines, HACCP plans, and "zero tolerance" policies on foodborne pathogens applied only to USDA regulated meat and poultry products, a group that comprises only about 20% of the foods regulated by the federal government. The remaining 80% of foods are regulated by the US FDA.

Since Riley's death in 1993, the math shows that some 75,000 American consumers have died from foodborne illnesses—a large portion of which could have been prevented (Mead et al., 1999).

References

Adu-Nyako, K., Kunda, D., & Ralston, K. (2003). Safe handling labels and consumer behavior in the southern U.S. American Agricultural Economics Association. Available from: http://ageconsearch.umn.edu/bitstream/21925/1/sp03ad01.pdf.

Best, D. (1993). 'Solution near on *E. coli* crisis. Prepared Foods. Available from: http://link.galegroup.com/apps/doc/A14123275/AONE?u=mlin_b_northest&sid=AONE&xid=ed1d188a.

Blake, J. (1994). USDA officials deny conflict of interest - promotional activities questioned. The Seattle Times. Available from: http://community.seattletimes.nwsource.com/archive/?date=19930602&slug=1704451.

Centers for Disease Control and Prevention. (1996). Outbreak of *Escherichia coli* O157:H7 infections associated with drinking unpasteurized commercial apple juice—British Columbia, California, Colorado, and Washington, October 1996. *Morbidity and Mortality Weekly Report 45*(44), 975. Available from: https://www.cdc.gov/mmwr/preview/mmwrhtml/00044358.htm.

Centers for Disease Control and Prevention. (2014). Estimates of Foodborne Illness in the United States. Available from: http://www.cdc.gov/foodborneburden/index.html#.

Clinton, W. (1998). Memorandum for the President's council on food safety. Available from: http://clinton6.nara.gov/1998/08/1998-08-25-memorandum-for-the-council-on-food-safety.html.

Clinton, W. (1997). Radio address of the President to the nation. Available from: https://www.gpo.gov/fdsys/pkg/PPP-1997-book1/pdf/PPP-1997-book1-doc-pg75.pdf.

Detwiler, D. (2014a). USDA food safety postcards – a father's different take on 'wish you were here'. Food Quality and Safety Magazine. Available from: http://www.foodqualityandsafety.com/article/usda-food-safety-postcards-a-fathers-different-take-on-wish-you-were-here/.

Detwiler, D. (2014b). Do meat and poultry handling labels really convey safety? Food Quality and Safety Magazine. Available from: http://www.foodqualityandsafety.com/article/do-meat-and-poultry-handling-labels-really-convey-safety/.

Egan, T. (1993). A year later, raw meat still lacks labels. The New York Times. Available from: http://www.nytimes.com/1993/12/20/us/a-year-later-raw-meat-still-lacks-labels.html?pagewanted=all&src=pm.

Flynn, D. (2009). Odwalla apple juice *E. coli* outbreak. Food Safety News. Available from: https://www.foodsafetynews.com/2009/09/meaningful-outbreak-4-odwalla-apple-juice-e-coli-o157h7-outbreak/.

FSIS. (1999). Beef products contaminated with *Escherichia coli* O157:H7. U.S. Department of Agriculture. Available from: https://www.federalregister.gov/documents/1999/01/19/99-1123/beef-products-contaminated-with-escherichia-coli-o157h7.

FSIS. (2002). *E.coli* O157:H7 Contamination of Beef Products. U.S. Department of Agriculture. Available from: https://www.federalregister.gov/documents/2002/10/07/02-25504/e-coli-o157h7-contamination-of-beef-products.

FSIS. (2011). Shiga toxin-producing *Escherichia coli* (STEC) in certain raw beef products. U.S. Department of Agriculture. Available from: https://www.fsis.usda.gov/wps/wcm/connect/1665f810-0723-4af8-b12f-78937585376a/2010-0023F_485.pdf?MOD=AJPERES.

FDA. (2015). Voluntary national retail food regulatory program standards. FDA Retail Food Policy Team. Available from: http://www.fda.gov/downloads/Food/GuidanceRegulation/RetailFoodProtection/ProgramStandards/UCM372399.pdf.

Liang, A. (2016). The increasing problem of outbreaks associated with produce. CDC. Presentation before the Conference for Food Protection Biennial Meeting, Boise, ID.

Mead, P., Slutsker, L., Dietz, V., McCaig, L., Bresee, J., Shapiro, C., et al. (1999). Food-related illness and death in the United States. Centers for Disease Control and Prevention. Available from: http://wwwnc.cdc.gov/eid/article/5/5/99-0502.

Odwalla Pleads Guilty. (1998). Odwalla pleads guilty, will pay $1.5 million in juice case. The Los Angeles Times. Available from: https://www.latimes.com/archives/la-xpm-1998-jul-24-fi-6616-story.html.

Oleck, J. (1993). "'War on pathogens' unites concerned industry. Restaurant Business Magazine. Available from: http://business.highbeam.com/137339/article-1G1-14347891/war-pathogens-unites-concerned-industry.

Strom, S. (2016). Odwalla founder tries a beverage comeback two decades after *E. coli* tragedy." The New York Times. Reprinted in The Seattle Times. Available from: https://www.seattletimes.com/business/odwalla-founder-tries-a-beverage-comeback-two-decades-after-e-coli-tragedy/.

Taylor, M. (1994). Change and opportunity: harvesting innovation to improve the safety of food. Speech before the American Meat Institute Annual Convention, San Francisco, CA. Available from: https://www.foodsafetynews.com/AMI%20Speech%20September%201994.pdf.

Tuttle, J., Gomez, T., Doyle, M., Wells, J., Zhao, T., Tauxe, R., & Griffin, P. (1999). Infectious dose and method of widespread contamination of hamburger patties. *Epidemiology Infection, 122*(2), 185–192 Available from: http://www.ncbi.nlm.nih.gov/pubmed/10355781.

US Department of Agriculture. (2015). Safe handling instructions. food safety inspection service. Available from: http://www.fsis.usda.gov/wps/wcm/connect/fa5e85b6-1f58-4af8-ab5e-3fef6c468eab/safe_handling_label_hi.jpg?MOD=AJPERES

US Department of Agriculture. (1993). News releases and other news material /United States Department of Agriculture, Office of Public Affairs. (Press Release). Available from: https://archive.org/stream/CAT10619378033/CAT10619378033_djvu.txt.

Webb, T. (1993). "Farm groups have beef with emotional USDA radio ad." The Seattle Times. Available from: http://community.seattletimes.nwsource.com/archive/?date=19931012&slug=1725681.

CHAPTER 5

Selected cases

"Stewart Parnell, you gave some people death sentences. Luckily, you are not being sentenced to death."
Peter Hurley, Testimony at PCA trial, 2015

"Even with all the required training and certifications, we still find violations of food handling. Employees don't think it is that big of a risk." Doug Beach, Manager
Ventura County (CA) Environmental Health, 2019

"Unfortunately for many Americans, falling ill from contaminated food has become all too regular."
Senator Harry Reid (D-NV), 2015

Since 1993, rarely have the owners or executive officers of major companies faced anything more than a fine after their companies had been found liable for criminal violations. Not one of the corporate executives related to the "Jack in the Box" *Escherichia coli* outbreak faced a single federal indictment for the illnesses and deaths caused by their actions. Historically, civil lawsuits ending in out-of-court settlements have been the only form of justice for victims of foodborne illness or death caused by corporations, retailers, or restaurants. Settlements, however, cannot erase the lifelong medical and emotional impacts of foodborne illnesses, nor can they bring back lives lost. If food company executives responsible for large-scale illnesses and deaths over the last 25 years had been prosecuted more often and more significantly, imagine the impact on the food industry and the likely prevention of many illnesses and deaths.

Peanut Corporation of America: *Salmonella*

Bobby Ray "Pete" Hullet, age 67, had recently retired after working for more than 30 years at a glove mill in North Carolina. During the morning of a late Sunday in November 2008, Pete became severely dizzy. By day's end, this soft-spoken man was unable to avoid complaining of excruciating abdominal cramps with vomiting and diarrhea. Early the next day, Pete's wife of 45 years, Shirley, and their son Tony found Pete on the floor—conscious but unable to stand. Tony drove his father to the nearest hospital,

http://dx.doi.org/10.1016/B978-0-12-818219-2.00005-3

where doctors immediately put Pete on IV fluids, oxygen, and antibiotics. They also collected urine, blood, and stool specimens for the lab to analyze (Detwiler, 2015c) (Pete Hullet, Personal communication, 2015).

As his condition continued to decline, the doctors told his family that every organ in Pete's body was shutting down. On Pete's third day in the hospital—and the day before Thanksgiving 2008—doctors met with the family to report that Pete had died (Detwiler, 2015c) (Pete Hullet, Personal communication, 2015).

Less than 2 weeks later, 72-year-old widow Shirley Mae Almer of Perham, MN, contracted a urinary tract infection. She had long relied upon assistance from her son Jeff, along with his two brothers and two sisters. Since 1990, after their father's death, the siblings helped out as much as they could when their mother took over running the family business, a bowling alley in Minnesota. They also helped their mother through her successful battles with lung cancer and a brain tumor. By December 2008, she was living in a short-term care facility near her home by her doctor's recommendation. Shirley made the best of it, often enjoying visits from her five children and grandchildren. Her health was stable, and when she contracted a urinary tract infection, the standard treatment was expected to take care of it easily. However, the infection was soon complicated by stomach cramps and diarrhea (Detwiler, 2015c) (Shirley Mae Almer, Personal communication, 2015).

Although Shirley had the will and the strength to survive lung cancer and a brain tumor, her immune system now was no longer strong enough to handle the infection and complications. The family's plan to bring Shirley home for Christmas had to be halted when doctors called for the family to gather by her bedside to say goodbye. Shirley's death from *Salmonella*—4 days before Christmas—caught everyone by surprise, even her doctors. Investigators would eventually learn that Shirley ate toast with peanut butter while trying to regain her health for the holidays. This finding fit into an emerging pattern (Detwiler, 2015c) (Shirley Mae Almer, Personal communication, 2015).

The pattern continued as new cases developed, such as 53-year-old Betty Shelander, who had performed as a professional actress/singer/dancer on stage and television in Los Angeles and New York before retiring to North Carolina. On December 27, 2008, Betty began suffering from extreme nausea and vomiting. The next morning, Betty's doctor prescribed some medicine for relief, but it was too late. That afternoon, Betty's husband, Albert, found her unconscious on the floor and called 911. Betty had no signs of life by the time an ambulance brought her to the emergency room. Doctors declared her as dead on arrival, soon listing her cause of death as pancreatitis (Detwiler, 2015c).

As similar cases continued to be reported, health officials informed Pete Hullet's family on December 23 that test results showed Pete died from "heavy growth" of *Salmonella typhimurium*, one of over 2500 types of the bacterium *S. enterica*. Shirley Mae Almer's children learned the cause of her death several days after burying their mother: *S. typhimurium*. During Betty Shelander's autopsy, the medical examiner identified the apparent cause of her pancreatitis as a *Salmonella* infection (Detwiler, 2015c).

The growing investigation

In early December 2008, the staff at the CDC's PulseNet (a national laboratory network that, since it began in 1996, connects foodborne illness cases across the nation to detect outbreaks) learned of 35 separate cases from 16 states of *S. typhimurium*—all with an unusual pulsed-field gel electrophoresis (PFGE) pattern. Established in 1996, CDC's PulseNet is a national laboratory network that has been investigating foodborne illness cases across the nation to detect outbreaks of foodborne illnesses.

After these first 35 cases, PulseNet, state, and local investigators soon had their hands full with a second group of 41 cases from 17 states displaying PFGE patterns similar to the first. By the beginning of 2009, investigators declared that the clusters shared the same DNA fingerprint and made up a single-strain outbreak. Through the collaboration of CDC and health officials from Minnesota, Connecticut, and Michigan, investigators linked all of the *Salmonella* infections to peanut butter.

Salmonella is one of the most common foodborne pathogens and among the most common causes of bacterial foodborne illness. An infection can cause diarrhea, fever, abdominal cramps, vomiting, bloodstream infections, reactive arthritis, and death. Symptoms generally appear 12–72 hours after eating contaminated food. The CDC estimates *Salmonella* causes about 1.2 million illnesses, 23,000 hospitalizations, and 450 deaths in the United States every year (CDC, 2019e).

When CDC officials asked Pete Hullet's wife about the foods he ate, she shared that his favorite treat was Austin-brand peanut butter crackers. "He ate it as a snack two or three times a day—usually just a few before he went to bed." An investigation into the foodborne illness that took the life of Betty Shelander tied her *Salmonella* infection to the consumption of a contaminated peanut product. When Minnesota State health officials asked Shirley Mae Almer's family about what she ate while in the long-term care facility, one of her daughters mentioned that during a family visit she served her mother some toast with peanut butter. According to Shirley's son, Jeff, "She was picky about what she ate, but she liked peanut butter on toast" (Detwiler, 2015c).

Tracing back to the source

The Connecticut Department of Public Health tested numerous peanut butter containers, identifying *Salmonella* in each container of products from King Nut. The CDC conducted a second study, finding prepackaged peanut butter crackers as another link in the illnesses. Austin and Keebler brand prepackaged peanut butter crackers, produced at a North Carolina facility, obtained their peanut butter paste from a single supplier: Peanut Corporation of America (PCA).

Simultaneously, the Minnesota Department of Health determined that the common denominator between the individuals infected was King Nut creamy peanut butter. FDA officials would soon identify PCA as the only company that produces King Nut brand peanut butter.

The fall of the peanut king

Hugh Parnell Sr. founded PCA, originally named Parnell's Peanuts, in Gorman, TX, during the late 1970s. The company provided its products to bakeries and manufacturers of candy, ice cream, and snacks, and also directly to consumers. The company caught the eye of the FDA in 1990 when the agency found that PCA was distributing peanuts with unacceptable levels of aflatoxins—a potential risk to public health caused by a mold that grows in nuts and seeds. Two years later, the American Candy Company sued PCA for lost inventory that included nuts because PCA falsely claimed that its product was free of aflatoxins.

In 2000, Hugh's son, Stewart Parnell, who owned a peanut plant in Blakely, GA, decided to purchase the Gorman facility, and within 3 years of ownership he successfully tripled PCA's revenue. By 2005, Stewart Parnell was able to add facilities in Suffolk, Virginia, and Plainview, TX. However, his success hit a roadblock in January 2006 when Nestlé completed an on-site audit of PCA's Plainview plant, giving it a "Does Not Meet Standards" score on nearly all 40 inspection areas.

Following the trail of the *Salmonella* cases, federal inspections of PCA's Blakely, GA, processing plant in early 2009 revealed problems that would seem to be the cause of all the illnesses and deaths: dirty conditions in the food processing plant, such as mold and grease, along with bird droppings, rats, and roaches. Inspectors noted leaks in the roof, and they found the PCA plant did not apply high enough roasting temperatures to kill *Salmonella* in their product.

Through the collaboration of CDC and health officials from Minnesota, Connecticut, and Michigan, investigators linked all of the infections to peanut butter. Although the FDA shut down PCA's Georgia plant, Stewart Parnell, PCA's owner, continued to operate his Suffolk, VA, plant. He stated early on that products were not shipped back and forth between PCA's various facilities in different states. However, this statement later proved to be a lie.

On January 28, 2009, Texas authorities ordered PCA to stop distribution and recall their product out of the Texas facility. At the time, the ingredients of more than 3600 products produced by numerous companies, such as King Nut and Austin, included PCA peanuts.

Further investigations by federal authorities conclusively identified PCA as the cause of the multistate *Salmonella* outbreak that sickened 714 consumers across 46 states and caused the deaths of 9 people between September 2008 and March 2009 (CDC, 2009).

Victims' families, including those of Pete Hullet, Shirley Mae Almer, and Betty Shelander, would wait almost 6 years to see Parnell and other executives from PCA brought to justice. Although the US Department of Justice (DOJ) indicted four executives from PCA in February 2013 on 76 criminal charges including the sale and distribution of adulterated food, none of the charges would technically involve PCA's sickening or killing of their consumers.

An eyewitness in the Plainview peanut plant

Despite inspections of PCA plants, and unbeknownst to investigators, there was one PCA peanut processing plant Stewart Parnell did not register with the state or with any county in Texas. It was at this PCA plant hidden (ironically) in Plainview, TX, where Kenneth Kendrick served as assistant plant manager for several months in 2006. PCA hired Kendrick after they failed an audit from Nestlé Foods. "When I was working there, [PCA had] nothing that resembled a quality assurance program," says Kendrick. "I came from a lab testing background in the meat industry. I thought there would be regular testing, like in the meat industry" (Detwiler, 2015b).

During his short time at the Plainview plant, Kendrick observed numerous problems, including rat infestations and excrement, bird nests, a roof leak, a false roof, and pools of rainwater in the basement—all of which alarmed his concern for feces in the product. According to Kendrick, "particularly with water leaking off a roof, bird feces can wash in and drip onto the peanuts" (Detwiler, 2015b).

A second Nestlé audit was scheduled for July 2006, but Kendrick commented to his plant manager that there was no way Nestlé would certify PCA with all its issues. As a result, Danny Kilgore, operations manager from PCA's facility in Georgia, flew out to the Plainview plant 2 days before Nestlé's second audit to allegedly hide the problems.

"Kilgore, Parnell, and everyone else in the plant were frantically patching holes in the walls, hiding roof leaks, pumping water out of the basement, and cleaning out mice traps, so the pest control guy would have a lower count," according to Kendrick. In addition, Kilgore had Kendrick rewrite the food safety and quality assurance policies as Kendrick recalls, "At the time, nobody at PCA knew any of the *Salmonella* standards as they applied to peanuts" (Detwiler, 2015b).

Although the second audit resulted in notations of "Much Improvement," the plant still did not pass Nestlé's inspection. Kilgore suggested to Kendrick that, in lieu of a third audit, Nestlé might look at improvements made after the July 2006 audit and approve PCA as a supplier. According to Kendrick, Kilgore insinuated that "microwaving the test sponges used for monitoring dangerous pathogens might gain better results, and if PCA gained Nestlé's business, [Kendrick] might get a raise in pay" (Detwiler, 2015b).

This type of skewing test results to make them look better is not unheard of. Jeremy Zenlea, Corporate Director of Food Safety at Cumberland Farms (a regional chain of over 550 convenience stores), recalls similar tactics he has seen during inspections. "It wasn't uncommon, years ago, if companies got possible *Listeria* results, they could just throw a white label over it, recopy it, make it say negative and then they would bury it (Jeremy Zenlea, Personal Communication, 2019).

According to Kendrick, Nestlé never did business with PCA; however, Frito-Lay and Kellogg's did purchase large amounts of peanuts from the company. These and other smaller companies decided to purchase products from PCA based upon inspections conducted by a third-party auditor that gave PCA the highest possible rating.

Kendrick sent anonymous emails and letters to the Texas Department of Health and to companies that purchased products from his plant—but he never received a response. In 2006, after only a few months on the job, Kendrick chose to resign from PCA because as he stated, "I knew it was a train wreck and something unethical and bad was about to happen" (Detwiler, 2015b).

From eyewitness to whistle-blower

Three years later while working at an orthopedic implants facility, Kendrick learned of the widespread *Salmonella* outbreak that traced to PCA's Georgia plant. In response, he spent "hundreds of hours" trying to contact the media and federal food or health agencies to get attention placed on the Plainview, TX, plant.

The only response he received was from the Chicago office of STOP Foodborne Illness (STOP), a nonprofit food safety organization. STOP convinced FDA officials to meet with Kendrick in January 2009, and they connected him with Gardiner Harris, a reporter at *The New York Times*. Harris' article, "After Tests, Peanut Plant in Texas Is Closed," appeared in the February 10, 2009, Health and Policy section of the paper (Harris, 2009).

Describing PCA's Plainview facility as a "disgusting plant" that "cut corners and had poor process controls" (Harris, 2009), Kendrick went on to explain how managers instructed workers to use tarps to direct water from ceilings away from peanuts and plant equipment and how this caused standing water in the basement. The article included statements from a second, anonymous former employee of the Plainview plant that confirmed Kendrick's statements. *The New York Times* article also revealed that the Plainview plant had not been inspected for 4 years since 2005, with Texas state officials blaming Parnell for failing to register the plant.

After that article appeared, STOP then connected Kendrick with a producer from ABC's show "Good Morning America." During a February 16, 2009, exclusive interview with the ABC show, Kendrick discussed how his granddaughter became ill with *Salmonella*-like symptoms for 3 weeks in December, a time when she only wanted to eat peanut butter crackers. "So I kept giving her the crackers and she kept getting sicker," Kendrick said. "I've had a lot of sleepless nights over that, a lot of crying over that issue" (Harris and Barrett, 2009). He then went on to describe in shocking detail the conditions he observed at the PCA plant in Plainview.

However, by these and other news outlets incorrectly calling Kendrick the "plant manager" as opposed to his real title of "assistant plant manager," the media cast doubt on his motives, implying he was only coming forward to exonerate himself since he was the so-called plant manager (Detwiler, 2015b).

On a positive note, investigators from the FDA did set up a personal meeting with Kendrick to get his side of the story. Kendrick gave them copies of emails he had sent to several companies warning of the dangers. He told of the lies that PCA's owner, Stewart Parnell, was selling to the public. According to Kendrick, Stewart Parnell knowingly made false statements claiming the peanut plant engaged in testing all the time. "What Parnell was saying was just not true," claims Kendrick. "Parnell would only do testing when a buyer requested one, and by 'testing' I mean that Parnell had an office worker simply change the dates on recent inspection sheets" (Detwiler, 2015b).

Kendrick also revealed how PCA was shipping product between production plants in different states. According to Kendrick, peanut meal, a sawdust-like product from chopping nuts, sat for over a year in large material containers until a full truckload was gathered—for the sake of saving money—before being shipped to Georgia for processing into peanut butter. He also said that the manager ordered employees to sweep the yearlong collection of dust and rat feces off the containers so that they did not look so bad upon arrival.

Kendrick even drew the FDA maps of the Plainview plant to show exactly where to find holes in the roof, evidence of the flooded basement, and where the dead rats could be found in a false ceiling.

The impact of the whistle-blower

Because of the Kendrick interviews, investigators shifted their focus to the unregistered Plainview plant. As a result of Kendrick's whistle-blowing, federal authorities and the Texas Department of Health investigated the Plainview plant as another source of the outbreak, and found the evidence they needed to pressure PCA to shut it down. Kendrick's information helped prove that peanut products were being shipped between PCA facilities in different states—contrary to what Parnell had told the public and investigators throughout the outbreak.

The CDC was also able to link the Plainview, TX, facility to the multistate *Salmonella* outbreak—but the outbreak had, by this time, already sickened 714 consumers in 46 states and caused the deaths of 9 people. PCA began recalling its products a month before *The New York Times* article in January 2009. At the time, PCA products were included as ingredients in more than 3800 different types of food produced by hundreds of companies (Goetz, 2013).

PCA also filed for bankruptcy on February 13, 2009, only a few days after *The New York Times* article was published. Four years later, the US DOJ indicted four PCA executives on 76 criminal charges related to adulterated and misbranded products that reached interstate commerce (DOJ, 2013). The charging documents allege that PCA executives defrauded their customers about the quality and purity of their peanut products, they misled their corporate customers and consumers about the existence of *Salmonella* in peanut products, and they participated in a scheme to fabricate certificates of analysis accompanying various shipments of peanut products (DOJ, 2013).

Investigators found *Salmonella* in PCA's processing environment, indicating inadequate sanitation controls. They found that PCA's peanut roasting process had not been validated for its effectiveness as a control measure or "kill step" for biological hazards, such as *Salmonella*. At the time, hundreds of companies used PCA's peanut ingredients in their products without an additional kill step (such as cooking, pasteurization, pathogen-killing washes, irradiation, etc.), thus the recall of over 3800 different types of products from more than 200 different companies.

The federal government filed criminal charges related to adulterated and misbranded products to reach interstate commerce, taking the following PCA executives to trial:

- Stewart Parnell, owner,
- Michael Parnell, peanut broker, and
- Mary Wilkerson, former quality control manager.

Daniel Kilgore and Samuel Lightsey, both of whom worked at the Blakely, GA, plant, took plea deals and cooperated with prosecutors.

Witness to the courtroom proceedings

In 2009, Jeff Almer sent a Mother's Day card to Stewart Parnell. Before he sent the card, however, Jeff checked with his attorney, who responded "Well, personally, I wouldn't do it, but I'm not the one who lost his mom, so—what the hell—go for it" (Almer, Personal communication, 2015).

Almer has a unique perspective of the American legal system, having witnessed the process as the family member of a victim, and through his collaboration with the prosecution team in advance and throughout the PCA trial. The two lead investigators from the US DOJ in DC and the lead prosecutor from Albany, GA, gave him a personal call when they handed down the 76 indictments for the PCA executives. Almer felt obligated to attend as much of the trial as he could, having attended 9 days of the trial in July and August 2014. He was also present when the verdicts came in on September 19, 2014.

Almer characterized the in-court tactics of Stewart Parnell's lead attorney, Thomas Bondurant, Jr., as that of playing the "government conspiracy game." Bondurant claimed the feds tried to "make an example of the little guy because it is easier than going after Kellogg's or the big companies." He also added that Parnell's team insinuated "the government was using Parnell to get more funding for the FDA" (Detwiler, 2015d).

"Bondurant also tried to make the jury sympathetic to 'a loving grandfather,'" said Almer. "He took a quote from Senator Patrick Leahy (D-VT) and twisted it around, claiming the senator said 'convict first, investigate later,' whereas what Sen. Leahy actually said was the responsible people needed to serve jail time" (Detwiler, 2015d).

On the day of the verdict, Almer prepared for the worst and hoped for the best. He went to the courtroom and sat in a front row seat at the side opposite of the Parnell family and listened as the courtroom clerk read the verdicts.

The jury foreman read, "Count one ... We the jury find the defendant—guilty."

The foreman proceeded to list the indictments and continued reading "guilty," "guilty," "guilty" (Detwiler, 2015a).

Together, the Parnell brothers received guilty verdicts on a total of 97 federal felony counts including conspiracy and fraud. The court also found Mary Wilkerson guilty on one of two counts (obstruction of justice).

Almer says he remembered his mother's last days as the clerk read the verdicts. He was overwhelmed with emotion sitting with tears in his eyes and feeling far too alone as his own family and other victims' families were not present due to the fluid nature of the court proceeding, making attendance near impossible.

He also watched as the three defendants' families reacted to the verdicts, recalling how Parnell's family members started sobbing; the sounds of their crying filled the courtroom. This emotional moment hit Almer hard—relief and closure for some, yet new pain and uncertainty for other families. He says he did not take any personal satisfaction as he watched another family become destroyed.

Almer could not help but notice that the prosecution team was emotional, too. He thanked them for their years of work on the case and putting their lives on hold for 5 years. "Sorry I was a pain in your butts for so long," he told attorney Patrick Hearn. The prosecutor's reply left Almer speechless, "Jeff, you made us care about this case" (Detwiler, 2015d).

Although the DOJ never called Kendrick to testify against PCA, he too expressed deep satisfaction that Parnell was indeed found guilty.

The aftermath of 2008–9 *Salmonella* outbreak

The 2008–9 PCA *Salmonella* outbreak and its related large recall illustrate the importance of process validation, sanitation controls, and supplier controls. Many policymakers viewed this event as one of the reasons why Congress later passed the FDA Food Safety Modernization Act (FSMA) in 2010.

Thousands of parents across this nation who have lost children to foodborne illnesses cannot ignore the fact that most of these outbreaks are preventable. CDC estimates of the millions of foodborne illnesses and thousands of deaths in this country each year are staggering. Many families of the victims from the 2008–9 *Salmonella* outbreak tied to PCA have spent the past few years testifying before legislators for stronger food safety policies and working to prevent such events from ever happening to other families.

Journalists and victims struggled with the fact that, since his conviction and before his sentencing hearing, Stewart Parnell spent many long hours working on his tennis swing at a country club in Virginia (Haughney, 2015). Unlike Stewart Parnell and PCA, the vast majority of companies in the food industry strive to make food safety a priority each and every day. Many dedicated food safety professionals and even some parents who lost children to foodborne pathogens work with some companies that invest in proactive measures to train employees and even indoctrinate their suppliers and distributors around their mission of food safety.

An important lesson out of this PCA outbreak and criminal trial is that our food industry includes only a very small percentage of companies whose low level of ethics and poor track record of food safety are so egregious. Perhaps the upcoming sentencing will serve as a warning to them.

Prior to the PCA sentencing, I talked with Stewart Parnell on the phone, even telling Parnell about his son, Riley's death from *Escherichia coli* in 1993. Parnell stated that while he believed that the executives at Jack in the Box should have been charged for their crimes and should have seen prison time, he and his brother should not have been charged for anything related to the illnesses and deaths related to PCA's products. Parnell also declared that this "whole mess" would be over in no time and suggested that he and I "meet up soon and talk over burgers and beer" (CNBC, 2017; *Food Republic*, 2015).

The sentencing hearing

Although the sentencing hearing was specifically for Stewart Parnell (former CEO of PCA), Michael Parnell (brother of Stewart and former broker for PCA), and Mary Wilkerson (former QA manager for PCA), the judge also ordered that Daniel Kilgore and Samuel Lightsey (both former plant managers for PCA) be present. Kilgore and Lightsey, also convicted for their roles in the *S. typhimurium* outbreak, were scheduled to receive sentencing the following week.

The lead prosecutor provided the judge with victims' testimonies. The defense team had earlier lost their challenge to prevent filing of written "Victim Impact Statements" and live testimony from any victims or their families (Flynn, 2015).

Gabrielle Meunier told the court that she did not want her son present to hear the tragic details of his 2008 illness. "My 7-year-old son told me that he was in so much pain that he wanted to die," she said.

Randy Napier, whose mother died as a result of eating tainted peanuts during the outbreak, shared with the court that his mother "taught us traits of love, respect, and forgiveness ... traits that are being tested today."

Jeff Almer, who attended most of the trial hearings the previous summer, stared at and talked directly to each of the defendants. In a haunting tone, he said, "Stewart Parnell, you killed my mom." Before ending his testimony, Almer stated before the court his appreciation for the efforts of Kenneth Kendrick in helping to make sure that the investigation, as well as the subsequent trial and sentencing, became possible.

Peter Hurley, whose son, Jacob, was sickened by PCA peanuts, flew in from Portland, OR, to say, "Stewart Parnell, you gave some people death sentences. Luckily, you are not being sentenced to death."

Ernest Clark had great difficulty controlling his emotions as he described the impact of the outbreak on his family. He told the court, "My grandmother suffered the maximum penalty anyone can pay for eating a food she loved."

The last to speak at the sentencing hearing was Al Shelander. In a solemn voice, he talked of how his life and the lives of his children were forever changed by the death of wife and mother Betty. "One day, the center of our family was gone," he said.

After hearing testimony from those impacted by the *Salmonella* outbreak, the court took statements from friends and family members of the convicted executives and comments from the prosecution and defense teams. They offered stories of their community involvement and dedication to family. These witnesses also described Stewart Parnell's many connections around the world and his hobby of being a licensed pilot and flying all over the country—even helping others with medical flights.

After a recess during the afternoon, the court reconvened and Judge Sands took his time remembering and discussing the victims and the courtroom testimony:

> *"We place faith that no one would intentionally ship products to market that are contaminated," the judge said. He continued, "Striking and strong testimony was heard today. Consumers are at the mercy of food producers for the safety of the products. These acts [of the convicted PCA executives] were driven by profit and the protection of profit . . . thus greed"*
>
> **(Detwiler, 2015e).**

Sands told Stewart Parnell that while this case "does not represent [his] entire life, the outcome affects a lot of people." He concluded that Stewart Parnell had clear "knowledge that there was *Salmonella* in the peanuts and that it was being shipped out of [his] plant." He noted that Parnell had "taken risks for years," that they were "eventually discovered and traced back" to his corporation, and that, unfortunately, "thousands of people suffered and nine died" from Parnell's knowing disregard for public health and safety (Detwiler, 2015e).

For Stewart Parnell's role, and after guilty verdicts on more than 60 criminal charges, Sands sentenced Parnell to a term of 336 months—28 years in prison.

When Michael Parnell stood before the bench, the judge made similar statements regarding how the case before the court reflected on only a small part of his life. Sands then sentenced Michael Parnell, following his conviction on more than 30 criminal charges, to a term of 240 months—20 years in prison.

Finally, the judge addressed defendant Mary Wilkerson, the former QA manager at PCA. "You were not a top executive in PCA, and your attorney painted a picture of you as a minor player in this case. You were aware of what was going on and played a role in concealing the problem. That was not actually a minor role in this case," he concluded. Sands acknowledged the testimony of Wilkerson's sister and husband regarding her spouse and two sons. "To have a strong family and still be able to care for them is a lot better than the reality for some of those in this courtroom," he said. The judge imposed sentence on Mary Wilkerson, after her conviction on one count of obstruction of justice, to the maximum possible term of 60 months—5 years in prison.

Judge Sands would, on a later date, impose a sentence on Daniel Kilgore (former plant manager for PCA) of 6 years in federal prison. He also imposed a sentence on Samuel Lightsey (former plant manager for PCA) of 3 years in federal prison.

In each instance, and especially for the lengthier sentences, the shock in the courtroom was evident. These sentencings account for the first time food executive had been sentenced to anything more than 3 months for their crimes.

The prosecution team asked the court to find that the Parnell brothers were flight risks and to deny them bail while they appeal their convictions. The prosecutors did not ask the same for Wilkerson. Judge Sands dismissed the defense team's allegations of prosecutorial misconduct and a less-than-unbiased jury. He also addressed defense objections to the victims' testimony, citing their constitutional rights. The judge then ordered that the Stewart Parnell and Michael Parnell be taken into custody of the US Marshals while allowing bail for Wilkerson until the Bureau of Prisons directs her to appear at a specified time and place to begin her sentence.

The PCA case, according to Judge Sands, was not about the "condemnation of peanuts or the peanut industry, but of a few individuals."

As stated at the beginning of this chapter, rarely have the owners or executive officers of major companies faced anything more than a fine since 1993. Corporate executives related to the "Jack in the Box" *E. coli* outbreak did not face a single federal indictment. The usual recourse for victims of foodborne illnesses or death has been civil lawsuits ending in out-of-court settlements. These settlements, however, cannot erase the lifelong medical and emotional impacts of foodborne illnesses, nor can they reverse the loss of lives.

The PCA case is different. Due to the unprecedented nature of the outbreak and sentencing of the judgments, the PCA case has and will likely continue to send strong messages throughout the food industry. Corporate boardrooms across America—those directly involved in, as well as ancillary to the food industry—will be talking about the legal implications of this case for many years to come.

For the first time, executives and others involved in allowing tainted food to enter the food chain will be facing potential personal criminal liability. That outcome has already gained a reputation as being a real wake-up call within the industry. For the victims and their families who played a key role in this trial at sentencing, and for the thousands of others across this country impacted by preventable foodborne illnesses, the outcome will hopefully serve to some degree as closure and vindication, as well as satisfaction in preventing future tragedies.

To some, these sentences were too long, while to others, they were not long enough.

The outcome of the sentencing sent strong messages.

Corporate boardrooms across America—those in the food industry and beyond—will be talking about the legal implications of this case for many years to come. For the first time, executives and others involved in allowing tainted food to enter the food chain will be facing potential personal criminal liability. That should be a real wake-up call.

The victims and their families played a key role in this trial at sentencing. For them, and for the thousands of others across this country impacted by preventable foodborne illnesses, the outcome should serve as some element of closure and vindication.

Nevertheless, this trial and the sentences should send a strong message of hope to American families, hope now that the justice system has tackled this in a meaningful and aggressive way.

Blue Bell Creameries: *Listeria monocytogenes*

During a random product sampling in February 2015, the South Carolina Department of Health and Environmental Control found some rare strains of *Listeria monocytogenes*, a bacteria found in foods, in Blue Bell Creameries' ice cream products. The discovery was by chance. It was an arbitrary choice by a lab assistant to select ice cream, as well as this particular brand of Chocolate Chip Country Cookie Sandwiches and Great Divide Bars for the department's protocol validation. In fact, the finding of high amounts of *Listeria* in these products prompted immediate retesting to validate the results. Upon validation, the department notified the FDA. This unusual finding—in a product that was chosen at random and one not normally associated with *Listeria*, due to its temperature—essentially initiated an outbreak response by authorities not triggered by consumers clinically proven to be infected, at least not yet.

The Texas Department of State Health Services responded to a request to collect and test products, manufactured at Blue Bell Creameries' facility in Brenham, TX. According to the CDC, Texas health officials sampled the same two products tested by South Carolina state lab, as well as another Blue Bell ice cream product, "Scoops," made on the same production line as the other two products. All of the Texas health officials testing yielded *Listeria*. PFGE performed on the *Listeria* isolated from the ice cream samples revealed seven different PFGE patterns, all of which were identified and uploaded to the PulseNet database.

In March 2015, Kansas health officials identified five people from the same hospital (admitted for unrelated problems prior to developing listeriosis) who were infected with *Listeria* bacteria. The PulseNet database was used to determine that six people from Arizona, Oklahoma, and Texas with listeriosis between 2010 and 2014 were exposed to these *Listeria* isolates (two isolates matched one PFGE pattern found in South Carolina and Texas, and three matched another identified from South Carolina and Texas). Available information from a number of the patients included the fact that they consumed milkshakes made with Blue Bell ice cream product while in the hospital (CDC, 2012).

In April 2015, the CDC and the Kansas Department of Health and Environment reported a total of 10 patients hospitalized in 4 states, including 3 who died in Kansas (FDA, 2016). Of note is that most of these cases took place before the issue in Blue Bell ice cream was identified. Between 2010 and 2015, at least eight people in two states became sickened and three died—but throughout that period, health officials investigating the illnesses were unable to find a common cause (Gillespie, 2015).

On April 20, Blue Bell recalled all its products. Within a week, the company stopped production at all their facilities to begin an intensive cleaning and retraining program.

Former employees of Texas-based ice cream maker Blue Bell Creameries described the factory's unsanitary conditions, including ice cream "all over the floor," oil leaking into barrels of ice cream, and rainwater dripping into the facility and standing on the floor (Miller, 2015). Although the company went on record to discredit the statements of former employees, the observations from FDA inspectors at all three of the company's production facilities supported the claims of unsanitary conditions.

On May 7, FDA released inspection reports on Blue Bell's facilities in Broken Arrow, OK, Brenham, TX, and Sylacauga, AL. The reports disclosed numerous food safety violations.

FDA Inspection Observations: (March 16, 2015–May 1, 2015) Blue Bell Creameries' Brenham, TX, Facility

1. Failure to manufacture foods under conditions and controls necessary to minimize the potential for growth of microorganisms.
2. The procedure used for cleaning and sanitizing of equipment has not been shown to provide adequate cleaning and sanitizing treatment.
3. The plant is not constructed in such a manner as to prevent condensate from contaminating food and food-contact surfaces.

4. Failure to clean food-contact surfaces as frequently as necessary to protect against contamination of food.
5. Failure to wear beard covers in an effective manner.
6. Failure to maintain buildings in repair sufficient to prevent food from becoming adulterated.

Source: US Department of Health and Human Services, Food and Drug Administration. (2015). FDA Inspection Observation of Facility Document: Brenham, TX. Available from: https://www.fda.gov/media/92059/download.

FDA Inspection Observations: (March 23, 2015–April 23, 2015) Blue Bell Creameries' Broken Arrow, OK, Facility

1. Failure to manufacture and package foods under conditions and controls necessary to minimize the potential for growth of microorganisms and contamination.
2. Failure to perform microbial testing where necessary to identify sanitation failures and possible food contamination.
3. The procedure used for cleaning and sanitizing of equipment and utensils has not been shown to provide adequate cleaning and sanitizing treatment.
4. Failure to provide running water at a suitable temperature for cleaning of equipment, utensils, and food-packaging materials.
5. The plant is not constructed in such a manner as to prevent drip and condensate from contaminating food, food-contact surfaces, and food-packaging materials.
6. Employees did not wash and sanitize hands thoroughly in an adequate hand-washing facility after each absence from the workstation and at any time their hands may have become soiled or contaminated.
7. Failure to store cleaned and sanitized portable equipment in a location and manner that protects food-contact surfaces from contamination.
8. All reasonable precautions are not taken to ensure that production procedures do not contribute contamination from any source.
9. The design of equipment does not allow proper cleaning and maintenance.
10. Failure to hold foods that can support the rapid growth of undesirable microorganisms at a temperature that prevents the food from becoming adulterated.
11. Failure to have smoothly bonded or well-maintained seams on food-contact surfaces, to minimize accumulation of food particles and organic matter and the opportunity for growth of microorganisms.
12. Failure to take apart equipment as necessary to ensure thorough cleaning.

Source: US Department of Health and Human Services, Food and Drug Administration. (2015). FDA Inspection Observation of Facility Document: Broken Arrow, OK. Available from: https://www.fda.gov/media/91871/download.

FDA Inspection Observations: (April 6, 2015–April 30, 2015) Blue Bell Creameries' Sylacauga, AL, Facility

1. Failure to perform microbial testing where necessary to identify possible food contamination.
2. Suitable outer garments are not worn that protect against contamination of food and food-contact surfaces.
3. Failure to maintain food-contact surfaces to protect food from contamination by any source, including unlawful indirect food additives.
4. The design and materials of equipment and utensils does not allow proper cleaning.
5. All reasonable precautions are not taken to ensure that production procedures do not contribute contamination from any source.
6. Employees did not wash and sanitize hands thoroughly in an adequate hand-washing facility at any time their hands may have become soiled or contaminated.
7. The plant is not constructed in such a manner as to prevent condensate from contaminating food-contact surfaces.
8. Nonfood-contact equipment in manufacturing areas is not constructed so that it can be kept in a clean condition.

Source: US Department of Health and Human Services, Food and Drug Administration. (2015). FDA Inspection Observation of Facility Document: Sylacauga, AL. Available from: https://www.fda.gov/media/91865/download.

These results highlighted specific deficiencies with plant construction, equipment maintenance, employee hygiene, testing, cleaning and sanitation protocols, and food holding temperatures. Furthermore, many of these observations were made at all three locations. Employees' actions alone could not have resulted in these observations, as failures (similar in some cases to those found at PCA facilities) stemmed from leadership, training, and facility/equipment issues.

As shocking as the findings are, these FDA observations were not new. The FDA released inspection reports from 2013 highlighting how the company had not only found *Listeria* on a variety of surfaces in its Broken Arrow, OK, plant, but also had not completed the necessary work to identify the source of the failures, taken action to solve the problem, or updated the agency (Elkind, 2015).

Not one of the company's executives or supervisors faced criminal charges, despite the hospitalizations and deaths. The Texas Department of State Health Services fined Blue Bell Creameries $850,000 as a penalty for the conditions that resulted in the outbreak, with $175,000 of that amount ordered to be paid within 30 days of signing an enforcement agreement.

However, the agreement allowed for the remaining $675,000 to be paid only if the company violates the terms of the agreement within 18-months of its signing (Robinson-Jacobs, 2016).

In June 2019, a video that went viral caused some to question the fairness of prosecutions related to food safety and, specifically, to Blue Bell Creameries. Dubbed the "Blue Bell licker," a female was featured in a video as she was filmed in the Lufkin, TX, Walmart licking an opened tub of Blue Bell's ice cream, resealing the ice cream, and placing it back in the store's freezer. In a statement emailed to media outlets, Blue Bell Creameries described this viral video incident as a "malicious act of food tampering" (Garcia, 2019).

Regardless of how random the choice of this brand of ice cream may have been for the "Blue Bell licker," her actions may come with legal consequences stricter than seen in response to the earlier, deadly food safety failures at the ice cream company. Before the Lufkin, TX, police determined that the suspect is a juvenile, authorities stated that she could face anywhere from 2 to 20 years in prison, as tampering with a consumer product is a second-degree felony in Texas (Matias, 2019). One journalist pointed out the irony of how "the first person to face criminal charges related to contaminated Blue Bell ice cream would be a kid who posted a video of herself pulling a dumb prank, and not any of the people who were at the company when their product literally killed people" (Solomon, 2019).

Chipotle Mexican grill: multiple outbreaks

According to the CDC and several states' regulatory agencies, Chipotle Mexican Grill is responsible for a rapid succession of six outbreaks, involving four different foodborne pathogens (*E. coli* O157:H7, *E. coli* O26, *Salmonella* Newport, and *Norovirus*) and sickening over 500 people starting in the fourth quarter of 2015 (Beach, 2016). Although the CDC has now declared the outbreak to be "over," the company's financial toll, as well as a possible criminal investigation, is still ongoing. The victims of the outbreaks also still live with uncertainty and, in some cases, long-term health complications.

Chipotle started in 1993, in the shadow of the landmark Jack in the Box *E. coli* outbreak. From the beginning they could have learned a great many lessons about mitigating food safety failures, but many experts and consumers who know far too much about food safety wondered how this chain—with 22 years of "post-Jack in the Box experience"—ended up at the center of multiple outbreaks.

Seattle, WA

In July 2015, Seattle & King County (WA) Public Health officials confirmed five victims sick with *E. coli* O157:H7, two of whom were hospitalized. They eventually tied the illnesses to a Chipotle restaurant in Seattle, WA. This outbreak took place well before the more publicized incidents, and came with criticism of the Seattle & King County Public Health department for not publicizing the fact that the series of illnesses were tied to Chipotle. Health officials justified their action, stating that the outbreak had ended before it was tied to the restaurant (Aleccia, 2016).

Simi Valley, CA

In August 2015, California Department of Public Health officials confirmed 234 victims sick with Norovirus from at least one sick employee at a Chipotle restaurant in Simi Valley, CA.

The father of a sickened customer filed an official report with the county health office, which is recognized as the first report in this outbreak on Thursday, August 20, 2015. On Saturday, August 22, the CBS News affiliate in Los Angeles broke the news on the norovirus outbreak after learning that about 11 Chipotle customers had posted on the crowdsourcing website "iwaspoisoned.com" about becoming ill at the same restaurant during the same period of time (Hopper, 2015).

Patrick Quade created the website "iwaspoisoned.com" in 2009, after he went through a very painful, violent case of food poisoning. Today, the website reports over 600,000 views per month between consumers, companies, and health officials, and has been noted as part of the detection of not only victims of foodborne illness, but also of outbreaks not previously reported. In recalling the 2015 incident, Quade underscored the importance of victims speaking up to draw attention to the outbreak.

> *"My assumption is that without the people posting to the website, the situation with Chipotle [in Simi Valley, 2015] may not have gained the additional attention. On the Saturday, we got six new reports that mentioned 23, so that was by Saturday were up to 34 persons reported sick on the site. Because of the website, the media ran with it and really put pressure on the company and on environmental health"*
>
> ***(Patrick Quade, Personal Communication, 2019).***

The use of social media has provided a new way in which consumers are becoming more involved as stakeholders. People are using crowdsourcing websites such as iwaspoisoned.com and Yelp to report illnesses. A year prior to these Chipotle outbreaks, the CDC reported how researchers found that these sites provided enough information to identify previously unreported illnesses and outbreaks. The New York City Department of Health and Mental Hygiene worked with Columbia University and Yelp on a project to examine restaurant reviews on Yelp that referred to foodborne illness. Ultimately, three previously unreported restaurant-related outbreaks linked to 16 illnesses met the department's outbreak investigation criteria. Furthermore, environmental inspections at restaurants identified in these outbreaks uncovered multiple food-handling violations (Harrison et al., 2014).

The CBS Los Angeles TV news report included an official statement from Chipotle that exposed a potential flaw that the local environmental health department would later note—the steps taken by the company up to that point did not include steps required by law.

> *"The safety and well-being of our customers is always our highest priority. When we were contacted by customers who reported feeling poorly after visiting our restaurant in Simi Valley, we immediately began a review of the incident, and have taken all of the necessary steps to ensure that it is safe to eat there"*
>
> ***(Hopper, 2015).***

It was on that same day as the CBS news report that Chipotle's corporate offices informed the public health department that 17 employees in Simi Valley were ill and that the company was sending in replacements for everyone who was working at that location.

Tipped off by the news report, the Ventura County (CA) Environmental Health Division inspected the Simi Valley restaurant on Monday, August 24, 2015. According to the report's comments:

> *"The area manager for Chipotle Mexican Grill .... reported they received their first customer complaint regarding a foodborne illness on August 20, 2015, via a computer complaint hotline. A second complaint was received on August 21, 2015, and, to date forty six customer complaints and another seventeen employee complaints have been received"*
>
> ***(Bassiri, 2015).***

According to the report, this inspection took place after the restaurant voluntarily closed, threw out all its food, cleaned and disinfected everything, and told all employees with symptoms to stay home. The comments section included an annotation that on August 20, 2015, rather than immediately contacting local public health officials to notify them and its customers of this foodborne illness outbreak, the restaurant remained in operation, selling food to customers until it unexpectedly closed its doors in the middle of the day on August 22, 2105. The employees then followed the chain's "corporate policy" to initiate the "Norwalk Protocol" after two or more customers complain of foodborne illness (Bassiri, 2015). Thus, in doing so on that date, "Chipotle knew it was highly likely that a Norovirus outbreak had occurred at its Simi Valley restaurant earlier that week" (Flynn, 2016).

According to Doug Beach, Manager at the Environmental Health Division of Ventura County's (CA) Resource Management Agency, Chipotle soon reopened, but during that time, this location was not listed on Environmental Health's online Food Facilities Closure Report because the restaurant voluntarily closed (Doug Beach, Personal Communication, 2019).

The report's comment section would go on to discuss the actions of the restaurant before the inspection:

> *"According to the area manager, after two or more complaints are received, the corporate policy is to initiate the 'Norwalk Protocol'... once the protocol was established, the facility was shut down to allow the facility to be cleaned and sanitized thoroughly by the existing staff members … all food (potentially hazardous food and non-potentially hazardous foods) that was [sic] handled by employees, prepped, handled, cooked, and/or cooled was (sic) discarded"*
>
> ***(Bassiri, 2015).***

Chipotle chose to try and conceal all evidence of the outbreak by disposing of all food items, bleaching all cooking and food-handling surfaces and replacing its sick employees with employees from other restaurants before notifying county health officials of the outbreak.

Of note is also the fact that an area manager put a sign on the door of the closed location stating "We are closed for the rest of the day due to a severe staffing shortage …" (Flynn, 2016). Thus, Chipotle, whose company motto had long been "food with integrity" (Petrak, 2007), was deceptive in how they communicated the situation to those who came to the door. Furthermore, instead of complying with California law and reporting an employee illness on August 18, Chipotle waited 4 more days until it had 17 sick food workers before it left health officials a phone message. In the meantime, it served about 3000 meals to unsuspecting customers.

The inspection report also noted information regarding the sick employees.

> *"The 17 employees who complained of gastro-intestinal symptoms are required to remain away from work for at least five days after they last experience any symptoms. They were replaced by staff members from other Chipotle restaurants, who are not allowed by the corporate office to return to their original facilities for a period of five days"*
>
> ***(Bassiri, 2015).***

According to the Environmental Health Division of Ventura County's (CA) Resource Management Agency, California has a mandatory notification law that requires the manager or person-in-charge of a food establishment to immediately file a report with the local environmental health agency if any employee is known to be ill with *E. coli* O157:H7, *Salmonella*, Shigella, Hepatitis A, *Norovirus*, Entamoeba histolytic, or any other illness that is transmittable through food (Doug Beach, Personal Communication, 2019).

In fact, California requires all employees and food managers to be trained and certified on foodborne illness, sick employees, and safety protocols beyond safe handling and cooking.

> *"Even with all the required training and certifications, we still find violations of food handling. One employee [at the Simi Valley Chipotle location] shared how he felt a duty to stay on shift, but did move to dishwashing. Employees don't think [being sick and working as a food handler] is that big of a risk"*
>
> ***(Doug Beach, Personal Communication, 2019)***

This lack of awareness pertains to the risk of handling food while ill is evidenced by the county documents from the 2015 incident. Beyond the employees' level of awareness, corporate sick employee policy can be seen as complicating the issue. The initial inspection report noted that while sick employees were prevented from working at that location or at other Chipotle locations, "two employees were confirmed to work at [a restaurant] two doors away" (Bassiri, 2015). Perhaps one good reason why sick employees would continue to work at a competitor restaurant is the fact that not all sick employees would be compensated for sick leave. An additional comment in the initial inspection report noted that while all "ill" employees "are being paid sick time above and beyond the normal sick day protocol," this cannot be said for all employees in other situations as, according to a statement from an area manager: "Under normal circumstances, effective July 1, 2015, all employees with at least one year of service time will receive five days of sick pay, and no pay with less than one year of service time" (Bassiri, 2015).

The absence of the suspect food (or potential evidence) rendered inspectors unable to take samples from food and the facility to extract and match isolates to those from confirmed victims. As a result, officials might never know exactly how the illness was contracted and spread (Von Quednow, 2015).

Ventura County (CA) Environmental Health Division Inspection Observations: (August 24, 2015) Chipotle Mexican Grill Simi Valley, CA, Facility

1 Management and personnel

- Food handlers employed at this facility do not possess a valid food handler card and/or records (as required by state law).

2 Pest control—flying insects
- Flying insects (fruit flies) observed within the food facility. (Multiple locations at facility.)

3 Equipment maintenance
- Accumulation of mildew on the deflector panel inside of the ice machine.
- Accumulation of mildew on the backsplash/wall junction above the ware-washing sink.
- Accumulation of grease and food debris in the lower compartment of the deep fat fryer.
- Damaged gasket to the tall one-door merchandiser at the front service counter.

4 Facility sanitation—unsanitary condition
- All floors not cleaned and maintained throughout the facility—especially below the ware-washing sink, at the cook's line, and below the storage racks throughout.

5 Restrooms—unclean/disrepair
- Plumbing and plumbing fixtures require maintenance and cleaning, as all food facilities shall provide clean toilet facilities in good repair for use by employees.
- Loose toilet base in the women's lavatory.

6 Facility maintenance—walls and ceilings
- Wall and/or ceiling surfaces are deteriorated and/or damaged.
- Portion of ceiling tile missing above the storage rack adjacent to the doorway from the customer service area to the preparation area.

7 Equipment maintenance—direct connection
- Equipment is connected directly to the sewer.
- Discharged liquid waste from equipment not drained by means of indirect waste pipes.
- All drained waste not discharged through a minimum 1-inch air gap into an open floor sink or other approved receptor that is properly connected to the sewer system.

Source: Bassiri (2015)

At the follow-up inspection 3 days later, Chipotle demonstrated that they corrected six of the seven violations it received during the first inspection. Inspectors continued, however, to observe food safety violations. They ordered the facility to immediately discontinue holding potentially hazardous foods at unapproved temperatures, noting that "a container of cooked beef was observed holding at 118 F at the steam table at the front service counter" (Bassiri, 2015).

The Ventura County Public Health Department issued an official statement on Saturday, August 29, 2015, that its lab had five positive results for Norovirus. The department also issued "exclusion notices" to prevent some employees from reporting for work until cleared. All employees were cleared to return to work by September 25, 2015 (Doug Beach, Personal Communication, 2019).

Beyond Norovirus in California

Chipotle would go on to experience another four outbreaks in different states, but this time the outbreaks were related to different pathogens.

During and just after the Simi Valley, CA, Norovirus incident, Minnesota State health officials reported 64 confirmed victims, sick with *Salmonella* Newport, in August through September of 2015, later tied to Chipotle restaurants.

Between September 2015 and January 2016, 55 confirmed victims sick with *E. coli* O26 (later tied to Chipotle restaurants) in the states of California, Delaware, Illinois, Kentucky, Maryland, Minnesota, New York, Ohio, Oregon, Pennsylvania, and Washington. Public health officials in Washington and Oregon first detected the initial outbreak. Through whole genome sequencing (WGS) and use of the so-called PFGE, a second, smaller outbreak of a different, rare strain of STEC O26 was identified in December 2015, with five ill reported from Kansas, North Dakota, and Oklahoma (CDC, 2016).

In December 2015, Boston, MA, health officials confirmed 151 victims sick with Norovirus from a sick employee at a Chipotle Mexican Grill near the campus of Boston College. The group of sick customers included 120 students at Boston College, many of whom were members of the college's men's basketball team. The administration at Boston College issued a warning, sent through email to students, warning them not to eat at the restaurant (Fuhrmeister, 2015a).

Massachusetts state health official stated, "Initial testing conducted by the State Public Health has shown the presence of Norovirus" (Fox, 2015). According to the report from the Boston Inspectional Services department, an employee at the store was sick while working at the location (Jenkins, 2015). With reports of customers sick from Norovirus, a sick employee worked, and an inspection having observed improper holding temperatures for cooked meat, city health officials ordered the location closed. Chipotle, however, said it had voluntarily closed the restaurant (Fox, 2015). The company fired the sick employee, identified as the source of the outbreak, along with the manager on duty at the time (Fuhrmeister, 2015b).

Chipotle ran print advertisements in 60 newspaper markets with an apology from Steve Ells, Chipotle's founder and co-chief executive. However,

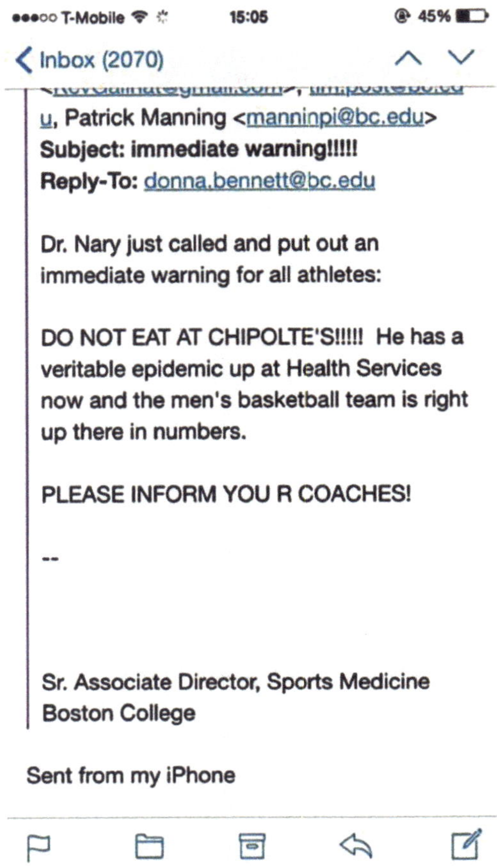
T-Mobile 15:05 45%

Inbox (2070)

u, Patrick Manning <manninpi@bc.edu>

Subject: immediate warning!!!!!

Reply-To: donna.bennett@bc.edu

Dr. Nary just called and put out an immediate warning for all athletes:

DO NOT EAT AT CHIPOLTE'S!!!!! He has a veritable epidemic up at Health Services now and the men's basketball team is right up there in numbers.

PLEASE INFORM YOU R COACHES!

--

Sr. Associate Director, Sports Medicine
Boston College

Sent from my iPhone

Image of text to team players. *Draper, K. (2015). Half the Boston College basketball team sick after eating chipotle, possibly* E. coli. Deadspin. *Available from: https://deadspin.com/half-the-boston-college-basketball-team-sick-after-eati-1746776378.*

his apology only went to the victims of the 11-state *E. coli* 026 outbreak and the Boston Norovirus outbreak. "From the beginning, all of our food safety programs have met or exceeded industry standards, but recent incidents, an *E. coli* outbreak that sickened 52 people and a norovirus outbreak that sickened approximately 140 people at a single Chipotle restaurant in Boston, have shown us that we need to do better, much better." This advertisement failed to mention the outbreaks in Seattle, Simi Valley, CA, or the ones unfolding in Kansas, Oklahoma, and Nebraska.

The CDC along with health officials in Kansas, Oklahoma, and Nebraska confirmed five victims sick with *E. coli* O26 between November 2015 and February 2016. All reported illnesses were eventually tied to Chipotle.

In its 2014 shareholder report, Chipotle executives argued that the chain may be at a higher risk for foodborne illness outbreaks "due to [the chain's] use of fresh produce and meats rather than frozen, and [the chain's] reliance on employees cooking with traditional methods rather than automation" (Chipotle, 2014). These claims had nothing to do with employees working while sick, nor the multiple times that inspectors found inadequate holding temperatures of cooked meat.

Recently, when asked about prioritizing and investing in blockchain for food safety and traceability purposes, a Chipotle company representative, in attendance at an industry group meeting, stated that with all of blockchain's hype, "we view it as a 'wait-and-see' technology. Quite honestly, we have many other issues to fix before we can invest in it" (stated in private industry meeting in 2019).

Similar to the 1993 Jack in the Box *E. coli* outbreak, Chipotle's reported profits in the last 3 months of 2015 plunged by 44% when compared to the same time a year prior, while the company's stock value decreased approximately 50% by the end of 2016, with an estimated loss value of $8 billion (Gillespie, 2015). In July 2019, Chipotle finally saw their NYSE stock value hit the pre-2015 outbreaks value (approximately $730) for the first time in 44 months. The lowest value during that time was $255 (down 65%).

Perhaps another way of looking at Chipotle's reputation is through the sentiments shared by executives and leaders in other parts of the food industry. During the panel of experts and participants discussing the Jack in the Box outbreak on its 25th anniversary, some industry attendees voiced their opinions of how leadership at Chipotle stopped participating in industry events and at one point actually left the table over a discussion on food safety.

Discussion about Chipotle by industry leaders also reflects observations that are not behind the scenes. The experience of visiting the restaurant shows just how the outbreaks have impacted customers. According to Jeremy Zenlea, Corporate Director of Food Safety at Cumberland Farms (a regional chain of over 550 convenience stores):

> *"When I went to Chipotle before all the outbreaks, there'd be a line around the block. You would take an hour just to get through there. I don't think I've waited in line once since, when we've gone there. So it's definitely has an effect. I know that Chipotle's doing a lot and trying to kind of market that they're getting all these sales back, but there's no way the average consumer has not forgotten. It's noticeable that they're their sales have dropped dramatically … and not to mention, I mean, come on, their brand name is now like kind of the butt of a lot of the jokes"*
>
> ***(Jeremy Zenlea, Personal Communication, 2019).***

Jimmy John's: *Salmonella* and *E. coli*

Although Chipotle struggled with multiple outbreaks of multiple pathogens, another major fast-food chain, Jimmy John's underwent state and federal health investigations of multistate outbreaks linked to the sprouts they included on their menu.

Jimmy John's is a sandwich chain, started in 1983, with more than 2800 locations across the United States. Its President and CEO James North said in a 2018 statement that "food safety and the welfare of our customers are top priorities and not negotiable in our business." North further stated that the company made the decision (in 2018) to stop serving sprouts across the country "after an investigation in the last 24 hours indicated that sprouts purchased from two growers in Minnesota … could be linked to seven food safety complaints received over a one-week period in December in Illinois and Wisconsin" (Bomkamp, 2018).

Problematic with this statement is the fact that, whereas "food safety and the welfare of our customers" are described as top priorities and not negotiable in our business, history tells us that perhaps they were negotiable or at least not a top priority when it came to sprouts. A clear pattern of concern (recalls and multistate outbreaks) over the past dozen or so years tied to one ingredient—sprouts—at a major, national fast-food restaurant chain even prompted the noted "*E. coli* Lawyer" Bill Marler (2018) to ask "would you buy sprouts from [Jimmy John's]?" (Flynn, 2018).

Year	Pathogen	Source	Ill	Hospitalized	Number of states
2018	*Salmonella* Montevideo	Sprouts	10	0	3
2014	*E. coli* 0121	Sprouts	19	7	6
2012	*E. coli* 026	Alfalfa sprouts	29	7	11
2010	*Salmonella* Newport	Clover sprouts	7	0	4 + Canada
2010	*Salmonella*	Alfalfa sprouts	140	0	Multiple
2009	*Salmonella* Saintpaul	Alfalfa sprouts	256	0	1
2008	*E. coli* 0157:H7	Alfalfa sprouts and iceberg lettuce	28	0	1

Chart by author, based on information from various sources, including Flynn (2018).

The problem with this 2018 decision, coming after so many opportunities to support their nonnegotiable top priority of food safety and the welfare of their customers, is also seen in the fact that their 2018 permanent ban on sprouts should be impossible: Jimmy John's had already made the permanent menu change to put an end to the restaurant's connection to outbreaks from raw sprouts. In 2012, owners and general managers of Jimmy John's franchises received an email sent by "Jimmy himself" ordering all franchise locations to permanently remove raw sprouts from their menus. According to one recipient, "Jimmy decided he was tired of the negative press from it" (Hunsicker, 2012). Apparently, after the negative press died down, the chain brought sprouts back, possibly due to demand, only to ban it again after continued illnesses.

Leafy greens/romaine lettuce

A 2015 study of leafy vegetable-associated outbreaks reported to the CDC between 1973 and 2012 revealed 606 leafy vegetable-associated outbreaks, with 20,003 associated illnesses, 1030 hospitalizations, and 19 deaths. On average, leafy vegetable-associated outbreaks were larger than those attributed to other food types. The pathogens that most often caused leafy vegetable-associated outbreaks were *Norovirus* (55%), Shiga toxin-producing *E. coli* (STEC) (18%), and *Salmonella* (11%) (Herman, Hall, & Gould, 2015).

Notable recent cases

Spinach: 2006

In 2006, some 200 *E. coli* O157:H7 illnesses tied to fresh spinach were reported to CDC from 26 states. A total of 100, or half of those reported ill, were hospitalized and 31 developed hemolytic uremic syndrome (HUS), a blood disorder characterized by, among other symptoms, kidney failure. Three deaths are attributed to this outbreak, including two elderly women and a 2-year-old child (CDC, 2006).

Bagged salads: 2016

Dole Food Co. knowingly produced and shipped salads from a contaminated facility in 2016, according to the FDA. Outbreak investigators in the United States and Canada linked cases of *L. monocytogenes* through PFGE DNA fingerprinting of victims' sample isolates. Investigators tied at least 33 illnesses in the United States and Canada to bagged salads from one of Dole's facilities. Four outbreak victims died, one in the United States and three in Canada. Although Dole closed the plant on January 21, 2016, several days after an FDA inspection, documents released by the FDA revealed that Dole officials knew of pathogens in the facility since at least July 2014 (Beach, 2016). Dole failed to take preventive steps against pathogen contamination of foods. Rosa DeLauro, (R-CT), the Ranking Member on the subcommittee responsible for funding the FDA has publicly criticized Dole, demanding that the executives "must be held accountable for their unconscionable actions" (DeLauro, 2016).

Romaine lettuce: 2017 and into early 2018

Late 2017, *E. coli* contaminated romaine lettuce in Canada, and leafy greens in the United States resulted in reports of 25 illnesses across 15 states, 9 hospitalizations, and 1 death (CDC, 2018b).

In spring, 2018, an *E. coli* outbreak—also involving romaine lettuce—resulted in 210 confirmed cases across 36 states, causing almost 100 hospitalizations. Five people died. The contamination was traced to the romaine lettuce from multiple farms in Yuma, AZ, with the source believed to be the use of canal water contaminated with cattle feces (CDC, 2018a).

What health officials first recognized as a restaurant-associated outbreak in New Jersey was linked to romaine lettuce within 8 days—but could not be traced back to any one source. By April 2018, the CDC warned the American public to avoid eating any brand of romaine lettuce grown or sold from any location in the country because of potential contamination with *E. coli*. As one common saying in food safety goes—"You don't cook salads." Some companies issued voluntary recalls of their products, but the FDA refrained from issuing mandatory recalls, because they could not find the exact source of contamination.

After eight inmates at Anvil Mountain Correctional Center in Nome, AK, became sick with *E. coli* O157:H7, the controlled environment at the Alaska prison helped state health investigators with their investigation. Seven of the eight sick inmates indicated through epidemiology interviews that they ate romaine lettuce. According to Dr. Robert Tauxe, Director of the CDC's Division of Foodborne, Waterborne, and Environmental Diseases, "this was way above baseline" (Tauxe, 2019).

What is unique about this Nome, AK, prison case is not that state health officials quickly able to identify whole heads of romaine lettuce as the culprit (DeMarban, 2018). Adding to this case is that, whereas many of the nation's other similar cases had been linked to chopped romaine lettuce that had been handled by multiple companies (and thus making it difficult to trace the lettuce back to the specific farm), the cases at this prison involved lettuce that came from only one supplier for the items, thus the state epidemiologists gained the ability to trace back and identify the exact Yuma, AZ, farm that provided romaine lettuce. Specifically, investigators traced the lettuce back to over 20 fields across the span of at least 50 miles in the Yuma, AZ, growing area.

The CDC's warning remained in effect until June 28, when the agency said tainted lettuce from Yuma "should no longer be available." In that update, the CDC said 210 people across 36 states were sickened by *E. coli* O157, and 5 people died, making it the worst outbreak in more than a decade. According to the CDC's Dr. Robert Tauxe, "This particular outbreak ... was a really catastrophic thing. It's right up there with the 1993 ground beef outbreak in the northwest" (Tauxe, 2019).

The CDC and the FDA would eventually release a very significant finding in this case: that the same *E. coli* strain found in sickened people across the country was also in Arizona's canal water used to irrigate crops. The CDC tested high-volume samples of the free-flowing water in the irrigation canal prompted the Leafy Greens Marketing Association (LGMA) to require farmers that are part of the LGMA to sanitize surface water sprayed on to leafy greens, whether for irrigation or for aerial crop-dusting-type applications (LGMA, 2015).

Although many scientists are quick to point out that *E. coli* 0157 is commonly found in the fecal matter of cattle and that it is easily possible that manure from one of Yuma County's many livestock operations ran off into the irrigation canals that fuel Arizona's agricultural system, the FDA Commissioner Scott Gottlieb holds that "More work needs to be done to determine just how and why this strain of *E. coli* O157 could have gotten into this body of water and how that led to contamination of romaine lettuce from multiple farms" (Gottlieb, 2018a).

According to a February 13, 2019, FDA report, the particular strain of *E. coli* O157:H7 was found in sediment from a water reservoir on a farm in Santa Maria, CA (about an hour's drive north west of Santa Barbara.) However, though the reservoir was only used by one farm, romaine from farms in all three counties tested positive for the same *E. coli* strain (FDA, 2019b).

The FDA report acknowledged uncertainty in terms of use of exactly how the lettuce came into contact with the contaminated water. The report went on to acknowledge that agricultural water from a reservoir is known for having a higher food safety risk than groundwater because pathogens are more likely to contaminate the surface.

Romaine lettuce: late 2018

Just two days before Thanksgiving 2018, the CDC issued a warning, advising Americans to avoid eating any romaine lettuce—no matter where it came from: "Consumers who have any type of romaine lettuce in their home should not eat it and should throw it away, even if some of it was eaten and no one has gotten sick" (CDC, 2019e). At the timing of this warning, no deaths had been reported, but 62 people in 16 states had become sick and 25 people were hospitalized (CDC, 2019e). The outbreak came at not only an inconvenient timing during the start of the holiday season, but also during a time when many other foods had been recalled (see Box below).

On November 5, 2018, the FDA announced a recall of Duncan Hines Classic White, Classic Butter Golden, Signature Confetti, and Classic Yellow cake mixes. Conagra Brands collaborated with health officials in connection with a positive finding of *Salmonella* in a retail sample of these cake mix that may be linked to a *Salmonella* outbreak currently being investigated by CDC and FDA. By the end of this outbreak, the CDC reported seven cases of illness across five states (CDC, 2019c).

On November 8, 2018, the CDC issued an investigation notice regarding a multistate outbreak of *Salmonella* infections linked to raw turkey products. The CDC reissued public warnings prior to the Thanksgiving holiday week. By the time the CDC declared the outbreak to be over, they reported 358 illnesses across 42 states and the District of Columbia, with 133 people hospitalized and 1 death reported from California (CDC, 2019b).

On November 16, 2018, the FDA issued an announcement that the Quaker Oats Company issued a voluntary recall of Cap'n Crunch's Peanut Butter Crunch Cereal distributed to Target Stores due to the potential presence of *Salmonella* (FDA, 2018).

On November 17, 2018, the USDA issued a "high-risk" recall of nearly 100,000 pounds of ground beef from Swift Beef Company due to possible *E. coli* O157:H7 contamination. This was a Class I recall—a "health hazard situation where there is a reasonable probability that the use of the product will cause serious, adverse health consequences or death" (Bell, 2018). This recall was unrelated to the 12.1 million pounds of ground beef involved in two other recalls (October 4, 2018 and December 4, 2018). Here, the CDC reported 403 consumers across 30 states and 117 hospitalized sick with *Salmonella* Newport in the outbreak. The USDA-FSIS and state partners traced the source of the ground beef eaten by ill people in this outbreak to JBS Tolleson Inc. (CDC, 2019d).

In late 2018, *E. coli* O157:H7 in romaine lettuce outbreak infected 62 people across 16 states in the United States and another 18 in Canada (Ontario and Quebec) hospitalizing 25 people, including 2 patients who developed HUS. Recorded illnesses dated as far back as October 7, 2018, and the CDC declared the outbreak over as of January 9, 2019. This outbreak sparked great media attention as the CDC issued a "stunning warning" from the CDC, issued just a few days before Thanksgiving, advising consumers to not eat any romaine lettuce—"no matter where it's from" (Atkin, 2018). Important to note is that, unlike the previous romaine lettuce outbreaks in 2017/18, this outbreak did result in a recall, with red leaf lettuce, green leaf lettuce, and cauliflower harvested from a farm in Santa Barbara County, CA, between November 27 and 30, 2018, being recalled (CDC, 2019a).

Leafy greens: aftermath?

With the last romaine lettuce outbreak over, perhaps it's less important where the *E. coli* initially came from than why the contaminated water was used on lettuce in the first place. The liability issue in this case, with implications for all farms, comes down water use practices: if farms are using contaminated water from open irrigation canals, and whether or not they are monitoring and testing it. Consumers started questioning the practice of using open irrigation canals in 2006, after the deadly *E. coli* O157:H7 outbreak tied to fresh spinach. Like the romaine outbreaks in 2018, the source of contamination was water polluted, traced to cattle fields near the spinach fields (Russell, 2006).

The Obama Administration's FDA passed "Standards for the Growing, Harvesting, Packing, and Holding of Produce for Human Consumption," commonly referred to as the 2010 FDA FSMA "Produce Safety Rule" (see Chapter 7 for an in-depth look at FAMS). The regulation, published in the Federal Register of November 27, 2015 (80 FR 74354) was supposed to have gone into effect in January 2018 and would have required farms to test their water for *E. coli* and other contaminants, thus reducing deadly outbreaks. However, in 2016 the Trump administration's FDA, responding to pressure from the farm industry over anticipated costs (and Trump's order to eliminate regulations), shelved the water-testing rules (except for sprouts) for another few years.

In September 2017, the then FDA commissioner Dr. Scott Gottlieb revealed before the National Association of State Departments of Agriculture (NASDA) that the FDA would issue a proposal to extend compliance dates for the agricultural water requirements by 2–4 years, based on feedback from farmers that the standards for agricultural water are "too complicated, and in some cases too costly, to be effectively implemented" (Gottlieb, 2017). One argument was that eliminating the water-testing rules would save growers $12 million per year (Shogren & Neilson, 2018). The costs of medical expenses that will be passed on to consumers, on the other hand, is potentially at least 8 times higher (see Chapter 6 for economic consideration).

Today, the FDA's rule: "Standards for the Growing, Harvesting, Packing, and Holding of Produce for Human Consumption; Extension of Compliance Dates for Subpart E," published in the Federal Register on March 18, 2019, states:

> *"As of March 18, 2019 the compliance dates for the agricultural water provisions (subpart E) in the Standards for the 'Growing, Harvesting, Packing, and Holding of Produce for Human Consumption' rule (November 27, 2015, 80 FR 74354), for covered produce other than sprouts, are delayed to January 26, 2024, for very small businesses, January 26, 2023, for small businesses, and January 26, 2022, for all other businesses (FDA, 2019).*

Just with leafy greens alone, the number of failures is not to be ignored. Social media posts, such as the @CDCgov posts on Twitter and memes on a variety of media, captured the frenzy over this string of concerns. Traceability will be the largest hurdle that the FDA and the industry will need to tackle going forward. FDA Commissioner Scott Gottlieb issued a statement in November 2018 in which he declared that "Complicating this already large-scale investigation, the majority of the records collected in this investigation were either paper or handwritten" (Gottlieb, 2018b). Thus, the FDA's emphasis on industry work to standardize record keeping adopt traceability best practices and state-of-the-art technologies.

At the 2019 meeting of the International Association for Food Protection (IAFP), many keynotes, panels, and symposia focused on these romaine lettuce outbreaks.

Robert Tauxe, MD, MPH, Director for the National Center for Emerging and Zoonotic Infectious Diseases at the Centers for Disease Control and Prevention in Atlanta, GA, delivered the annual John H. Silliker lecture and showed how WGS, new ways of using data, and strong investigative work were key to finding the source of and ending these romaine lettuce outbreaks (Tauxe, 2019).

Frank Yiannas, FDA's Deputy Commissioner for Food Policy and Response, took office during the November 2018 romaine lettuce outbreak. He dedicated a significant portion of his IAFP 2019 speech "Helping to Ensure the Safety of Leafy Greens" to the issue and stated that the FDA's investigation "highlighted the need for better management of agricultural water as well as the need for better traceability" (Yiannas, 2019).

After discussing the compliance extension for the agricultural water provisions for all produce (other than sprouts) covered by FSMA's Produce Safety Rule, Yiannas addressed the concerns about the delay in the compliance dates, stating that the FDA's priority now is working with the produce industry and industry groups to make agricultural water as safe possible.

> *"Routine inspections of large farms, under the Produce Safety Rule, began this spring. States are conducting the majority of the domestic inspections under a cooperative agreement with FDA. FDA is inspecting farms in other countries that export produce to the United States.*
>
> *We are engaged in collaborative research investigations with government and academic groups to sample agricultural water in the U.S. and internationally. These environmental water surveys are designed to increase our understanding of pathogen contamination and inform preventive measures that mitigate the risks. Water quality standards, inspections and testing—you see there's a lot of good work underway"*
>
> ***(Yiannas, 2019).***

Yiannas went on to discuss the need for greater traceability, focusing on "best practices for real-time, farm-to-fork traceability and state of-the-art technology to assure quick and easy access to key data elements when leafy greens are involved in a potential recall or outbreak" (Yiannas, 2019).

Not even one month after these remarks, Dole Fresh Vegetables, Inc. announced a voluntary recall of some of its Baby Spinach over possible *Salmonella* contamination. In a statement, the company acknowledged that the "precautionary recall" came after notification of a positive result for *Salmonella* in a random sample test conducted by Michigan State's Department of Agriculture (Silverman, 2019). This news reawakened some food safety experts' criticism that too many food companies are operating only at the "compliance" level with their sampling and testing programs. To prevent the frequently recurring incidents of failure, all food operators would operate at a more effective, higher level than simply compliance.

Before the industry and regulators can focus on technology, however, the legal, economic, and political concerns pertaining not only to the safety of specific food commodities, but also to the larger picture of our food supply system, must be prioritized.

References

Aleccia, J. (2016). Seattle man sues Chipotle; fell ill months before big outbreak. The Seattle Times. Available from: https://www.seattletimes.com/seattle-news/health/seattle-man-sues-chipotle-fell-ill-months-before-big-outbreak/.

Atkin, E. (2018). All Romaine Lettuce is Unsafe to Eat—Again. Here's Why. The New Republic. Available from: https://newrepublic.com/minutes/152362/romaine-lettuce-unsafe-eatagain-heres-why.

Bassiri, R. (2015). Food program inspection report. Ventura County Environmental Health Division. Available from: https://foodsafetynewsfullservice.marlersites.com/files/2015/12/CHIPOTLE-NOROVIRUS-Ventura-County-EH-inspection-re.pdf.

Beach, C. (2016). Updated: CDC declares Chipotle *E. coli* outbreaks over; cause unknown. Food Safety News. Available from: http://www.foodsafetynews.com/2016/02/cdc-declares-chipotle-e-coli-outbreaks-over-cause-unknown/#.Vw1acvkrLIU

Bell, B. (2018). News Release: Swift Beef Company Recalls Ground Beef Products due to Possible *E. coli* O157:H7 Contamination. USDA. Available from: https://www.fsis.usda.gov/wps/portal/fsis/topics/recalls-and-public-health-alerts/recall-case-archive/archive/2018/recall-114-2018-release.

Bomkamp, S. (2018). Jimmy John's Sprouts Linked to Multistate *Salmonella* Outbreak. The Chicago Tribune. Available from: https://www.chicagotribune.com/business/ct-biz-jimmy-johns-sprouts-salmonella-20170120-story.html.

CDC. (2006). Multistate Outbreak of *E. coli* O157:H7 Infections Linked to Fresh Spinach [Final Update]. Available from: https://www.cdc.gov/ecoli/2006/spinach-10-2006.html.

CDC. (2009). Multistate Outbreak of *Salmonella typhimurium* Infections Linked to Peanut Butter, 2008-2009 [Final Update]. Centers for Disease Control and Prevention. Available from: https://www.cdc.gov/salmonella/2009/peanut-butter-2008-2009.html.

CDC. (2012). Multistate Outbreak of Listeriosis Linked to Whole Cantaloupes from Jensen Farms, Colorado [Final Update]. CDC. Available from: https://www.cdc.gov/listeria/outbreaks/cantaloupes-jensen-farms/index.html.

CDC. (2016). Multistate Outbreaks of Shiga Toxin-Producing *Escherichia coli* O26 Infections Linked to Chipotle Mexican Grill Restaurants [Final Update]. Available from: https://www.cdc.gov/ecoli/2015/o26-11-15/index.html.

CDC. (2018). Multistate Outbreak of *E. coli* O157:H7 Infections Linked to Romaine Lettuce [Final Update]. Available from: https://www.cdc.gov/ecoli/2018/o157h7-04-18/index.html.

CDC. (2018). Multistate Outbreak of Shiga Toxin-Producing *Escherichia coli* O157:H7 Infections Linked to Leafy Greens [Final Update]. Available from: https://www.cdc.gov/ecoli/2017/o157h7-12-17/index.html.

CDC. (2019). Outbreak of *E. coli* Infections Linked to Romaine Lettuce [Final Update]. Available from: https://www.cdc.gov/ecoli/2018/o157h7-11-18/index.html.

CDC. (2019). Outbreak of Multidrug-Resistant *Salmonella* Infections Linked to Raw Turkey Products [Final Update]. Available from: https://www.cdc.gov/salmonella/reading-07-18/index.html.

CDC. (2019). Outbreak of *Salmonella* Infections [Final Update]. Available from: https://www.cdc.gov/salmonella/agbeni-11-18/index.html.

CDC. (2019). Outbreak of *Salmonella* Infections Linked to Ground Beef [Final Update]. Available from: https://www.cdc.gov/salmonella/newport-10-18/index.html.

CDC. (2019). *Salmonella*. Available from: https://www.cdc.gov/salmonella/index.html.

Chipotle. (2014). 2014 Annual Report and Proxy Statement. Available from: https://ir.chipotle.com/download/2014+Annual+Report_Color.pdf.

CNBC (2017). American Greed: From Peanuts to Sick Millions [News Documentary]. Kurtis Productions, CNBC. Episode AG 141 (Original Air Date July 3, 2017). Available from: https://vimeo.com/259271860.

DeMarban, A. (2018). Illness Among Nome Prison Inmates Exposed to Lettuce is Key to Solving Nationwide *E. coli* Outbreak. The Anchorage Daily News. Available from: https://www.adn.com/alaska-news/health/2018/04/20/illness-among-nome-prison-inmates-exposed-to-lettuce-is-key-to-solving-nationwide-e-coli-outbreak/.

DOJ. (2013). Former Officials and Broker of Peanut Corporation of America Indicted Related to *Salmonella*-Tainted Peanut Products. Office of Public Affairs Press Release. Available from: https://www.justice.gov/opa/pr/former-officials-and-broker-peanut-corporation-america-indicted-related-salmonella-tainted.

DeLauro, R. (2016). DeLauro Demands that Dole Answer for Distributing Contaminated Salads that Killed Americans. [Press Release]. Available from: https://delauro.house.gov/media-center/press-releases/delauro-demands-dole-answer-distributing-contaminated-salads-killed.

Detwiler, D. (2015a). Bearing Witness to Justice at the PCA Sentencing. Food Safety News. Available from: http://www.foodsafetynews.com/2015/09/bearing-witness-to-justice-at-the-pca-sentencing/#.VgKDMN9Viko.

Detwiler, D. (2015b). Blowing the Whistle on Wrongdoings: PCA *Salmonella* Outbreak. Food Quality and Safety Magazine. Available from: http://www.foodqualityandsafety.com/article/blowing-the-whistle-on-wrongdoings/.

Detwiler, D. (2015c). Cracking the Case of a Multi-State *Salmonella* Outbreak: The Victims' Stories. Food Quality and Safety Magazine. Available from: http://www.foodqualityandsafety.com/article/cracking-the-case-of-a-multi-state-salmonella-outbreak/.

Detwiler, D. (2015d). Holding Food Companies Accountable. Food Quality and Safety Magazine. Available from: http://www.foodqualityandsafety.com/article/holding-food-companies-accountable/.

Detwiler, D. (2015e). Final Sentencing for PCA Case. STOP Foodborne Illness News. Available from: http://www.stopfoodborneillness.org/sofs-final-sentencing-for-pca-case/.

Elkind, P. (2015). How Blue Bell Blew It. Fortune 172(5), 122-126. Available from: http://fortune.com/2015/09/25/blue-bell-listeria-recall/.

FDA. (2016). FDA Investigated Multistate Outbreak of *Listeria* in Dole Leafy Greens Products Produced in the Dole Facility in Springfield, Ohio. Outbreaks of Foodborne Illness. Available from: https://www.fda.gov/food/outbreaks-foodborne-illness/fda-investigated-multistate-outbreak-listeria-dole-leafy-greens-products-produced-dole-facility.

FDA. (2018). Company Announcement: The Quaker Oats Company Issues Voluntary Recall of a Small Quantity of Cap'n Crunch's Peanut Butter Crunch Cereal Distributed to Five Target Stores Due to Possible Health Risk. Available from: https://www.fda.gov/safety/recalls-market-withdrawals-safety-alerts/quaker-oats-company-issues-voluntary-recall-small-quantity-capn-crunchs-peanut-butter-crunch-cereal.

FDA. (2019a). Standards for the Growing, Harvesting, Packing, and Holding of Produce for Human Consumption; Extension of Compliance Dates for Subpart E. Available from: https://www.federalregister.gov/documents/2019/03/18/2019-04652/standards-for-the-growing-harvesting-packing-and-holding-of-produce-for-human-consumption-extension.

FDA. (2019b). Investigation Summary: Factors Potentially Contributing to the Contamination of Romaine Lettuce Implicated in the Fall 2018 Multi-State Outbreak of *E. coli* O157:H7. Available from: https://www.fda.gov/food/outbreaks-foodborne-illness/investigation-summary-factors-potentially-contributing-contamination-romaine-lettuce-implicated-fall.

Flynn, D. (2015). Government Wants PCA Victims to Testify at Sept. 21 Sentencing. Food Safety News. Available from: https://www.foodsafetynews.com/2015/08/government-wants-pca-victims-to-testify-at-sept-21-sentencing/.

Flynn, D. (2016). Letter from the Editor: It's Always the Cover-Up. Food Safety News. Available from: https://www.foodsafetynews.com/2016/01/letter-from-the-editor-23/.

Flynn, D. (2018). Record Shows Jimmy John's Sprouts Repeatedly Sicken Patrons. Food Safety News. Available from: https://www.foodsafetynews.com/2018/01/record-shows-jimmy-johns-sprouts-repeatedly-sicken-patrons/.

Food Republic. (2015). Food Crimes: P.B. & Jail [Video]. Available from: https://www.youtube.com/watch?v=rzYtI9xEmyg.

Fox, M. (2015). Norovirus Caused Chipotle Outbreak in Boston, Officials Say. NBC News. Available from: https://www.nbcnews.com/health/health-news/chipotle-outbreak-grows-80-boston-college-students-n476316.

Fuhrmeister, C. (2015). Tests Show Norovirus to Blame for Illnesses Linked to Boston Chipotle [Updated]. Eater. Available from: https://www.eater.com/2015/12/8/9873194/chipotle-boston-college-norovirus.

Fuhrmeister, C. (2015). Norovirus-Stricken Chipotle Plans to Reopen in Boston. Eater. Available from: https://www.eater.com/2015/12/23/10661646/chipotle-boston-norovirus-reopening.

Garcia, S. (2019). Blue Bell Ice Cream Licker in Viral Video Is Found, Police Say. The New York Times. Available from: https://www.nytimes.com/2019/07/06/us/blue-bell-licker-lufkin-tx.html.

Gillespie, C. (2015). Blue Bell Ice Cream Listeria Outbreak Timeline. Food Poisoning Bulletin. Available from: https://foodpoisoningbulletin.com/2015/blue-bell-ice-cream-listeria-outbreak-timeline/.

Goetz, R. (2013). Peanut Corporation of America from Inception to Indictment: A Timeline. Food Safety News. Available from: https://www.foodsafetynews.com/2013/02/peanut-corporation-of-america-from-inception-to-indictment-a-timeline/.

Gottlieb, S. (2017). Speech to the 2017 NASDA Annual Meeting. FDA. Available from: https://www.fda.gov/news-events/speeches-fda-officials/speech-2017-nasda-annual-meeting-09122017.

Gottlieb, S. (2018). Statement from FDA Commissioner Scott Gottlieb, M.D., on Developments in the Romaine Outbreak Investigation, Recent Outbreaks and the Use of Modern Tools to Advance Food Safety. FDA. Available from: https://www.fda.gov/news-events/press-announcements/statement-fda-commissioner-scott-gottlieb-md-developments-romaine-outbreak-investigation-recent.

Gottlieb, S. (2018). Statement from FDA Commissioner Scott Gottlieb, M.D., on Findings from the Romaine Lettuce *E. coli* O157:H7 Outbreak Investigation and FDA's Efforts to Prevent Future Outbreaks. FDA. Available from: https://www.fda.gov/news-events/press-announcements/statement-fda-commissioner-scott-gottlieb-md-findings-romaine-lettuce-e-coli-o157h7-outbreak.

Harris, G. (2009). After Tests, Peanut Plant in Texas Is Closed. New York Times. Available from: https://www.nytimes.com/2009/02/11/health/policy/11peanut.html.

Harris, D., & Barrett, K. (2009). Former Manager Says Peanut Plant Complaints Ignored. ABC News. Available from: https://abcnews.go.com/GMA/story?id=6888169.

Harrison, C., et al. (2014). Using online reviews by restaurant patrons to identify unreported cases of foodborne illness—New York City, 2012-2013. CDC, Morbidity and Mortality Weekly Report 63(20), 441–445. Available from: https://www.cdc.gov/mmwr/preview/mmwrhtml/mm6320a1.htm.

Haughney, C. (2015). Deadly Peanuts, Foodborne Pathogens and the Possibility of Life in Prison. Food Republic. Available from: https://medium.com/@chaughney/deadly-peanuts-foodborne-pathogens-and-the-possibility-of-life-in-prison-36c2992a5e4e.

Herman, K., Hall, A., & Gould, L. (2015). Outbreaks attributed to fresh leafy vegetables, United States, 1973-2012. National Institutes of Health Journal of Epidemiological Infections. 143(14), 3011–3021, doi:10.1017/S0950268815000047.

Hopper, B. (2015). Dozens Fall Ill after Eating at Simi Valley Chipotle. CBS News, Los Angeles. Available from: https://losangeles.cbslocal.com/2015/08/22/dozens-fall-ill-after-eating-at-simi-valley-chipotle/.

Hunsicker, J. (2012). Jimmy John's Permanently Pulls Sprouts from Menu. The Kirksville Daily Express. Available from: https://www.kirksvilledailyexpress.com/article/20120217/NEWS/302179941.

Jenkins, N. (2015). 80 Boston College Students Fall Sick after Eating at Chipotle. Time Magazine. Available from: https://time.com/4140147/chipotle-ecoli-boston-college/.

LGMA. (2015). The Why Behind Food Safety [Video]. Available from: https://www.youtube.com/watch?t=4&v=AE9G818uJsQ.
Marler, B. (2018). After 7 Sprout Outbreaks, Would You Buy Sprouts from Jimmy John Liautaud? Marler Blog. Available from: http://www.marlerblog.com/legal-cases/after-7-sprout-outbreaks-would-you-buy-sprouts-from-jimmy-john-liautaud/.
Matias, D. (2019). Police Identify The 'Blue Bell Licker' In Viral Video. NPR. Available from: https://www.npr.org/2019/07/05/738938037/police-identify-the-blue-bell-licker-in-viral-video.
Miller, K. (2015). Blue Bell Workers Describe Unsanitary Conditions before Listeria Outbreak. Yahoo Health. Available from: https://www.yahoo.com/health/blue-bell-workers-describe-unsanitary-conditions-165449479.html.
Petrak, L. (2007). Food with Integrity. Available from: https://www.provisioneronline.com/articles/95183-food-with-integrity-1.
Robinson-Jacobs, K. (2016). State Health Department Fines Blue Bell $850,000 Following *Listeria* Outbreak. Dallas News. Available from: https://www.dallasnews.com/business/retail/2016/07/29/state-health-department-fines-blue-bell-850000-following-listeria-outbreak.
Russell, S. (2006). Spinach *E. coli* Linked to Cattle/Manure on Pasture had Same Strain as Bacteria in Outbreak. SF Gate. Available from: https://www.sfgate.com/health/article/Spinach-E-coli-linked-to-cattle-Manure-on-2550111.php.
Shogren, L., & Neilson, S. (2018). The Science is Clear: Dirty Farm Water is Making Us Sick. Wired Magazine. Available from: https://www.wired.com/story/the-science-is-clear-dirty-farm-water-is-making-us-sick/.
Silverman, H. (2019). Dole Recalls Baby Spinach Over *Salmonella* Concerns. CNN. Available from: https://www.cnn.com/2019/08/13/health/dole-spinach-recall-salmonella/index.html.
Solomon, D. (2019). Worse Things have Happened to Blue Bell Ice Cream than a Gross Prank at Walmart. Texas Weekly. Available from: https://www.texasmonthly.com/the-culture/worse-things-have-happened-to-blue-bell-ice-cream-than-a-gross-prank-at-walmart/.
Tauxe, R. (2019). From outbreak catastrophes to Clades of concern, how whole genome sequencing can change the food safety landscape. Silliker Lecture presented at the annual Meeting of International Association for Food Protection, Louisville, KY.
Von Quednow, C. (2015). Dozens report feeling sick after eating at Chipotle in Simi Valley. The Ventura County Star. Available from: http://archive.vcstar.com/news/local/simi-valley/dozens-report-feeling-sick-after-eating-at-chipotle-in-simi-valley-ep-1243518085-351108681.html.
Yiannas, F. (2019). Remarks by Frank Yiannas to the International Association for Food Protection, Louisville JULY 22, 2019. FDA. Available from: https://www.fda.gov/news-events/speeches-fda-officials/remarks-frank-yiannas-international-association-food-protection-louisville-07222019.

CHAPTER 6

Legal and economic factors impacting reform

"Our food safety system is fragmented, outdated, and in desperate need of repair."
Senator Dick Durbin (D-IL), 2019 in a press release for reintroducing the Safe Food Act

"With foodborne illness and outbreaks—public fear drives a lot of reform."
Thomas Gremillion, 2019
Director of Food Policy, Consumer Federation of America's Food Policy Institute

The types of foods involved in foodborne illnesses have changed radically over the last two decades. When the concerns back in 1993 over *Escherichia coli* focused on beef, the majority of the federal government's response took place within the US Department of Agriculture (USDA), which has authority over meat and poultry. Over the last several years, however, fewer illnesses and deaths have been attributed to meat and poultry, whereas growing numbers of recalls and multistate outbreaks have stemmed from foods that fall under the regulatory authority of the US Food and Drug Administration (FDA). Two major concerns plagued food safety regulation at the federal level in the early 2000s: the large number of agencies that played various roles in food or food-related regulations and the FDA's lack of authority over inspections of nonmeat and poultry food items.

Too many agencies

The USDA and the FDA are 2 of the 15 federal agencies playing a role in food safety regulation or enforcement. These agencies include two from the Department of Health and Human Services (HHS), seven from the USDA, two from the Department of Commerce, one each from the Department of Treasury and the Department of Homeland Security, as well as the Federal Trade Commission and the Environmental Protection Agency. At times, additional departments may also take on some of these food safety responsibilities. In 2013 US Senator Richard Burr (R-NC) introduced a bill that

Food Safety
http://dx.doi.org/10.1016/B978-0-12-818219-2.00006-5

would move the National Oceanic and Atmospheric Administration and its seafood inspections from the Department of Commerce to the US Department of the Interior (Food Safety News, 2014) (For a list of acronyms associated with each agency, see Table 6.1)

Table 6.1 List of major federal agencies and their food-related responsibilities.

Agency	Food-Related Responsibilities
Department of Health and Human Services (HHS)	
Food and Drug Administration (FDA)	Domestic and imported foods, except processed egg products and major types of meat and poultry
Centers for Disease Control and Prevention (CDC)	Monitors, identifies, and investigates communicable diseases, including foodborne diseases
US Department of Agriculture (USDA)	
Agricultural Marketing Service (AMS)	Establishes and certifies quality standards and marketing grades for dairy products, produce, meat, poultry, seafood, and shell eggs
Agricultural Research Service (ARS)	Conducts in-house USDA research on agricultural and food topics, of which food safety is one of many
Animal and Plant Health Inspection Service (APHIS)	Oversees animal and plant health, including the prevention / containment / eradication of foreign diseases and domestically
Food and Nutrition Service (FNS)	Encourages and coordinates efforts to ensure the safety of foods in school lunch and other targeted domestic programs
Food Safety Inspection Service (FSIS)	Regulates the safety, wholesomeness, and proper labeling of domestic and imported meat and poultry, and processed egg products
Grain Inspection, Packers and Stockyards Administration (GIPSA)	Sets quality standards for and tests grains and related commodities, primarily for marketing purposes
National Institute of Food and Agriculture (NIFA)	Coordinates and administers federal funding for agricultural and food (including food safety) research, education and extension activities
Department of Commerce	
National Marine Fisheries Service (NMFS)	Seafood inspection and grading program that focuses on marketing and quality attributes of US fish and shellfish
National Oceanic and Atmospheric Administration (NOAA)	Voluntary seafood safety and quality inspection services

Table 6.1 List of major federal agencies and their food-related responsibilities. (*Cont.*)

US Environmental Protection Agency (EPA)	
	Regulates the use of certain chemicals/substances/pesticides. Sets water standards quality criteria for rivers, lakes, and streams
Federal Trade Commission (FTC)	
	Enforces federal prohibitions against unfair or deceptive acts or practices in trade, including consumer deception regarding foods
Department of the Treasury	
Alcohol and Tobacco Tax and Trade Bureau (ATF)	Administers and enforces laws on the production, safety, distribution and use of alcoholic beverages
Department of Homeland Security (DHS)	
US Customs and Border Protection (CBP)	Food security activities, including inspecting imports of food, plants, and animals at the border, and agricultural border inspection

Source: Table modified by Author; Johnson, 2014.

Though the Department of HHS is the "principal agency for protecting the health of all Americans," (US Department of Health and Human Services, 2018), only two agencies listed earlier are part of this department, whereas half of the agencies belong to the USDA, and the rest belong to other agencies. As a result, the division of authority and funding is imbalanced. The USDA's Food Safety Inspection Service (FSIS) is responsible for the safety of approximately 20% of the US food supply, and the FDA has been responsible for the remaining 80%, but the food safety budget of the FSIS has equaled approximately 60% of the two agencies' combined budget, with the FDA receiving about 40% (Johnson, 2014). The division of responsibility has also caused a lack of resources, obstructions to successfully collaborate as needed, and inconsistencies in regulatory capabilities. These organizational inefficiencies have created obstacles too big for the variety of experts in these organizations to overcome alone.

Taking a step back, a look at the history of changes at the executive branch level offers an aerial view of how the USDA and the FDA became two different agencies. The US Patent Office (known today as the United States Patent and Trademark Office) existed within the Department of State from 1802 until 1849. The US Patent Office established their Agricultural Division in 1839. In 1849 the US Patent Office was transferred to the Department of

Interior. Shortly after Congress created the USDA in 1862, the Patent Office's Agricultural Division transferred to the USDA (Griesbach & Camarota, 2016).

The Agriculture Division went through a series of name changes, from Division of Chemistry to the Bureau of Chemistry between 1890 and 1901. In 1927, Congress transformed the Bureau of Chemistry into United States Food, Drug, and Insecticide Administration. In total, three years later, it became the US FDA. In 1940 Congress placed the FDA under the Federal Security Agency, then moved to in 1953 to under the Department of Health Education and Welfare, known today as the US Department of HHS.

1839	Agricultural Division established within the US Patent Office
1862	The USDA created and inherited the Patent Office's Agricultural Division
1890	The Agricultural Division became the Division of Chemistry
1901	The Division of Chemistry became the Bureau of Chemistry
1927	The Bureau of Chemistry became the United States Food, Drug and Insecticide Administration
1930	The United States Food, Drug, and Insecticide Administration became the US FDA
1940	The FDA transferred from the USDA to the Federal Security Agency
1953	The Federal Security Agency became the Department of Health Education and Welfare
1979	The Department of Health Education and Welfare became the US Department of HHS

Between 1947 and 1949, the Hoover administration's Commission on Organization discussed consolidation as a necessary solution to a fractured US food safety system. As consolidations did not occur as recommended, the two key agencies have operated as separate entities for many decades.

In 1997 the Senate Committee on Governmental Affairs concluded that America's food regulatory system was "marred by duplication and inconsistency" and suggested the creation of a single food safety agency (Merrill & Francer, 2000). In 1998 the National Academy of Science committee recommended a change in the organization of federal food safety responsibilities. Specifically, they recommended that Congress establish, by statute, a unified, and central framework for managing federal food safety programs, headed by a single official and which has the responsibility and control of resources for all federal food safety activities. The committee proposed three options for who should have responsibility over all food—the USDA, the FDA, or the Consumer Product Safety Commission (Institute of Medicine, National Research Council, 1998).

In 1999 Senate Subcommittee on Oversight of Government Management heard testimony from Lawrence J. Dyckman, then US General Accounting Office Director, Food, and Agriculture Issues. Dyckman (1999) argued not only that the structure of the current food safety system was too expensive, but that it ultimately "hampers efforts to address public health concerns associated with existing and newly identified food safety risks."

In his March 14, 2009, Weekly Address, President Barack Obama expressed his concerns about a "troubling trend" in which the average number of outbreaks from contaminated produce and other foods increased some 350% since the early 1990s. One specific reason President Obama pointed to is the underfunded and understaffed state of the FDA "leaving the agency with the resources to inspect just 7,000 of our 150,000 food processing plants and warehouses each year. That means roughly 95% of them go uninspected" (Obama, 2009).

Later that year, FDA Commissioner Dr. Margaret Hamburg testified before the Senate Subcommittee on Health, Committee on Energy and Commerce, that the federal government has registered approximately 378,000 food facilities (Hamburg, 2009). To do this, FDA Commissioner Hamburg discussed implementing a facility registration fee of $1000 per year to increase FDA funding and staffing (Hamburg, 2009). However, the committee also heard opposition to that idea of a facility registration fee, as Pamela G. Bailey, president of the Grocery Manufacturers Association (GMA), raised concerns over the size of the proposed fees. Bailey acknowledged that the industry is "ultimately responsible for the safety of its products," but she went on to stress that, at a larger scale, "securing the safety of the food supply is a government function which should be largely financed with government resources" (Harris, 2009).

Two years later, President Obama would continue to voice his concerns, such as when, during a press conference on June 29, 2011, President Obama discussed how the tough consequence of keeping tax breaks for millionaires and billionaires included compromising food safety (Obama, 2011). The president, as well as the committees, was not alone in their concerns.

The Proposed Safe Food Act

US Senator Dick Durbin (D-IL), a member of the Senate Oversight of Government Management Subcommittee, and US Representative Rosa DeLauro (D-CT) have long advocated for a single, independent food safety agency at the federal level to solve for the disparities at the state level. In his 2004 paper "Food safety oversight for the 21st century: the creation of a single, independent federal food safety agency," published in *Food and Drug Law Journal*, Senator Durbin notes that his efforts on this change date back to 1996 (Durbin, 2004).

Senator Durbin introduced, without success, a Safe Food Act Bill into Congress in 1999, 2001, 2004, 2005, 2007, and in 2015 intending to consolidate the responsibilities of food safety, labeling, and inspection into a single independent agency in the executive branch (Durbin, 2015). In June 2019 Senator Durbin and Congresswoman DeLauro introduced the Safe Food Act of 2019, which would create a single, independent food safety agency.

> *"Our food safety system is fragmented, outdated, and in desperate need of repair... as it stands, our nation's broken food safety system sickens 48 million Americans every year. The Safe Food Act would modernize federal food safety laws to protect and improve public health, giving families peace of mind that the food in their refrigerators, pantries, and on their dining room tables won't harm them."*
>
> ***(Durbin, 2019)***

The Consumer Federation of America (CFA) expressed strong support for the Safe Food Act of 2019, as it would bring about the consolidation of federal food safety activities into "one independent single food safety agency, with broad jurisdiction to address food safety hazards wherever they may emerge" (Consumer Federation of America, 2019). The CFA is an association of nearly 300 nonprofit consumer organizations that advances the consumer interest through research, advocacy, and education.

Thomas Gremillion, who serves as the Director of Food Policy for CFA's Food Policy Institute, pointed out that one of CFA's concerns is over the USDA's many conflicts of interests. He adds that The Safe Food Act, with the concept of the single, independent food safety agency could reduce this conflict of interest:

> *"That's why it's the gold standard for that matter. With an independent food safety agency, even if we had a change of administration, we would have that independent agency keep on going and we wouldn't have to worry about them under investing in this, or are they still committed to doing the surveillance and are they measuring things the way they are supposed to be."*
>
> ***(Thomas Gremillion, Personal communication, 2019)***

While Gremillion calls the Safe Food Act "ideal, our positive vision," some members of Congress, unfortunately, likely see the threat of the independent agency as something that would get in the way of the Safe Food Act becoming a reality.

The Safe Food Act would presumably benefit American consumers by streamlining the powers of multiple agencies to better coordinate and communicate facts to improve how they prevent, detect, and respond to outbreaks (Zuraw, 2015). Durbin's view was also shared by the Obama Administration. Only a few weeks after Senator Durbin last introduced the bill in 2015, President Obama's February 2015 budget proposal for fiscal year 2016 included his own recommendation for a "single overseer agency for food safety" housed within the Department of HHS (Nixon, 2015).

In his budget proposal for the fiscal year 2016, President Obama recommended a single food agency. The White House cited "fractured oversight" and confusing "disparate regulatory approaches" in the current food regulatory system. "Although the United States has one of the safest food supplies, the administration said, "consolidating food safety functions is an essential step to reforming the federal food safety system overall" (OMB, 2015).

According to a 2015 federal report involving the survey of over 1,000 outbreaks from 1998 to 2012, most cases of foodborne pathogens and related strains of concern did not come from food or food products regulated by any one federal agency (IFSAC, 2015). This first-of-its-kind report took the combined efforts of the Interagency (USDA, FDA, and CDC) Food Safety Analytics Collaboration to gather and evaluate all the data and conclude that this regulatory problem can only be rectified by establishing an independent, single overseer agency for food safety and inspection. However, the proposed agency has not gained enough congressional support to progress toward becoming law.

Though the United States has seen much change in the food regulatory agencies, the likelihood of significant change any time soon is low. "This administration, particularly the USDA, is only interested in what the industry wants. There will be no meaningful meat and poultry inspection reform, as long as this [current] administration is in office" (Thomas Gremillion, Personal communication, 2019).

Unfortunately, some members of Congress likely see the threat of the independent agency as something that would get in the way of the Safe Food Act becoming a reality.

> *"[The Safe Food Act] is a nonstarter because it would be creating a whole new bureaucracy from a bunch of existing ones. So you've got many who are vested in the current system. They don't want to leave their turf... get moved over into somewhere else. You've got people that think this would just add a bunch of added bureaucracy."*
>
> ***(Thomas Gremillion, Personal communication, 2019).***

Some have argued that it will take another 9/11 in the food industry, like the 1993 Jack in the Box *E. coli* outbreak or the 2008–09 Peanut Corporation of America (PCA) *Salmonella* outbreak for really progressive change, such as the Safe Food Act, to make it through Congress. "With foodborne illness and outbreaks—public fear drives a lot of reform" (Thomas Gremillion, Personal communication, 2019).

But what if fear alone is not enough? According to former FDA Associate Commissioner for Foods, Dr. David Acheson stated that "We need, I hate to say it, but bodies in the street before we get it" (Acheson, 2015).

The significance of the Safe Food Act would be comparable to the passage of the Homeland Security Act of 2002, which established the Department of Homeland Security. In fact, Senator Durbin's office noted that in 2015 that his bill gained increased support when they reframed the issue of an independent, single overseer agency for food safety and inspection as benefiting national security in the face of an intentional attack on American people through the nation's food supply.

Though the United States has seen much change in the food regulatory agencies, the likelihood of significant change any time soon is low. "This administration, particularly the USDA, is only interested in what the industry wants. There will be no meaningful meat and poultry inspection reform, as long as this [current] administration is in office" (Thomas Gremillion, Personal communication, 2019).

Increasing the FDA's regulatory authority

More than 25 years ago, both Canada and the European Union made significant modifications to their national food regulatory systems to adapt to improvements in science and industry. In contrast, the US Congress has not adopted any new significant food safety policies for the FDA in over 70 years since the passage of the 1938 Food Drug and Cosmetics Act.

Many changes in industry have gone virtually unchecked by US regulators, whereas significant public health issues have not only increased and persisted, but also encompassed many pathogens and many sources of contaminated foods. However, many upgrades in the United States have taken place, adopting advances in both science and computer technologies to enhance data collection and analysis for outbreak investigations.

In the late 1990s the CDC and other agencies began using pulse field gel electrophoresis (PFGE) as a new means of identifying bacterial strains (DNA isolates from product and patient samples), allowing labs to compare patterns to deduce if the strains are the same or different. PFGE allows public officials to connect otherwise seemingly random and unconnected illnesses, making it easier for them to identify outbreaks, and often an outbreak's source. The data allow regulators to inform the public, work with industry to stop the source of an outbreak, and initiate recalls. Using data from PFGE, CDC has noted that the incidents of illnesses have decreased, despite the fact that the number of identified outbreaks has increased. The reason for the change is that an increase in the early detection of pathogens in nonmeat foods allows for outbreak sources to be identified and stopped sooner (Liang, 2016). Today, an additional, newer technology, whole genome sequencing has proven to be more effective in connecting sample isolates to their source.

FDA standards programs

In keeping with the goals and mission of President Clinton's Food Safety Initiative, the FDA took steps in 1996 to improve its retail food protection program. Meeting with personnel from the FDA's Center for Food Safety and Nutrition, state, and local regulatory officials from the six FDA regions, the Association of Food and Drug Officials, the Conference for Food Protection (CFP), and industry representatives, the FDA established a goal of "providing national leadership, being equal partners, being responsive, providing communication, and promoting uniformity" (FDA, 2019b).

The collaboration of the many stakeholders produced the "Voluntary National Retail Food Regulatory Program Standards." After pilot testing in each of the FDA regions in 1999, pilot participants reported the results at the 2000 biennial meeting of the CFP, which endorsed improvements and refinements to these voluntary standards 2 years later. During this time, the HHS Office of the Inspector General, June Gibbs Brown, released a report of FDA's oversight of state contracts, recommending that the FDA take steps to promote "equivalency among Federal and State food safety standards, inspection programs, and enforcement practices" (Brown, 2000).

The FDA established the Manufactured Food Regulatory Program Standards (MFRPS) in 2007 as a uniform foundation for measuring and improving the performance of manufactured food regulatory programs in the United States. This was the FDA's first major attempt to implement a modern, risk-based food safety program. The MFRPS are comprised of 10 standards (Table 6.2) that establish requirements for the critical elements of a regulatory program designed to improve the safety and security of the

Table 6.2 Manufactured Food Regulatory Program Standards (MFRPS) areas of focus.

Standard	Title
1	Regulatory Foundation
2	Training Program
3	Inspection Program
4	Inspection Audit Program
5	Food-related Illness and Outbreaks and Response
6	Compliance and Enforcement Program
7	Industry and Community Relations
8	Program Resources
9	Program Assessment
10	Laboratory Services

Source: Table modified by Author; FDA (2016). Regulatory Program Standards: Manufactured Food Regulatory Program Standards (MFRPS). Available from http://www.fda.gov/ForFederalStateand-LocalOfficials/ProgramsInitiatives/RegulatoryPrgmStnds/ucm475064.htm

United States food supply and, thus, protect the public from foodborne illness and injury. The FDA updated MFRPS in 2010 and 2013 and has essentially used MFRPS as a tool to improve contracts with states and to better direct their regulatory activities toward reducing foodborne illness hazards in food plants (FDA, 2016).

Still in use, Voluntary National Retail Food Regulatory Program Standards are only what the title indicates: voluntary. Similarly, while 42 states are currently participating in the MFRPS program (FDA, 2016), the idea of uniformity across the United States has not come to fruition. As of April 2019, according to the FDA, 66 state or territory level jurisdictions have enrolled, as have 75 district-level agencies; 483 county level jurisdictions; 183 city or town level jurisdictions; and 26 other types of agencies, such as tribe, village, etc. (FDA, 2019a). While these numbers may complicate trying to determine the level of participation of the program and its impact on consumer safety, the FDA also reports that 69.02% of the US population resides in a locality (city, county, parish, etc.) in which the local-level food regulatory agency has enrolled in the standards (FDA, 2019a).

These programs provide a means for guidance and evaluation, but they are not subject to enforcement by the FDA's legal authority.

Legal authority

From a legal perspective, foodborne illness outbreaks caused by the illegal actions of those in the food industry are not only being identified by the investigations conducted by state and federal authorities, but are, of recent, being prosecuted by the US Department of Justice (DOJ). As stated earlier, rarely have the owners or executive officers of major companies faced anything more than a fine for their actions that resulted in recalls, outbreaks, hospitalizations, and even deaths of American consumers. For the most part, the FDA's regulatory powers (and the USDA's) involve enforcing food policy violations as civil, rather than criminal and crimes.

For example, in 1998 Odwalla was indicted and held criminally liable for the 1996 *E. coli* outbreak tied to their apple juice products (Chapter 4). The company pleaded guilty to 16 federal criminal charges of shipping an adulterated food product and agreed to pay a $1.5 million fine. While this was the largest such fine at that time in a food-poisoning case, no individuals received sentences of jail time for their role in this outbreak.

Perhaps this is not a surprise seeing as how not one single corporate executive related to the 1993 "Jack in the Box" *E. coli* outbreak faced a single federal indictment for the illnesses and deaths caused by their actions—though the company admittedly broke the law related to minimum cooking temperatures. Ironically, Stewart Parnell, the now convicted CEO of the PCA, stated before his sentencing that "those [Jack in the Box] guys definitely should have gone to jail" (Parnell, personal communication, 2015).

The PCA case—*US v. Stewart Parnell, Michael Parnell, and Mary Wilkerson*, as well as Daniel Kilgore and Samuel Lightsey (Chapter 6) is not only a landmark court case for foodborne illness outbreaks, but is also one of only a few examples of court cases where the executives of a food company have been prosecuted in court for its actions involving the Responsible Corporate Officer doctrine of criminal liability that resulted from the Supreme Court's decision in *US v. Park* 412 US 658 (1975).

The roots of the "Responsible Corporate Officer (RCO) Doctrine" stretches back to 1943. RCO imposes strict liability on corporate officers based solely on their area of responsibility within the corporation, regardless of their knowledge of the underlying criminal activity or their participation in it. This doctrine pertains specifically to those industries governed by public health and welfare regulations, such as the pharmaceutical industry, the retail sector of the food industry, and the agricultural sector of the food industry.

In *US vs. Dotterweich*, 320 US 277 (1943), involving allegations of shipping in interstate commerce adulterated and misbranded drugs, the US Supreme Court held that a corporate officer in an industry directly affecting the safety of the public health could be held criminally liable for a misdemeanor violation of the Federal Food, Drug, and Cosmetic Act (FDCA) simply by reason of his position in the corporation. Though the defendant in that case was not directly responsible for violating the FDAC, he was in a position to prevent or correct the activity of the corporation.

In *US vs. Park* (1975), the president of a large national food chain was charged with violating § 301(k) of the FDCA in that they had allegedly caused interstate food shipments being held in their warehouse to be exposed to rodent contamination. The company, but not its president, pleaded guilty. At his trial, respondent conceded that he was "responsible for the entire operation of the company," and that, as Acme's president he was responsible for any result that occurred in the company. The Court found Park *strictly* liable for the unsanitary conditions that his company had created, arguing for strict liability under the rationale that the FDCA was a 'public welfare' statute.

The Court's decision ultimately strengthened the RCO Doctrine, in that their ruling held that if someone were to willingly be in charge of a company, and therefore its problems, then he or she willingly accepts the consequences of any illegal practices that his or her company or organization is involved in. An exception is made if the problem is impossible to fix.

While the Supreme Court's decision in *US v. Park* (1975) established the RCO Doctrine of criminal liability, only a few historical examples exist of court cases where the executives of a food company have been prosecuted over the last 40 years.

US v. Eric Jensen and Ryan Jensen (2013) involved the 2011 *Listeria* outbreak tied to improperly cleaned cantaloupe from their Colorado farm. This outbreak ranks among the deadliest US outbreaks, sickening 147 people in 28 states, resulting in the 43 deaths (CDC, 2012). The Jensen brothers pled guilty to six counts, including Introducing an Adulterated Food into Interstate Commerce [21 U.S.C. §§ 331(a) and 333(a)(1)] and Aiding and Abetting (18 U.S.C. § 2). In 2014 they received 5 years of probation, 6 months of home detention, and 100 hours of community service and were ordered to pay a total restitution of $300,000 to victims' families (DOJ, Office of Public Affairs, 2014)

US v. Quality Egg, LLC (2014) involved the 2010 outbreak of *Salmonella* that sickened nearly 2000 consumers nationwide and resulted in the recall of over one half of one billion eggs. The defendants, Austin DeCoster and his son Peter DeCoster, and the company pled guilty in June 2014 to introducing an Adulterated Food into Interstate Commerce [21 U.S.C. §§ 331(a) and 333(a)(1)]. In 2015 the court sentenced the two owners to serve 6-month jail terms, pay a $100,000 fine each, as well as pay restitution to victims. The court placed the corporation on 3 years' probation and ordered it to pay a fine of $6.79 million (DOJ, Office of Public Affairs, 2015). The two convicted felons appealed all the way to the US Supreme Court, asking the Justices to determine whether (1) the due process clause prohibits the imposition of a term of imprisonment as punishment for a supervisory liability offense, such as the one described in *US v. Park* and (2) whether *Park* and its precursor, *United States v. Dotterweich* (1943), should be overruled. Their efforts, had they been successful, would have greatly undermined the RCO Doctrine. On May 22, 2017, however, the US Supreme Court denied the DeCosters' petition for appeal (SCOTUS Blog, 2017).

Marchand v. Barnhill et al., No. 533, 2018 (Delivered June 19, 2019) is a recent case in which the Delaware Supreme Court reversed a lower court's dismissal of a stockholder lawsuit against the members of the board of directors and two officers of Blue Bell Creameries. The plaintiff filed this lawsuit in the wake of the 2015 *listeria* outbreak tied to the company's ice cream products. At least eight people in two states became ill and three died (Gillespie, 2015).

The Delaware Supreme Court went further, however, with the court's Chief Justice Strine writing, in the court's unanimous opinion. The justices held that the board of directors "failed to implement any system to monitor Blue Bell's food safety performance or compliance and applied the "duty to monitor" doctrine enunciated the *In re Caremark Int'l Inc. Derivative Litig.,* 698 A.2d 959, 971 (Del. Ch.1996). Chief Justice Strine quoted *Caremark,* in adding that "A board's 'utter failure to attempt to assure a reasonable information and reporting system exists' is an act of bad faith in breach of the duty of loyalty."

After concluding that "In Blue Bell's case, food safety was essential and mission critical," the Supreme Court ruled that the complaint pled facts supporting a fair inference that no board-level system of monitoring or reporting on food safety existed. Specifically, the court noted that the plaintiff found facts supporting a fair inference that:

- no reasonable compliance system and protocols were established as to the obviously most central consumer safety and legal compliance issue facing the company;
- the board's lack of efforts resulted in it not receiving official notices of food safety deficiencies for several years; and
- as a result of their failure to take remedial action, the company exposed consumers to *listeria*-infected ice cream, resulting in the death and injury of company customers.

The Court thus declined to dismiss a claim that the directors breached their duty of loyalty, potentially exposing directors to monetary damages. While the outcome of a stockholder lawsuit against Blue Bell remains to be seen, one must wonder about how the FDA's findings have not yet resulted in any major fines or federal charges being brought against the company or any of its executives (Table 6.3).

The "PCA" effect

More so than the convictions, the sentencing of Stewart Parnell, along with his brother Michael, the QA Manager Mary Wilkerson, and two other company employees sent shockwaves far beyond the courtroom. For those whose work in quality assurance (far from the board rooms and executive offices), the 5-year federal prison sentence handed to the QA manager for her guilty verdict on one (of two charges) hit much closer to a reality check than the lengthy sentences handed by the judge to the Parnell brothers. Jeremy Zenlea, Corporate Director of Food Safety for over 550 regional convenience stores, has observed this effect.

> *"Since the whole PCA case went down, nowadays, someone like the QA manager would be maybe a little tougher than they were 10 years ago in terms of a recall or something like that. And because they know, [they are likely to say to their supervisors]* 'If you decided not to recall, that's fine. That's a business decision but leave my name out of it. I'm leaving the company because there's no way I'm putting my reputation on the line or my personal liability on the line for this.' *I've sat in meetings and heard people say that before. And that's the feeling now."*
>
> ***(Jeremy Zenlea, Personal Communication, 2019)***

Economic impacts

During, and for a short while after the landmark 1993 *E. coli* O157:H7 outbreak, several newspapers and magazines focused on the economics of the event, as Jack in the Box's stock fell 30% (Roberts, 2018). Some did not view the economic impact on the company and on the industry nearly as important as the costs associated with the outbreak's public health impact.

Tanya Roberts, PhD, author of *Food Safety Economics: Incentives for a Safer Food Supply* (2018) retired after 33 years as a Senior Economist for the USDA's Economic Research Service. She recalls: "The 1993 outbreak came along and we had better data, more data, and that raised the importance of economic research into food safety" (Roberts, T., Personal Communication,

Table 6.3 Overview of selected outbreaks and legal action.

Outbreak	Year	Ill	Hospitalized	Deaths	Fines	Convictions	Sentencings
Jack in the Box ground beef *E. coli*	1993	732 across 4 states	> 150	4	None	None	None
Odwalla Apple juice *E. coli*	1996	66 across 3 states and in Canada	14	1	$1.5 million	1998: Pleaded guilty to 16 criminal counts of distributing adulterated juice	None
Jensen Brothers Cantaloupe *Listeria*	2011	147 across 28 states	143	33	$300,000 restitution to victims	2014: Pleaded guilty to misdemeanor counts of introducing adulterated food into interstate commerce	6 months home detention, 100 hours of community service, 5 years' probation
DeCosters Quality Egg *Salmonella*	2010	1936 confirmed, (CDC estimates over half a million)	Unknown	Unknown	$200,000 in personal fines, $6.8 million in company fines	Various federal misdemeanor charges	Father and son (owners) 3 months in prison each
Peanut Corporation of America (PCA) *Salmonella*	2008	714 across 46 states	171	9	Millions in forfeitures	2014: Found Guilty of nearly 100 combined criminal counts, including conspiracy, fraud and other federal charges	CEO—28 years, partner—20 years, Plant Manager—6 years, QA Manager—5 years, Plant Manager—3 years
Blue Bell Creameries Ice cream *Listeria*	2015	At least 8, but total unknown	At least 8	3	$850,000[a]	None—However, the Delaware Supreme Court reversed a lower court's dismissal of a stockholder lawsuit against the members of the board of directors and two officers of Blue Bell Creameries	None

a. $675,000 to be paid only if the company violates the terms of the agreement within 18-months of signing

2019). Her research into the cost of foodborne illnesses in the United States changed over time.

> *"At first, economic evaluations focused on acute health concerns and deaths. Soon, economists added the long-term health outcomes, such as renal failure and young children survivors dealing with arthritis. The long-term items soon became recognized as being the most expensive. In 1995, economists spent a great deal of time chasing down factors and data related to long-term health outcomes."*
>
> ***(Tanya Roberts, Personal Communication, 2019)***

In 2014, the USDA's Economic Research Service published "Cost Estimates of Foodborne Illnesses", an economic report that took into account such factors as associated outpatient and inpatient expenditures for medical care and lost income. The report provides data sheets for the top 15 foodborne pathogens and shows that foodborne illnesses impact the US economy by more than $15.5 billion each year (Hoffmann, 2015). These estimates do not take into consideration the economic impact of lost profit, stock values, fines, fees, legal costs, and out-of-court settlements to victims.

Foodborne illness outbreaks cause significant health and economic hardship and an enormous burden on the economy with medical and legal costs. Furthermore, absenteeism at work and school create further economic impact.

The Center for Science in the Public Interest is a nonprofit organization based in Washington, DC that works to improve the public's health, largely through its work on nutrition and food safety issues. In their 2005 report "Global and Local: Food Safety Around the World" the authors highlight that in the US "a government estimate of seven foodborne pathogens reported a cost of between U.S. $5.6 billion to $9.4 billion in lost work and medical expenses" (DeWaal & Robert, 2005).

Economically, foodborne illness costs are estimated to range between $51 billion and $77 billion using a basic and enhanced model for calculating total health costs of foodborne illness in the United States based upon in disease-incidence estimates from the CDC (2016). Other estimates place this range at $61 billion–$90 billion annually (Roberts, 2018).

A variety of sources outline different economic costs associated with foodborne illness events in the United States with varying figures from 1999 to 2015. In 2011 Robert Scharff compared the 1999 and 2011 US cost estimates of foodborne illness in his paper "Economic burden from health losses due to foodborne illness in the United States". The reported costs were estimated ranging from $51 billion (US) to $77 billion (US) using a basic and enhanced model for calculating total health costs of foodborne illness in the United States based upon in disease-incidence estimates from the CDC revised models for calculation (Scharff, 2012). The USDA estimates are significantly lower.

In 2013 the USDA's Economic Research Service estimated $14.1 billion based upon reports by Hoffman and Anekwe (2012) arguing that the Scharff, (2012) methodology included the enhanced models monetized quality-adjusted life years to account for pain and suffering caused by foodborne illness and illness impact on daily activities, which they claimed to be flawed. In 2014 the USDA estimated the cost to be $15.6 billion; Scharff estimated $55.5 billion; both estimate higher than the 2013 estimates. The estimates in all these studies did not include regulatory or industry costs associated with foodborne illness.

According to Bill Marler, a prominent Washington State attorney who has represented foodborne illness victims for decades, the Jensen Farms case could have cost $150 million if claims did not progress to court (Marler, 2011). He also noted that Jensen Farms was culpable but so were other parties involved in the distribution, sales, and the third-party auditor of the tainted cantaloupe (Marler, 2011). That was the cost for victims, not the cost of the associated outbreak for the Jensen brothers with fines estimated to be $1.5 million, nor the approximately $12 million in medical expenses as of 2012 (Marler, 2011).

Though the aftermath of the attacks on September 11, 2001, resulted in considerable investment in public health preparedness, that same funding declined 38% between 2005 and 2012 (Levi, Segal, & Vinter, 2009). In 2007 a hearing the House Energy and Commerce investigations subcommittee learned from the FDA's data highlight how a shrinking inspection staff examines less than 1% of all imported food (Zhang, 2007).

Funding constraints place an undue burden on regulators and our regulatory systems, including staffing. Another impact on staffing, albeit in the short term, is a government shutdown. One needs only look as far back as the Trump administration's long government shutdown from December 22, 2018 to January 25, 2019, in which some 800,000 federal employees were reported to have been prevented from doing their jobs and from receiving their paychecks (Rein and Whoriskey, 2019).

Budget constraints hinder inspection in the food supply both domestic and imported, thus failing to reduce the occurrences of foodborne illnesses in the retail and wholesale sectors of the food supply. In addition to state and local boards of health, the FDA and the USDA have experienced a decline in funding for inspection over past decades. Inadequate funding presents a stumbling block for maintaining sufficient staffing of qualified inspectors for these regulatory segments.

Economic impacts on industry

The Jensen Farms outbreak and recall severely impacted cantaloupe farmers across the nation. Cantaloupe sales after the recall dropped 53%, and it was estimated that the California Central Valley cantaloupe acreage would drop by 30% in 2012 by the California Cantaloupe Advisory Board (Marcum, 2012; Bailin, 2013) "Since consumers who had trusted the U.S. food safety system to protect them had gotten sick and died, public uncertainty about food safety increased, which resulted directly in cantaloupe industry losses" (Bailin, 2013).

A Purdue University study on "The impact of food safety events on the value of food-related firms: An event study approach" (Seo et al., 2013), looking at 20 years of food safety events, showed how a large food crisis can impact a company's stock value. The study specifically examined six notable cases:

- After the landmark 1993 *E. coli* O157:H7 outbreak, the "Jack in the Box" fast food hamburger chain in the western states lost millions of dollars in sales revenue. Health officials reported that the outbreak resulted in some 700 ill across several states, over 120 hospitalizations, and the deaths of four young children (Marler, 2017).
- After its 1996 *E. coli* O157:H7 outbreak (resulting in at least 65 ill across many states and in Canada, 12 patients developing HUS, and one death) the "Odwalla" juice drink company faced bankruptcy, eventually being bought by the Coca Cola company. In January 2001, the FDA issued juice regulations based on the principles of Hazard Analysis and Critical Control Point to ensure safe processing and importing of juice (Marler, 2016).
- The 2000 *E. coli* O157:H7 outbreak in Wisconsin led to "Sizzler's" (a chain of steakhouse restaurants) bankruptcy. Health officials reported 64 lab-confirmed cases with notations of over 550 additional probable cases, dozens of hospitalizations; four patients developing HUS, and one child's death (Marler, 2015).
- The 2003 hepatitis A outbreak at a "Chi-Chi's" restaurant in Pennsylvania, tied to green onions, in which tainted brand image and negative publicity was blamed for the close of the company. The outbreak resulted in at least 565 confirmed cases, including at least 13 employees and residents of seven states, and three deaths. More than 9000 people were given hepatitis A shots (Outbreak Database, n.d.a).
- The 2002 *E. coli* O157:H7 outbreak tied to ground beef from a production plant. Dozens of cases of *E. coli* O157:H7 infection across six states prompted "ConAgra" to voluntarily recall over 18 million pounds of

ground beef, then the third largest recall in US history. This recall was an expansion of a ConAgra 354,000-pound voluntary recall from the month prior (Roos, 2002).

- 2005 *E. coli* outbreak tied to "Dole" triple-washed, prepackaged lettuce impacted the entire leafy green industry. Health officials reported 25 lab-confirmed illnesses, 12 hospitalizations, and 1 death. (This incident would not only be followed with a similar outbreak in spinach the following year, but also a series of outbreaks involving Romaine lettuce in late 2017 through 2018) (Outbreak Database, n.d.b)

The Purdue study found that:

- The role of media/social media was the #1 factor (informing consumers).
- On average, a company's stock continued to drop for 57 trading days after an event (one quarter of the year).
- On average, a company's stock required 264 total trading days to return to pre-event value (total of over four quarters after trigger event). Note: a typical trading year on the New York Stock Exchange (NYSE) is only 252 days (See diagram as follows).

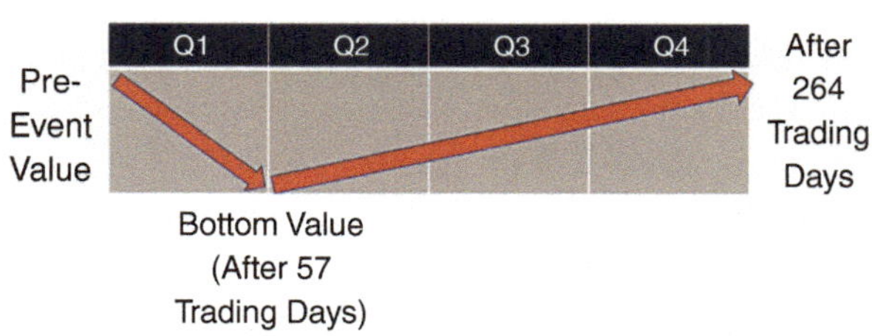

Diagram by Author, based on findings from Seo et al. (2013)

In the first quarter after Chipotle's series of multistate and multipathogen outbreaks in fourth quarter 2015, their NYSE stock values predictably fell during the first quarter of 2016. Specifically, they fell by 43%, at a loss of nearly $8 billion. For a while, the second quarter 2016 started to look like the economic model from the study. That similarity did not last, however. While Chipotle's pattern of first quarter losses spiraling to a new bottom point mirrored that of the model, so did much of the second quarter's return to pre-event value. At some point during the second quarter, amid additional outbreaks tied to the chain, the company's stock value failed to continue to rise. Worse, it hit new, lower points before the end of 2016 and again before the end of 2017. The stock values showed and increasing tend through the second quarter of 2018 and a rapid rise through the first quarter of 2019. Finally, on June 12, 2019, almost 15 quarters after the outbreaks of 2015, Chipotle's NYSE stock value reached the company's preoutbreak amount for the first time (see diagram as follows).

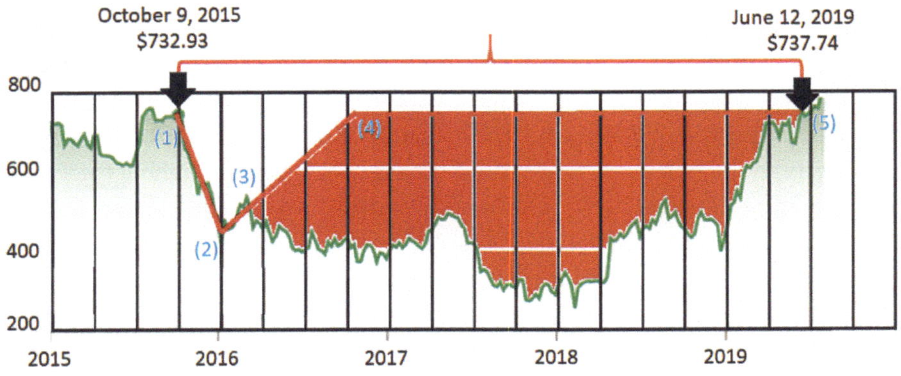

Diagram by Author, combining 2015–19 NYSE data from Market Summary for Chipotle Mexican Grill, Inc. (NYSE: CMG) with the model from Seo et al. (2013)

The numbered points on the diagram indicate the following:

1. Highest NYSE value ($732.93) at the start of 2015's fourth trading quarter and start of Chipotle's outbreaks.
2. One NYSE trading quarter later, Chipotle's stock value appeared to be at its bottom mark ($413.29) on January 16, 2016.
3. Chipotle's NYSE stock value started to deviate from the patterns found in the Perdue University model.
4. Somewhere just after the start of 2016's fourth quarter was the point at which Chipotle's NYSE stock value should have returned to its pre-event value, based on the trends seen in the Perdue University model.
5. June 12, 2019, over 10 NYSE trading quarters after the Perdue model would have placed it, Chipotle's stock value reached the company's pre-outbreak value for the first time in over 14 quarters.

To summarize, after a cluster of outbreaks, Chipotle Mexican Grill experienced a drop in profit stock value and announced changes in policies related to food safety and training. These changes were not caused by recalls, litigation (which did come later), legislation, or changes in regulation/oversight.

The cause for the company's stock value and profits to decrease and then fail to rebound as per studied patterns was two-fold. First, Chipotle did experience a change in consumer behavior, as their reputation took a significant hit. A balance of opposing memes, videos, and other elements of social media exposed that, in addition to consumers professing their undying affection for Chipotle, many consumers across the nation became aware of these outbreaks and now associated the restaurant chain with failures in food safety. Also, after learning of all the outbreaks tied to Chipotle, a significant number of customers voted with their dollars and chose to spend elsewhere.

Second, investors rethought their confidence in Chipotle as a dependable stock. Investment firms reached out to experts to reevaluate the questions they asked and how they measured the company's ability to avoid future outbreaks and bad publicity.

During a December 2016, conference call with investors, however, Mark Crumpacker, their Chief Marketing Officer, used their company's data to argue that "there are not large numbers of customers staying away from Chipotle" because of food-safety problems (Dewey, 2017).

Meanwhile, a US Attorney for California and the FDA opened a criminal investigation earlier that year, looking into Chipotle's 2015–16 outbreaks, with the company revealing that the government had subpoenaed their records as part of its investigation.

During the 2015 and 2016 outbreaks, Chipotle CEO Steve Ells promised that the company would revise their training materials and prioritize employee training. The company even gained headlines when it closed all their locations across the country on the same date for mandatory training. This commitment to solving the outbreak problems at the location and employee levels reflected a failure to commit 100% to solving the larger, corporate-wide problems, as evidenced by the numerous outbreaks and incidents at a variety of Chipotle locations.

In July 2017 a customer's video went viral of several mice spotted inside a Dallas, Texas, Chipotle (CNN, 2017). Later that month a sick employee caused a norovirus outbreak at a Chipotle restaurant in Sterling, Virginia, with multiple customers developing symptoms. The company closed that restaurant temporarily after several customers reported becoming sick from eating at that location on the crowdsourced website "I Was Poisoned." Blaming a breakdown in the company's sick policy was the culprit, (then) CEO Steve Ells reported that the company's employees will undergo more " comprehensive communication and…relentless training" to prevent another outbreak (Goldman, 2017).

July of 2017 also saw the NYSE value of Chipotle's stocks fall from $413.89 on July 7, 2017, down to a low of $255.46 on February 9, 2018. The stock value did not return above that July, 2017 value until April 27, 2018. During this low value period, with a low that took the company back to its November 2012, price, Chipotle again took center stage during another major outbreak—perhaps it worst.

In August, 2018 the CDC confirmed that over 700 Chipotle customers who ate at a single location in Powell, OH, in late July, became infected with the foodborne pathogen clostridium perfringens. This pathogen typically occurs when food is held at unsafe temperatures. Again, the company's response was predictable. In a press release, Chipotle CEO Brian Niccol stated at the time that "Chipotle Field Leadership will be retraining all restaurant employees nationwide ... on food safety and wellness protocols" (Flager & McDowell, 2018). At industry events and even at international food safety conferences, experts discussed how Chipotle's annual statement about retraining employees is now seen as an empty response similar to the sending of "thoughts and prayers."

The costs of recalls

Recalls represent regulators and industries removing adulterated products from commerce to prevent foodborne illness events. In 2011 The GMA, a Washington, DC-based trade association representing the food, beverage, and consumer product companies, published "Capturing Recall Costs Measuring and Recovering the Losses" (Grocery Manufacturers Association, 2011) This report focused on the experiences of US-based companies and under US law dealing with Class 1 recalls (see table below).

Types of recalls

Class	FDA definition	USDA definition
Class I	"A situation in which there is a reasonable probability that the use of or exposure to a violative product will cause serious adverse health consequences or death."	"Involves a health hazard situation in which there is a reasonable probability that eating the food will cause health problems or death."
Class II	"A situation in which use of or exposure to a violative product may cause temporary or medically reversible adverse health consequences or where the probability of serious adverse health consequences is remote."	"Involves a potential health hazard situation in which there is a remote probability of adverse health consequences from eating the food."
Class III	"A situation in which use of or exposure to a violative product is not likely to cause adverse health consequences."	"Involves a situation in which eating the food will not cause adverse health consequences."

Source: Created by author based on information from US Food and Drug Administration (2014) and US Department of Agriculture (2015)

The report was based on survey responses from 36 GMA member companies using an online survey of 20–25 questions. Of the participating companies, 91% reported themselves as being in the food and beverage segment and 58% had experienced a recall within 5 years at the time of the survey. Approximately three quarters of the participants reported earning between $500 million and $5 billion annually. Within the companies who faced a recall, 77% of the respondents estimated the cost to be up to $30 million with 23% citing higher costs (Grocery Manufacturers Association, 2011). Considering this survey was to 36 firms the estimated average cost of $10 million dollars per recall represents only a fraction of the cost of US recalls within a 5-year period.

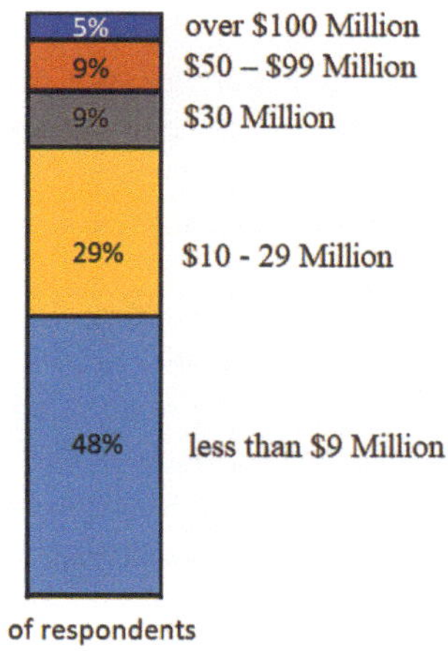

Responses (N = 36 firms)	Financial impact from direct recall costs, sales losses, etc.
5.00%	>$100 million
9.00%	$50–99 million
9.00%	$30 million
29.00%	$10–29 million
48.00%	<$9 million

Figure by author, based on the data from Grocery Manufacturers Association (2011)

Jeremy Zenlea, Corporate Director of Food Safety at Cumberland Farms (a regional chain of over 550 convenience stores) describes a normal recall situation in his stores:

"What happens is the manufacturer will do the recall. They'll give us a call, they'll say, *'Hey, Jeremy, we found a lot of extraneous matter in our hotdogs. So we're going to do a recall.'* And what I'll tell them is, okay, this is what we do. And then I submit a claim to them and they'll pay you back 100% because they're the one basically having you get their product out. And we won't just charge them back for the product itself. We'll charge you for all the shipping costs and if any labor had to go into it at the store, to prepare at the store, they'll take care of all of it. And there's no questions asked because they're the ones that called the recall. In a situation where they don't call the recall, but there's a pending recall, like the Romaine lettuce situation, where there's a huge gray area. That money that we're saying that we lost, there's maybe a 25% chance we're going to actually get it back. So we really are taking the hit. But that hit is so much less, in terms of value than what would happen if all of our consumers started equating any symptoms they have to our brand.

The symptoms of foodborne illness are common to many, many other things, and they can be caused by many other things, not necessarily related to the last thing you ate. And one of the biggest misconceptions is that foodborne illness, the onset of it, is like right away, like you eat the salad and one second later, you are puking all over the place.

The last thing [a retailer] needs is something where that's our brand, then we're going to get a claim and just to handle the claim, even if it's nothing, could be like $100 per claim though. And that's not resulting in anything. It's just that we sit down and we complete the investigation. Obviously, I take every single claim of foodborne illness seriously, because you have to, because there are surprises out there. We use our own internal labor to go through the investigation. So it really comes down to that, that quarter million dollars, it's such a drop in the bucket. Even if we're not going to get it back compared to what we would have to face, even if there was no health risk with that Romaine lettuce, we would still have to face it no matter what. Cause that's just as a retailer, we're the ones where they're representing the industry to that consumer. So we kind of have to take the brunt of it.

A recall may cost a quarter of a million dollars to do. If I'm talking to the owner of the company, that quarter million dollars is negligible to him. He's like, *Okay, it's a drop in the bucket compared to what we could lose if we don't handle this correctly*. And remember that, especially like in the Romaine [lettuce] situation, we don't know if we're going to get any of that back.

Recalls are money. Money definitely plays a huge, huge role in the decision-making. For example, some operations guy versus the QA guy: the operations guys saying it costs a lot of money to do a recall, and then the QA guy says, *Yeah, but if we don't do it and something really, really happens, then we could go to jail."*

To the food company, especially to retailers, brand awareness and brand integrity are definitely important, but recalls can be seen as playing a role in maintaining that integrity.

References

Acheson, D. (2015). E. Coli Outbreaks Changed Food Production, But How Safe Are We? [Video Transcript] The New York Times Retro Report. Retrieved from https://www.retroreport.org/transcript/chasing-outbreaks-how-safe-is-our-food/.

Bailin, D. (2013). The consequences of killer cantaloupes. Union of Concerned Scientists. Center for Science & Democracy. Available from: https://blog.ucsusa.org/deborah-bailin/the-consequences-of-killer-cantaloupes-257.

Brown, J. (2000). Work Plan: Fiscal Year 2000. Health and Human Services, Office of Inspector General. Available from: https://oig.hhs.gov/publications/docs/workplan/2000/workpl.pdf.

Center for Disease Control (CDC). (2012). Multistate Outbreak of Listeriosis Linked to Whole Cantaloupes from Jensen Farms, Colorado (FINAL UPDATE). Available from: https://www.cdc.gov/listeria/outbreaks/cantaloupes-jensen-farms/index.html.

Center for Disease Control (CDC). (2016). Estimate of Foodborne Illness in the United States. Available from: https://www.cdc.gov/foodborneburden/index.html.

CNN. (2017). Watch: Mice caught on tape in Dallas Chipotle. CNN. Available from: https://www.cnn.com/videos/cnnmoney/2017/07/20/chipotle-dallas-mice.cnn.

Consumer Federation of America. (2019). CFA and CFI Applaud Introduction of the Safe Food Act [Press Release]. Available from: https://consumerfed.org/press_release/cfa-and-cfi-applaud-introduction-of-the-safe-food-act/.

Dean, L. (2015). FSMA Federalism. *Produce Processing Magazine*. Available from: http://produceprocessing.net/fsma-federalism/.

In re Caremark Int'l Inc. Derivative Litig., 698 A.2d 959, 971 (Delivered 1996).

DeWaal, C, & Robert, N. (2005). Global and Local: Food Safety Around the World. The Center for Science in the Public Interest. Available from: https://cspinet.org/sites/default/files/attachment/global.pdf.

Dewey, C. (2017). Economic Policy: A Chipotle Restaurant is Closed After Yet Another Foodborne Illness Outbreak. *The Washington Post*. Available from: https://www.washingtonpost.com/news/wonk/wp/2017/07/18/a-chipotle-restaurant-is-closed-after-yet-another-foodborne-illness-outbreak/?utm_term=.1204f8df828c.

DOJ. (2014). Statements Regarding the Sentencing of Eric And Ryan Jensen. Press Release. Available from: https://www.justice.gov/usao-co/pr/statements-regarding-sentencing-eric-and-ryan-jensen.

Durbin, D. (2004). Food safety oversight for the 21st century: the creation of a single, independent federal food safety agency. *Food and Drug Law Journal*, *59*(3), 383–385.

Durbin, D. (2015). Safe Food Act of 2015, S-287, 114th Congress. Available from: https://www.congress.gov/bill/114th-congress/senate-bill/287/text.

Durbin, D. (2019). Durbin Reintroduces Food Safety Act: Legislation Would Improve Nation's Food Safety System [Press release]. U.S. Senator (D-IL), Office of the Press Secretary. Available from: https://www.durbin.senate.gov/newsroom/press-releases/durbin-reintroduces-food-safety-act.

Dyckman, L. (1999). Food Safety: U.S. Needs a Single Agency to Administer a Unified, Risk-Based Inspection System. Testimony Before the Subcommittee on Oversight of Government Management, Restructuring and the District of Columbia, Committee on Governmental Affairs, U.S. Senate. U.S. General Accounting Office. Available from: https://www.gao.gov/assets/110/108064.pdf.

FDA (2016). Regulatory Program Standards: Manufactured Food Regulatory Program Standards (MFRPS). Available from: http://www.fda.gov/ForFederalStateandLocalOfficials/ProgramsInitiatives/RegulatoryPrgmStnds/ucm475064.htm.

FDA. (2019a). Retail Food Program Standards Enrollments (as of 3/31/2019). Available from: https://www.fda.gov/food/voluntary-national-retail-food-regulatory-program-standards/listing-jurisdictions-enrolled-voluntary-national-retail-food-regulatory-program-standards.

FDA. (2019b). Voluntary National Retail Food Regulatory Program Standards—Introduction. Available from: https://www.fda.gov/media/86636/download.

Flager, M., & McDowell, M. (2018). UPDATE: This Is What Caused Chipotle's Worst Food Poisoning Outbreak Yet. Delish. Available from: https://www.delish.com/food-news/a22667902/chipotles-food-poisoning-outbreak-ohio/.

Food Safety News. (2014). Senate Bill Would Send NOAA's Seafood Inspection Program to Interior. Available from: https://www.foodsafetynews.com/2014/01/senate-bill-would-send-noaa-to-interior-department/.

Gillespie, C. (2015). Blue Bell Ice Cream Listeria Outbreak Timeline. Food Poisoning Bulletin. Available from: https://foodpoisoningbulletin.com/2015/blue-bell-ice-cream-listeria-outbreak-timeline/.

Goldman, D. (2017). Chipotle says sick employee responsible for latest outbreak. CNN Business. Available from: https://money.cnn.com/2017/07/26/news/companies/chipotle-sick/index.html.

Griesbach, R., & Camarota, A. (2016). Putting Down Roots at the Patent Office. Inventors' Eye: A Newsletter of the U.S. Patent and Trade Office. Available from: https://www.uspto.gov/learning-and-resources/newsletter/inventors-eye/putting-down-roots-patent-office.

Grocery Manufacturers Association. (2011). Capturing Recall Costs Measuring and Recovering the Losses. Available from: https://cdn2.hubspot.net/hub/288450/file-606071909-pdf/Capturing_recall_costs.pdf.

Hamburg, M. (2009). Testimony before subcommittee on health, committee on energy and commerce. Washington, DC: U.S. Senate.

Harris, G. (2009). F.D.A. Chief Lauds Food Safety Bill as the 'Right Direction'. *The New York Times.* Available from: https://www.nytimes.com/2009/06/04/health/policy/04fda.html.

HHS. (2018). About Us. Available from: https://www.hhs.gov/about/strategic-plan/introduction/index.html.

Hoffmann, S., & Anekwe, T. (2013). Making sense of recent costof-foodborne-illness estimates. USDA Economic Research Service Economic Information Bulletin No. (EIB-118). Available from: https://www.ers.usda.gov/webdocs/publications/43796/40344_eib118.pdf?v=0.

Hoffmamn, S. (2015). Quantifying the impacts of foodborne illnesses. U.S. Department of Agriculture, Economic Research Service. Available from: https://www.ers.usda.gov/amber-waves/2015/september/quantifying-the-impacts-of-foodborne-illnesses/.

IFSAC. (2015). Foodborne Illness Source Attribution Estimates for *Salmonella, Escherichia coli* O157 (E. coli O157), *Listeria monocytogenes* (Lm), and *Campylobacter* using Outbreak Surveillance Data. USDA. Available from: https://www.fsis.usda.gov/wps/wcm/connect/df7eebf6-911c-47c4-aee6-36b60ea04663/IFSAC-Project-Report-022415.pdf?MOD=AJPERES.

Institute of Medicine, National Research Council. (1998). *Ensuring Safe Food: From Production to Consumption.* Washington, DC: National Academy Press. Committee to Ensure Safe Food from Production to Consumption.

Johnson, R. (2014). The Federal Food Safety System: A Primer. Congressional Research Service. Available from: https://www.fas.org/sgp/crs/misc/RS22600.pdf.

Levi, J., Segal, L. M., & Vinter, S. (2009). *Ready or Not?: Protecting the public's health from diseases, disasters, and bioterrorism*. Washington, DC: Trust for Americas Health.

Liang, A. (2016). The Increasing Problem of Outbreaks Associated with Produce. CDC. Presentation before the Conference for Food Protection Biennial Meeting, Boise, ID.

Marchand v. Barnhill et al., No. 533, 2018 (Delivered 2019).

Marcum, D. (2012). California cantaloupe farms regroup after listeria outbreak. The Los Angeles Times. Available from: https://www.latimes.com/business/la-xpm-2012-jan-05-la-fi-cantaloupe-crop-20120106-story.html.

Marler, B. (2011). Listeria cantaloupe outbreak could cost $150 million. Food Safety News. Available from: https://www.foodsafetynews.com/2011/10/listeria-cantaloupe-outbreak-could-cost-150-million/.

Marler, B. (2015). Sizzler E.coli Outbreak. *About E.coli*. Available from: https://about-ecoli.com/ecoli_outbreaks/sizzler-e-coli-outbreak.

Marler, B. (2016). Chipotle – Parallels with Jack-in-the-Box and Odwalla. Food Safety News. Available from: https://www.foodsafetynews.com/2016/01/publishers-platform-chipotle-parallels-with-jack-in-the-box-and-odwalla/.

Marler, B. (2017). Jack in the Box E. coli Outbreak – 25th Anniversary. Food Safety News. Available from: https://www.foodsafetynews.com/2017/12/jack-in-the-box-e-coli-outbreak-25th-anniversary/.

Merrill, R. A., & Francer, J. K. (2000). Organizing Federal Food Safety Regulation. *Seton Hall Law Review, 31*(1), 61–173. Available from: https://scholarship.shu.edu/cgi/viewcontent.cgi?referer=http://theconversation.com/&httpsredir=1&article=1334&context=shlr.

Nixon, R. (2015). Obama Proposes Single Overseer for Food Safety. *New York Times*. Available from: http://www.nytimes.com/2015/02/21/us/obama-proposes-single-overseer-for-food-safety.html?_r=0.

O'Hagan, M. (2009). Food-safety Lawyer's Wish: Put Me Out of Business. *The Seattle Times*. Available from: http://www.seattletimes.com/seattle-news/food-safety-lawyers-wish-put-me-out-of-business/.

Obama, B. (2009). Weekly Address. The Obama White House. Available from: https://www.youtube.com/watch?v=WjX0iJU3vtY&feature=youtu.be.

Obama, B. (2011). President Obama Talks about Budget Negotiations. MSNBC. Available from: https://www.youtube.com/watch?v=rV1KO01mrqc.

OMB (2015). Fiscal Year 2016 Budget of the U.S. Government. Washington, DC: Office of Management and Budget.

Outbreak Database. (n.d.a). Chi Chi's Restaurant Green Onions 2003. Outbreak Database. Available from: http://outbreakdatabase.com/details/chi-chis-restaurant-green-onions-2003/?

Outbreak Database. (n.d.b). Dole Food Company Triple-Washed, Ready-to-Eat, Lettuce 2005. Outbreak Database. Available from: http://outbreakdatabase.com/details/dole-food-company-triple-washed-ready-to-eat-lettuce-2005/?

Rein, L., & Whoriskey, P. (2019). While federal workers go without pay, senior trump administration officials are poised to get $10,000 raises. The Washington Post. Available from: https://www.washingtonpost.com/business/2019/01/04/while-federal-workers-go-without-pay-senior-trump-administration-officials-are-poised-get-raises/.

Roberts, T. (2018). Food safety economics: incentives for a safer food supply. Switzerland: Springer.

Roos, R. (2002). ConAgra Recalls 18 Million Pounds of Ground Beef Because of E coli O157:H7 Risk. The University of Minnesota Center for Infectious Disease Research and Policy. Available from: http://www.cidrap.umn.edu/news-perspective/2002/07/conagra-recalls-18-million-pounds-ground-beef-because-e-coli-o157h7-risk.

Scharff, R. (2012). Economic burden from health losses due to foodborne illness in the United States. Journal of Food Protection 75(1):123-131. doi: 10.4315/0362-028X.JFP-11-058.

Scharff, R.L. Economic burden from health losses due to foodborne illness in the United StatesJournal of Food Protection7512013Available from: http://www.marlerblog.com/uploads/image/s18.pdf

Scharff, R.L. Economic burden from health losses due to foodborne illness in the United StatesJournal of Food Protection 75(1)201-131 doi: 10.4315/0362-028X.JFP-11-058.

Scharff, R. (2015). State estimates for the annual cost of foodborne illness. *Journal of Food Protection, 78*(6), 1064–1071. doi: 10.4315/0362-028X.JFP-14-505.

SCOTUS Blog. (2017). DeCoster v. United States. Available from: https://www.scotusblog.com/case-files/cases/decoster-v-united-states/.

Seo, S., et al. (2013). The impact of food safety events on the value of food-related firms: an event study approach. *International Journal of Hospitality Management, 33*, 153–165.

US Department of Agriculture (2015). FSIS Food Recalls. Food Safety Inspection Service. Available from: https://www.fsis.usda.gov/wps/portal/fsis/topics/food-safety-education/get-answers/food-safety-fact-sheets/production-and-inspection/fsis-food-recalls/fsis-food-recalls.

US Food and Drug Administration (2014). Recalls Background and Definitions. Available from: https://www.fda.gov/safety/industry-guidance-recalls/recalls-background-and-definitions.

Zhang, J. (2007). FDA food inspections are seen as inadequate. The Wall Street Journal. Available from: https://www.wsj.com/articles/SB118463989137768585.

Zuraw, L. (2015). Lawmakers Introduce Bills to Create Single Food Safety Agency. Food Safety News. Available from: http://www.foodsafetynews.com/2015/01/lawmakers-introduce-legislation-to-create-single-food-safety-agency/#.VRL6WJ7TDIU.

CHAPTER 7

The 2010 FDA Food Safety Modernization Act (FSMA)

"Put me out of business—Please!"
Bill Marler, 'The* E. coli *Lawyer' addressing the Agriculture Forum, 2007

"No parent should have to worry that their child is going to get sick from their lunch ..."
President Barack Obama Weekly Address, March 14, 2009

"We have gone from a period where people got sick only at church suppers or potluck dinners to a global situation where foods come to us from all over the world, and it's just a completely different situation that we deal with now."
Joe Corby, former Executive Director, Association of Food and Drug Officials, 2019

New post-9/11 realities

Not even a year had passed since the September 11, 2001, attack on New York's World Trade Center buildings and on the Pentagon when the World Health Assembly, the decision-making body of the World Health Organization (WHO), adopted a 2002 resolution expressing serious concern about threats against civilian populations by deliberate use of agents disseminated via food. Later that year, WHO published 'Terrorist threats to food"—a food safety/food terrorism document for national government policy makers (WHO, 2002). Focusing on food, food ingredients, and water (in the forms of food ingredients and of bottled water), the document classifies food safety as an essential element of modern, global public health security. It goes on to define "food terrorism" as follows:

> *"an act or threat of deliberate contamination of food for human consumption with biological, chemical, and physical agents or radionuclear materials for the purpose of causing injury or death to civilian populations and/or disrupting social, economic or political stability."*

In outlining the potential effects of food terrorism, the WHO utilized data from "unintended" foodborne disease outbreaks to describe the toll of

Food Safety
http://dx.doi.org/10.1016/B978-0-12-818219-2.00007-7

potential disease and death. The document looks at how a single incident of "unintentional contamination" of just one kind of food can infect hundreds of thousands of people with a "serious debilitating disease," then goes on to extrapolate the effects of some more deliberate and dangerous attack on our food supply.

The impact on trade and the economy is discussed as a "primary motive" for food terrorism. Recalls in American markets of foreign fruits resulted in bankruptcy of international growers and shippers after consumers around the globe shunned such products. The WHO document details specific events in recent history when individual US recalls of domestic ground beef contaminated with *Escherichia coli* O157:H7 and lunch meats contaminated with *Listeria* numbered in the 20= millions of pounds of affected product each.

The US Department of Agriculture's Food Safety Inspection Service (FSIS) lists on its webpage a great amount of information online for each recall issued in the United States. The number of entries for individual recalls is staggering. Not only are the examples listed by the WHO the tip of the iceberg in terms of the numbers of recalls and the quantity of food products adulterated, but a look at data from the Bureau of Labor Statistics shines more light on scope of this economic impact. When analyzing consumer price index average price data specific for the products and the year of the recalls, one learns that the approximate dollar value loss of just the two beef recalls listed in the WHO document come in at $44 million and $61 million, respectively.

Again, the WHO points to the significant financial impact on the market and related stakeholders. Beyond the loss of profit and the closing of businesses and the financial toll on individual countries, however, the WHO uses lessons learned from outbreaks and recalls over the last 20 years to emphasize that foodborne diseases have the potential of causing the disruption of global trade and economic stability and may even impact political stability.

While the WHO published "Terrorist Threats to Food" to provide member governments with guidance on preventing the deliberate contamination of food, some of this document's main points hold significant meaning for unintentional food problems. The understanding of those in the industry of every facet of the food chain, from farm to table, is critical in identifying and preventing failures and violations of the system.

In the United States, The Public Health Security and Bioterrorism Preparedness Response Act of 2002 (Public Law 107–188—June 12, 2002) is described as an Act "To improve the ability of the United States to prevent, prepare for, and respond to bioterrorism and other public health emergencies."

Introduced in the House as H.R. 3448 on December 11, 2001, the Public Health Security and Bioterrorism Preparedness Response bill passed the House the next day almost unanimously. It passed the Senate unanimously on December 20, 2001, and then signed into law by President George W. Bush, the Department of Health and Human Services (HHS), and the USDA on June 12, 2002.

The Act established procedures for preparation for bioterrorism and public health emergencies, as well as the National Disaster Medical System, comprised of teams of health professionals. Furthermore, the rules under this Act include security risk assessment of individuals who have access to the select agents and toxins, with the purpose being to restrict access from any person who meets the criteria of a "restricted person" as defined in the USA Patriot Act of 2001 (PL 107-56—October 26, 2001) signed into law by President George W. Bush the previous year.

A subpart of the Public Health Security and Bioterrorism Preparedness Response Act of 2002, the Agricultural Bioterrorism Protection Act of 2002 (80 FR 10627, 7 CFR 331, 9 CFR 121) provides for the regulation of certain biological agents and toxins that have the potential to pose a severe threat to human, animal, and plant health, or to animal and plant products.

Growing concerns behind new legislation

Some experts point out that the momentum for modernizing the FDA really started with the 2006 spinach *E. coli* O157:H7 outbreak, involving at least 199 ill across 26 states, 102 being hospitalized, 31 developing Hemolytic Uremic Syndrome (HUS), and at least three confirmed deaths (CDC, 2006). In California the leafy green produce industry took responsibility for the event and made an unprecedented, formalized commitment to protect public health through the creation of the California Leafy Green Products Handler Marketing Agreement (LGMA). The program's goal is to assure safety and confidence in California-grown lettuce, spinach, and other leafy greens. Since then, they have partnered with a sister program in Arizona to include approximately 90% of the leafy greens grown in the United States.

LGMA collaborated with STOP Foodborne Illness to enlist the involvement of Rylee Gustafson and Lauren Bush—two young *E. coli* victims—

to produce a video training tool called "The WHY behind Food Safety" (LGMA, 2015) as part of their training program.

Rylee Gustafson became ill in the 2006 *E. coli* outbreak tied to spinach just days after her ninth birthday. She experienced kidney failure, loss of vision, loss of hearing, and swelling around her brain and heart. She also developed HUS, a condition that damages the kidneys and which will likely require that she have a kidney transplant in the future (Rutledge, 2016). Kathleen Chrismer described her daughter's battle *E. coli* as "very emotional.... Watching Rylee in that hospital bed was the worst thing I have ever been through in my life. The pain that she went through, the distress that comes with not knowing the likely outcome" (Rutledge, 2016).

Rylee, now a student in university, still deals daily with long-term health conditions, including Type 1 diabetes and kidney disease.

> *"When I first got ill, I wanted to know 'Why me?' After getting sick, finding out that I was a part of a national outbreak made me question how food can make someone very ill. I wanted to know why food safety wasn't being looked at as a huge problem."*
>
> ***(Rylee Gustafson, Personal Communication, 2019).***

Lauren Bush was a junior in college when she ate the contaminated spinach in 2006. "I almost died," Lauren later testified. After a series of misdiagnoses, two day of hemorrhaging finally convinced her doctors to search for the real cause of her suffering. She ultimately spent several weeks in two hospitals, two emergency rooms, and three different urgent treatment facilities. She would describe her state upon returning home as being "Unable to feed and care for myself... in complete emotional and physical turmoil. I spent the next five months on a continuous regimen of antibiotics and vitamins" (Bush, 2014).

The (then) FDA Deputy Commissioner, Michael Taylor called this new video project a great example of the "spirit of partnership which characterizes today's food safety landscape" (Mike Taylor, Personal Communication, 2016.) Aimed at farm workers, this industry video features Gustafson and Bush, who explain, in vivid detail, about their illnesses to illustrate why it is so important for workers on leafy green farms to follow proper food safety practices. The video stresses not only what farms should be doing, but why.

During this time, outbreaks tied to a variety of produce, and even cookie dough captured the headlines across the country. This string of high-profile food incidents prompted the House Energy and Commerce investigations subcommittee to hold a 2007 hearing to discuss the perceived inability of the FDA to conduct an adequate amount of food inspections—specifically, the agency's shrinking staff and large inspection load (Zhang, 2007).

In his March 14, 2009 Weekly Address, President Barack Obama listed a number of food safety concerns at the time, including contaminated spinach in 2006, *Salmonella* in peppers and tomatoes in 2008, in how, in 2009, "bad peanut products led to hundreds of illnesses and costs nine people their lives" while describing these events as a "painful reminder of how tragic the consequences can be when food producers act irresponsibly and government is unable to do its job" (Obama, 2009).

Caroline Smith DeWaal, then the Director of Food Safety at the Center for Science in the Public Interest (CSPI), refers to these multiple outbreaks as the "Little Shop of Horrors" that resulted in her testifying before legislators some 20 times in a short period (DeWaal, personal Communication, 2019). Another way she looked at these events presented an open "Policy Window."

A "Policy Window" is defined as "the opportunities for action on given initiatives" (Kingdon, 2011). But it is through this window of opportunity where "policy entrepreneurs" want to be able to couple a policy proposal to a problem (such as failures in food safety) and gain political support for movement on a piece of legislation (Kingdon, 2011). Public concern from the recalls and outbreaks, along with an increase in print and broadcast media attention to these incidents, added to the clear presence of a problem. Aligning the awareness and support of policymakers, various nonprofit organizations and coalitions of consumers interest groups brought victims to meet with their legislators in their state offices and in Washington, DC.

The Pew Charitable Trusts began its focus on food safety in 2009 after a person in senior leadership (who had been at the FDA) convinced the board that food Safety is an area that was ripe for reform and one where Pew could have an impact on public health. Sandra Eskin has served as the Project Director for Food Safety for 10 years.

> *"… one of the major issues that prompted this particular person to make the push on food safety was the 2006* E. coli *in Spinach outbreak. There had been spinach outbreaks before, but, for some reason, that one captured public attention. At the time, I was at a PEW grantee that worked only on produce safety. Our focus was just on pushing FDA within its existing authority to do produce safety standards to which very arguably they could have, but politically they didn't. Pew brought me in and we said 'Okay, where do we start? Do we look at FDA or USDA'? And through the discussion, I think we all agreed that it made sense to focus on the FDA first, because these outbreaks of spinach were freaking people out. The FDA did not have as*

comprehensive an inspection program. There were no standards at all for produce. Safety obviously went beyond produce safety to processed foods and imports."

(Sandra Eskin, Personal Communication, 2019)

Once Pew made the decision to focus on food safety and identified their legislative priorities, they aligned mostly with the legislation that became Food Safety Modernization Act (FSMA). "I think it was the Senate bill, but initially, not knowing which would go forward, we were also pushing [Connecticut Congresswomen (D)] Rosa DeLauro's bill" (Sandra Eskin, Personal Communication, 2019).

Moving forward on legislation, Pew took out their whole "tool chest" (Sandra Eskin, Personal Communication, 2019). They took out full-page advertisements in major magazines that highlighted foodborne illness victims. Various contractors produced materials, including a lunch bag that had a little board book in it about all the things that could be wrong with lunch. Pew also conducted, at great expense, a nationwide poll to highlight concerns about food safety and support for the type of reforms that were reflected in the bill that ultimately was passed.

"We brought victims, I think two or three times to DC for, lobbying visits and that required a lot of work on the end of putting together a lobbying training and other materials and escorting them around and having them follow up. And that was hugely impactful."

(Sandra Eskin, Personal Communication, 2019)

These efforts brought constituents to their representative in face-to-face opportunities to share real stories and faces, as well as emotional accounts of the true burden of disease. One of the key "victim advocates" was a teenage girl.

"Riley Gustafson was just a little girl when she got sick from the spinach outbreak back in 2006. She was from Nevada. Ooh. And guess what? The majority leader of the Senate, Harry Reid was from Nevada .... He was absolutely instrumental in the passage of that bill."

(Sandra Eskin, Personal Communication, 2019)

Now, in addition to the federal government's nationwide warning not to eat spinach, members of Congress also had to come to grips with the fact that this outbreak demonstrated how the FDA did not have the adequate tools to keep the food supply safe. Finding the right fit legislation that could help give FDA those tools became a top priority.

One proposal that had long been at the ready was that of changing the structure of the nation's top food agencies. For many years, US Senator

Dick Durbin (D-IL) and US Representative Rosa DeLauro (D-CT) had been filing a bill for a single food safety agency.

> *"This was legislation that CSPI had been very actively engaged with. We worked on the bill every single year . . . improving it...making it better."*
>
> ***(Caroline Smith DeWaal, personal communication, 2019).***

The 2006 version of the legislation included a provision for creating a single food safety agency. Ultimately, this bill would not progress through Congress. However, those behind the intent of the legislation decided that they "couldn't wait for Congress to get behind a full vision of the way food safety was managed and the FDA needed immediate attention" (DeWaal, 2019). Senator Durbin and Representative Delauro and would continue to introduce new bills for a single food safety agency.

The next year, they filed legislation for the first FDA modernization bill. The bill went through the normal process of revisions and ownership and getting feedback from industry. The House Energy and Commerce Committee, chaired by John Dingell, took over by the bill, putting it through multiple revisions before it went over to the Senate. There, Senator Kennedy's staff rewrote it more. On June 8, 2009 Representative Betty Sutton, D-OH, introduced the first version of the Act, H.R. 2749, "The Food Safety Enhancement Act," and it passed the House without amendments one day later, on June 9, 2009.

> *"The legislation that CSPI had been pushing, both through an FDA modernization bill and through a single agency bill, had been comprehensive. It included food register, registration of facilities. It included inspection [and] microbial monitoring. It was a really comprehensive set of tools that are needed for modern food safety deregulation. That that comprehensive bill was what was taken up in both the house and the Senate. There were a few additions. One of the additions was in the area produce safety. And in the area of imported food safety, especially in the area of the addition of the foreign supplier verification program. But other aspects of the bill really had been part of the original legislation."*
>
> ***(DeWaal, 2019)***

While the comprehensive nature of the legislation remained, changes resulting in the final product being more comprehensive made sense as they were written during a series of outbreaks between 2006 and 2010. "These incidents demonstrated the need for an even more comprehensive approach. So that was the key to the FSMA is how comprehensive it was" (DeWaal, 2019).

After being introduced in the Senate, concerns over some of the line items, as well as the dominant focus of the Senate on passing the Affordable Care Act jeopardized the passage of any significant food safety bill during that session. As an alternative, members of the House chose to take the route of passing a more senate friendly bill, H.R. 2751, the "FDA FSMA." Though H.R. 2751 passed the House, the bill passed with less support from Republican members than the earlier version, H.R. 2749.

The new bill drew great opposition in the Senate, mostly from Republican Senators. Advocacy groups, namely the PEW Charitable Trusts, the CSPI, and STOP Foodborne Illness, brought young victims and their parents to Washington, DC to meet with legislators in their offices and provided testimony on panels and on the Senate floor. Even Bill Marler, "The *E. coli* Lawyer" notable for his unparalleled work in representing victims since the 1993 outbreak, testified on behalf of passing new food safety legislation stating his famous quote "Put me out of business" (O'Hagan, 2009).

The work to gain buy-in from legislators is best characterized as the cumulative, Herculean efforts from a wide range of interest groups, advocacy organizations, industry experts, lobbyists, and regulatory officials.

> *"I was working with a lot of all my favorite people in Washington, including the people at CSPI and at PEW. Then, you know, the, the whole nine yards of people who were involved in this, all played a part. And there's a cliché with Washington that success has many parents, and I think this is a situation where it really is true. We had a lot of folks both on and off the hill play an important role and pushing this forward ...."*
>
> ***(Brian Ronholm)***

After a year and a half and numerous revisions, on December 19, 2010, the Senate passed their own version of the Act. The first version of the law was the Food Safety Enhancement Act of 2009, H.R. 2749, 111th Cong. (FSEA), which borrowed several provisions from the FSMA and the Food and Drug Administration Globalization Act. FSEA passed the House on June 9, 2009. However, negotiations with the Senate led to the final product, the "FSMA."

Working with the nonprofit consumer advocacy organization STOP Foodborne Illness (then known as "Safe Tables Our Priority"), The PEW Charitable Trusts paid for a July, 2010 full-page ad in Consumer Reports magazine featuring a photo of an empty hospital bed with a photo of Rylee Gustafson from her ninth birthday. In large font, the ad read: "How Many More? Rylee almost died from foodborne illness. It's time for the US

Senate to act." This included a letter from her mother, Kathleen Chrismer, addressed to US Senator Harry Reid (D- NV), who was, at the time, the Senate Majority Leader and represented the same state in which Rylee lived.

> *"Dear Senator Reid:*
>
> *In 2006 my daughter Rylee became violently ill and almost died from eating bagged spinach contaminated by a deadly strain of* E. coli. *She will have serious health problems for the rest of her life, but she was one of the lucky ones. Every year, thousands of Americans die because our food safety system is dangerously outdated and fails to prevent or detect such outbreaks before it's too late. In July 2009, the US House of Representatives passed a strong food safety modernization bill, but despite strong bi-partisan support, and support from food industry leaders, the Senate has still not acted. While we appreciate your support for the Senate version of the bill, it won't become law until the Senate approves it. For Rylee and millions of others whose health is at stake, please make food safety a priority and schedule S. 510 for a vote.*
>
> *Sincerely,*
>
> *Kathleen Chrismer*
>
> *Senator Reid, please schedule a vote on the FDA Food Safety Modernization Act (S. 510)" (Chrismer, 2010).*

"It was pretty dramatic"

The Senate passed the FSMA bill in November 2010. However, because of an export certification provision added to the bill, (which is constitutionally required to begin in the House), the vote did not count. There was concern that with the short time left in the session, the bill would not get the time needed to be voted on and passed before the next Congress (which would see Republicans take the majority of the House seats.) Eventually, however, the Senate moved to pass the fixed bill by unanimous consent on December 19, 2010. The House approved the bill two days later (the last day of the session) only to have the Senate send it back to the House for a revision on a budget item.

Brian Ronholm, then the USDA's Deputy Undersecretary of Food Safety, witnessed the events play out from his role within the executive branch. He describes December 21, 2010 as being "crazy" and with a great deal of "uncertainty."

> *"I remember we all were anxious and very nervous whether it was really going to happen. whether it was going to pass ... i f it even was going to be discussed. We did reach a point where we were worried that a lot of the key stakeholder groups would be disappointed because it looked like [passage of the bill] was not going*

to happen. I think we were all trying to process the disappointment, and then whether we could get over that, whether we can make another push at some point."

(Ronholm, Personal Communication, 2019)

For those who worked with legislators and regulators to bring this act to fruition, this last day of the session, right before legislators were about to go home, was equally dramatic. Caroline Smith DeWaal recalls:

"It was very stressful. We sat all afternoon watching CSPAN. We were waiting, but it never came up. When CSPAN stopped broadcasting, the bill still hadn't passed, and we were all on pins and needles, thinking that [legislators] were all going home."

(DeWaal, Personal Communication, 2019)

Late that day, however, the legislative processes jumped into high gear. According to Ronholm:

"... we got word from the floor that the discussion was renewed and it happened so quickly that there wasn't really much time to galvanize the stakeholder groups and push anything over the finish line. There wasn't any time where we could let people know that something was afoot."

(Ronholm, Personal Communication, 2019)

One of the very last acts of the 111th Congress was to pass the FDA FSMA (FSMA, P.L. 111-353).

"When it did pass, after going through this whole day of uncertainty and anxiety—it was just so unbelievable that we, I think we were just stunned. And then we kind of like, 'Oh wow: we have got to tell people."

(Ronholm, Personal Communication, 2019)

About 30 or 40 minutes after Congress passed FSMA, Brian Ronholm texted the news to Caroline Smith DeWaal. Almost speechless, Caroline thought simply: "Wow... just, just the sheer enormity of it."

Brian Ronholm was the USDA's Deputy Undersecretary for Food Safety. He recalled the day that Congress passed FSMA:

"It was such an intense process overall for a sustained period of time. This was a moment where a lot of folks came together. When it finally did pass, all of these emotions come to the forefront simultaneously. There's validation, there's relief, there's immense pride: it's one of those moments where you feel proud to be part of the institution. A lot of what can be good about Washington, a lot of what can be good about government and Congress (as dysfunctional as it has shown itself to be over the years)—this good all came to the forefront. And I think there's a lot of people who can legitimately claim credit and feel proud of what was accomplished ... getting it to pass and become law."

(Ronholm, Personal Communication, 2019).

Caroline Smith DeWall recalled her work on this piece of legislation, as it was impacted by many.

> *"I've worked with so many people who played a role in that: seasoned veterans and young victims and, and families and Oh yeah ... the effort made by the families. I mean, I always talked about CSPI as the technical arm ... the people in the back [editing and revising] the right words we needed to fix this problem or that problem. But the families themselves were right out front, and building the case, and creating the groundswell of support that got the bill through."*
>
> ***(DeWaal, Personal Communication, 2019)***

President Obama signed the FSMA into law on January 4, 2011. This was done with no ceremony, no official event—simply a signing while aboard Air Force One on a flight back from Hawaii. The celebration around that moment, however, was deafening. Most consumers will never truly understand how much hard work went into getting FSMA passed and to bring about these long-needed improvements to the safety of America's food supply. While this victory may be remembered for the final few steps taken by elected representatives, it would not have happened without the marathon of work by organizations, by many victims and their families, and by the people who lost loved ones due to food safety failures.

The FDA Food Safety Modernization Act

The 2010 FDA FSMA (Pub. L. 111-353) aims to "reduce risk of illness attributed to food from facilities subject to preventive controls rule under the act" (Milazzo, 2015). This public law is a modification to the Federal Food, Drug, and Cosmetic Act (21 U.S.C. 301 et seq.). Specific sections of FSMA focus on improving "capacity to prevent food safety problems," "capacity to detect and respond to food safety problems," and "the safety of imported foods." In passing this Act, Congress directed the FDA to coordinate inspection and compliance efforts through state agencies and resources. This poses a concern in terms of how the Act is impacted by Federalism.

Federalism is a balance between federal powers, enumerated in Article I, Section 8 of the Constitution, and States' powers, reserved in the 10th Amendment. Another way to look at this balance of power is to consider the role of food as a part of state and cultural identity, not to mention the will of the people, with the fact that pathogens do not discriminate, nor do they care about political lines. The complications of federalism have long been, ironically, compared to the differences between a layered cake—a metaphor for a perfect and uniform division of powers, and a marbled cake, where ideal and uniformity are not realistic. Within states can be found federal lands, tribal lands, national borders, interstate commerce, federal farm subsidies, and companies with ownership in other states.

The capacity and effectiveness of county and state regulatory agencies depend on their level of funding which, these days, is tempered by the access of federal money that comes with increased federal regulation. The Produce Marketing Association (PMA) offered a different take on FSMA and the idea of federalism (Dean, 2015). In his Produce Processing editorial, Editorial Director Lee Dean explores PMA as it identifies how state agencies implementing and enforcing this Act as participants in a federal-state partnership mirrors federalism, thus encouraging industry to recognize the roles of both the federal government and the states' agencies. Evidence for the need to recognize states' agencies can be found in how corporate perspectives of the challenges this new federal food policy places on many stakeholders ignore completely the role of the states' agencies as the critical regulatory and investigatory arms of the federal government. Defining food safety policies under the concept of federalism is not the only issue that requited defining.

Similar to the advances in food industry technology over the last 50 years, the definitions terms "food" and "farm," as well as others in the Act, held a wide range of interpretations from the use of the same words in the 1938 Food Drug and Cosmetics Act, which Congress intended FSMA to update. As a result, drafting and publishing of final rules would need to wait until after the FDA established modern definitions.

FSMA rules redefining terms and exemptions

A series of FDA meetings, visits, and listening events held across the country, many of which attended by FDA Deputy Commissioner of Food and Nutrition Michael Taylor, allowed for the agency to publish parameters around their working definitions of "farm," "facility," "raw agricultural product," and, later, "exemption criteria." Exemptions to farms came about as the result of an amendment to the bill prior to passing in the Senate. Referred to as the "Tester Amendment," Senator Jon Tester (D-MT), himself a small family farm owner, added that small-scale food producers should not be subject to any new federal requirements if they "sell the majority of their food directly to consumers within the state, or within a 275-mile radius of where it was produced," and have "less than $500,000 per year in sales" (Tester, 2010). This amendment to FSMA does not supersede existing food safety regulation tied to local and state food safety and health agency policies.

With exemptions required from the Tester Amendment, the FDA's work in redefining "farms" and "facilities" resulted in the agency's work with stakeholders to redefine the specific parameters for exemption. The FDA's definition for "very small farms" came with the exemption modification for $250,000 as a sales cap. This decision brought about not only a great amount of resistance from legislators and industry, but the Office of Management and Budget ultimately pushed back and determined that a definition for "small business" of less than $1 million in sales would be required. Further complicating exemptions and the definition of "small farm" and "small businesses" are the cottage food industry (home-based food production programs), the variety (or lack) of laws and levels of restrictions from state to state regarding cottage foods, and the growth of internet sales of foods, specialty foods, niche foods, and cottage foods.

In 2012 after 2 years of the FDA's delays in writing, the Center for Food Safety (CFS), a national non-profit public interest and advocacy organization, filed suit under the Administrative Procedure Act (APA), alleging that the FDA had failed to publish the rules by their statutorily mandated deadline. In "*Center for Food Safety et al. v. Hamburg et al.*," 4:12-CV-04529 (US DIST. N. D. CA.), CFS sought a declaratory judgment that the FDA violated the purpose of the Act, violated the APA by failing to issue the rules by the deadline, and sought an injunction ordering the FDA to issue the regulations as soon as possible. The organization alleged that the FDA's delay increased the risk that their members and the public at large might contract a foodborne illness.

Though FSMA mandated an aggressive implementation schedule to promulgate regulations in seven key areas by 2012. Many stakeholders referred to this timeline as "unrealistic," (The War Over FSMA, 2013) and were not surprised when the FDA did not meet the deadline. In August 2012, the CFS filed suit in US District Court for the Northern District of California under the APA to force the FDA to propose and implement FSMA food safety regulations within the time limits set by Congress. In response, the FDA's top officials stated that "The enormity and scope of the task given to FDA cannot be overstated" (Gillam, 2012).

The court granted summary judgment in favor of CFS, making the decision to "compel agency action" because the Act set out specific statutory deadlines (*Center for Food Safety v. Hamburg*, 2013). Specifically, the court ordered that:

- the FDA must publish all proposed regulations by November 30, 2013;

- for each regulation, the close of the public comment period shall be no later than March 31, 2014; and
- all final regulations shall be published in the Federal Register no later than June 30, 2015.

Even with that the FDA sought and gained an extension on that deadline.

In 2013 Rylee provided not only testimony through the PEW Charitable Trusts in which she went beyond sharing the true burden of her disease, but also voiced support for the FDA's Produce Safety Rule with the message to "finalize it quickly with the hope that fewer people, young and old, are forced to suffer because of foodborne illness" (Gustafson, 2013).

One further roadblock was the funding needed for FSMA implementation in the states. Nobody, especially all the consumer advocacy groups and victims themselves, wanted to see FSMA become an unfunded mandate. Again, the PEW Charitable Trusts and other advocacy groups called upon victims to persuade their elected representatives in DC to act.

In 2014 PEW called upon Rylee again for help, but she was not alone in these efforts. Joining her were other victims and their families, including Dana Dziadul. At three years of age, Dana became ill from *Salmonella* Poona after eating contaminated cantaloupe in 2001. After weeks in the hospital, she returned home with long-term health consequences including reactive arthritis, a debilitating, inflammatory condition (Dziadul, 2014). Rylee and Dana testified before state and federal legislators, raised awareness about food safety through local and nationwide events, shared personal accounts of illness and efforts with media, and collaborated with industry to improve food safety training.

In 2015 Rylee Gustafson and her mother, along with Lauren Bush, traveled to Washington, DC, to meet with legislators, including the Senator Reid (D-NV) to push Congress to fully fund the FSMA. In his remarks on the floor of the US Senate, Senator Reid stated that "Unfortunately for many Americans, falling ill from contaminated food has become all too regular" (Zuraw, 2015).

In 2016 the FDA awarded $21.8 million to the states through cooperative agreements to develop FSMA implementation plans. In 2017 FDA funding for state implementation increased to $30.9 million (National Sustainable Agriculture Coalition, 2017). Unfortunately, this amount is only a fraction of the predicted amount of needed funding. In 2017 the National Association of State Departments of Agriculture (NASDA), a bipartisan organization built around the appointed and elected state agricultural directors and commissioners, sent a letter to congressional budget leadership in which they estimated that state governments need an annual additional $100 million per year for "sufficient funding" for FSMA implementation (Flynn, 2017a, 2017b).

Publishing final FSMA rules

The FDA supplemental rules for the Act include a set of seven preventive controls, standards, and program specifics. See Table 7.1 for a list of the rules and a timeline of their proposals and publishing.

Though the rules' delay resulted in court ordered adherence to a publishing timeline, the FDA's road to complete this and other rules included an "unprecedented level of outreach" by the agency, including public meetings, webinars, listening sessions, and visits to farms and food facilities across the country. These events allowed the FDA to hear input from nearly every possible type of stakeholder, including representatives from industry, consumer groups, the agency's federal, state, local and tribal regulatory counterparts, academia, and more (FDA, 2016).

Table 7.1 Seven rules under FDA Food Safety Modernization Act.

Rule	Title	Date proposed	Date published
Final rules			
1	Preventive Controls for Human Food (21 CFR Parts 1, 11, 16, 106, 110)	January 16, 2013	September 17, 2015
2	Preventive Controls for Animal Food (21 CFR Parts 11, 16, 117, 500, 507, 579)	October 29, 2013	September 17, 2015
3	Standards for Produce Safety	January 16, 2013	November 27, 2015
4	Foreign Supplier Verification Program	July 29, 2013	November 27, 2015
5	Accredited Third-Party Certification	July 29, 2013	November 27, 2015
6	Sanitary Transportation of Human and Animal Food	February 5, 2014	March 31, 2016
7	Intentional Adulteration (21 CFR 11 and 121, 81 FR 34165)	December 24, 2013	May 27, 2016

Source: Based on the data from FDA (2016). FSMA Fact Sheet. Retrieved from http://www.fda.gov/Food/GuidanceRegulation/FSMA/ucm247546.htm

Rules #1 and #2: preventive controls for human food and preventive controls for human food

Under the Preventive Controls for Human Food rule, and very similarly for Animal food, food production or related facilities that fall under the regulatory control of the Act must establish and implement a written food safety plan to include:

- hazard analysis (for reasonably foreseeable biological, chemical, and physical hazards that may affect the safety of food);
- preventive controls (process, food allergen, and sanitation controls, supply-chain controls, and a recall plan); and
- oversight and management of preventive controls
  - monitoring,
  - corrective actions and corrections, and
  - verification (validating with scientific evidence, calibration of process monitoring and verification instruments, and reviewing records to verify that monitoring and corrective actions are being conducted).

This rules also required a new definition of a "farm" to include primary and secondary production facilities to discern which types of establishments are subject to the preventive controls rule or not. Similar implications for regulatory application can be found in the Produce Safety Rule. This rule also updated Current Good Manufacturing Practices for clarifications and alignment with the rule. Furthermore, these rules clarified implications for the food supply chain, with a look for further implications from a Sanitary Transportation rule.

Rule #3: standards for produce safety

The FDA FSMA Final Rule on Produce Safety (21 CFR Part 112) embraces science-based minimum standards for the safe growing, harvesting, packing, and holding of fruits and vegetables grown for human consumption. This is a departure from how the FDA previously.

Key requirements of the Produce Safety Rule include criteria for microbial agricultural water quality (based on the presence of generic *E. coli)*, that is, directly applied to growing produce (other than sprouts), as well as testing untreated water used for certain agricultural purposes. Another area of focus for this rule pertains to standards for "biological soil amendments" including raw manure and stabilized compost. These are microbial standards that set limits on detectable amounts of bacteria (to minimize the potential for contact of pathogens with produce during and after application). The Produce Safety Rule also includes new requirements to help prevent the contamination of sprouts, which have been frequently associated with forborne illness outbreaks. These requirements specify water treatment and testing standards. Water and soil, however, are not the only environmental concerns for produce safety.

The Produce Safety Rule addresses concerns about contamination from domesticated and wild animals. Standards regarding grazing distances and waiting times allow farms to take measures reasonably necessary to minimize potential contamination of harvest produce. Other areas of concern covered in this rule include worker training, health, hygiene, as well as standards related to equipment, tools, and buildings to prevent these sources from contaminating produce.

Business types	Compliance date
Large businesses—over $500,000 in produce sold annually	January 26, 2018
Small businesses—$250,000 but not more than $500,000 in produce sold annually	January 28, 2019
Very small businesses—over $25,000 but no more than $250,000 in produce sold annually	January 27, 2020

Businesses refer to covered farms based on the calculated average annual monetary value (see values shown earlier) of produce the farm sold during the previous 3-year period.

Rule #4: Foreign Supplier Verification Program

> *"The FDA FSMA rule on Foreign Supplier Verification Programs (FSVP) for Importers of Food for Humans and Animals ... requires that importers perform certain risk-based activities to verify that food imported into the United States has been produced in a manner that meets applicable U.S. safety standards .... In order to facilitate compliance FDA will provide guidance, outreach and training."*
>
> ***(FDA, 2018c)***

Essentially, the FSMA Section 301, the Foreign Supplier Verification Program (FSVP), requires importers of food to verify that food they import is not adulterated or misbranded with respect to allergen labeling before the food product arrives at the dock in the United States Importers are required to verify that foreign suppliers produce food "in a manner that provides the same level of public health protection as required in FSMA's first three rules." This is a first for the FDA, in that it is now making importers responsible prior to the product or commodity's arrival to the states.

To be compliant, an importer must establish written procedures (developed by a "qualified individual" as defined by FSMA) and follow them as part of conducting appropriate supplier verification activities to ensure that food is only imported from approved foreign suppliers. Importers are also required to take appropriate corrective measures when needed to prevent less than compliant importation of food.

Compliance with FSVP began on September 31, 2017, 18 months after the rules' publishing on March 31, 2016. In July of 2019, after a *Salmonella* outbreak linked to imported tahini, the FDA issued its first ever-warning letter to an importer for failure to follow the FSVP food safety rule (Beach, 2019).

Rule #5: Accredited third-party certification

"The FDA Food Safety Modernization Act (FSMA) rule on Accredited Third-Party Certification .... establishes a voluntary program for the accreditation of third-party certification bodies, also known as third-party auditors, to conduct food safety audits and issue certifications of foreign entities and the foods for humans and animals they produce. These requirements are intended to help ensure the competence and independence of the accreditation bodies and third-party certification bodies participating in the program".

(FDA, 2018b).

FSMA rules #4 and #5 (accredited third-party certification) go hand-in-hand as the FDA is extending its reach to improve the safety of foods by proactively preventing potentially harmful imported food from reaching the United States. This rule, which began implementation in June of 2017, specifies two uses for certifications under this program:

1. importers who wish to participation in the Voluntary Qualified Importer Program (VQIP), for expedited review entry of food; and
2. certification (from an accredited third-party certification body) to accompany a food offered for import, as required in specific circumstances by the FDA.

Rule #6: Sanitary transport of human and animal food

"The FDA Food Safety Modernization Act (FSMA) rule on Sanitary Transportation of Human and Animal Food ... [advances the] FDA's efforts to protect foods from farm to table by keeping them safe from contamination during transportation. The goal of this rule is to prevent practices during transportation that create food safety risks, such as failure to properly refrigerate food, inadequate cleaning of vehicles between loads, and failure to properly protect food."

(FDA, 2018a).

Understanding of this rule requires one to look at a bit of history behind it. In June 1990 the precursor to the Government Accountability Office (GAO) released a report *Truck transport: little is known about hauling garbage and food in the same vehicles*. In its executive summary, the report opens stating how:

> *"Press accounts in spring 1989 first alerted the public that some trucks that hauled garbage from the New York/New Jersey area to midwestern landfills were then used to carry meat, poultry, and produce. Concerned over the food contamination risk of alternately hauling, or 'crosshauling,' garbage and foodstuffs, the Subcommittee on Investigations and Oversight, House Committee on Public Works and Transportation, investigated and held hearings, concluding that the practice was occurring.*
> ***(US General Accounting Office, 1990).***

This GAO report resulted in Congress enacting the Sanitary Food Transportation Act in 1990, instructing the Department of Transportation to establish regulations for safe transportation of food products. This did not, however, prevent a 1994 *Salmonella* outbreak tied to cross contamination of Schwan's pasteurized ice cream transported in tanker trailers that had previously hauled non-pasteurized liquid eggs. The CDC collected reports of over 400 ill, whereas a study published in the *New England Journal of Medicine* estimated that 224,000 people became sick across at least 35 states (AP, 1994; Hennessy et al., 1996). With that article in the *New England Journal of Medicine*, the conclusion of the 11 authors was that "To prevent further outbreaks, food products not destined for repasteurization should be transported in dedicated containers" (Hennessy et al., 1996).

More recently, a 2013 outbreak of *Salmonella* affected 261 people across 24 states and caused three deaths. Investigation results indicated *Salmonella typhimurium* and *Salmonella* Newport contamination in an Owensville, Indiana, farm's cantaloupe crop likely was likely caused initially in the field, then later amplified during storage and transportation (Schnirring, 2013).

Ultimately the goal of this FSMA rule is to reduce the risks to human or animal health associated with the transportation of food under conditions that may render it adulterated. Though not 100% new, as the rule serves as a means to incorporate into FSMA safeguards for prevention of food safety problems throughout the food chain as envisioned in the 1990 law and in the 2005 Sanitary Food Transportation Act which specified how US Department of HHS regulations, pertaining to sanitary transportation practices (including equipment, records, transportation operations, training, and waivers) for those entities engaged in food transport via motor vehicle and rail; however, this rule does not apply to transportation of food by ship or air.

Rule #7: Intentional adulteration

"The FDA FSMA final rule is aimed at preventing intentional adulteration from acts intended to cause wide-scale harm to public health, including acts of terrorism targeting the food supply. Such acts, while not likely to occur, could cause illness, death, and economic disruption of the food supply absent mitigation strategies."

- The incident commonly referred to as the first and single largest bioterrorist attack in US history is the 1984 "Rajneeshee bioterror attack" carried out by followers of Bhagwan Shree Rajneesh in The Dalles, Oregon. In their attempt to incapacitate the local voting population so that their own candidates would win the county elections, the group deliberately contaminated water glasses, salad bars, and salad dressings at 10 local restaurants with *Salmonella enterica typhimurium*. At least 750 people became ill, 45 of whom were hospitalized, with no deaths as a result.
- More recently, just 1 month after the FDA issued this final rule, a court sentenced a Cold Spring, Minnesota woman to 90 days in jail and $200,000 in restitution after convicted her of two felony counts of causing damage to property in the first degree for her actions in 2016 in which she contaminated chicken with sand and dirt from the parking lot. The company recalled nearly 28 tons of chicken products (Flynn, 2017a, 2017b).
- Also in 2016 a Michigan man was charged with two criminal counts of poisoning unpackaged food by spraying a mixture of hand sanitizer, mouse poison, and water on fresh food at grocery stores in the Ann Arbor. A judge later found him not guilty by reason of insanity (Associated Press, 2017).
- In October, 2017, a disgruntled South Carolina man sprayed a mixture of his own feces and urine on a Harris Teeter supermarket's salad bar, sushi bar, fresh produce section, deli food, and prepared food bar, ruining approximately $3,000 worth of food (Burke, 2017).

Almost every food fraud risk demands vigilant actions regarding food safety. Impact on public health typically takes place long before any regulator or court will determine whether an act is intentional, economically motivated, or worse. The FDA's (then) Deputy Commissioner for Foods and Veterinary Medicine, Stephen Ostroff, MD, stated at a 2016 food industry conference that the FDA will only focus on food fraud when it affects food safety. Unfortunately, before any fraudulent or other intentional act gains classification is when such acts are identified—typically after public health threats have become a reality. As a result, regulators must focus on authenticity to (as FSMA's mission states) "reduce risk of illness attributed to food from facilities subject to preventive controls rule under the act."

Specific sections of FSMA focus on improving "capacity to detect and respond to food safety problems," and "the safety of imported foods," but, perhaps more importantly, the "capacity to prevent food safety problems." Authenticity is a key component of FSMA's mission beyond the intentional adulteration rule, including both preventive controls rules and even the foreign supplier verification rules.

According to the FSMA Intentional Adulteration rule, each covered facility is required to prepare and implement a food defense plan. This written plan must identify:

- A "Vulnerability Assessment"—required for each type of food manufactured, processed, packed, or held at the food facility. Elements to be evaluated include: the severity and scale of the potential impact on public health, the degree of physical access to the product, and the ability to successfully contaminate the product.
- "Mitigation Strategies" (tailored to the facility and its procedures) that should be identified and implemented at each actionable process step to provide assurances that vulnerabilities will be minimized or prevented.
- "Mitigation Strategy Management Components" which shall include monitoring, corrective actions, and verification.
- "Training and Recordkeeping" related to training for personnel assigned to the vulnerable areas, as well as records for food defense monitoring, corrective actions, and verification activities.

Compliance dates

Business types	Compliance date
Large businesses—a business that is not small or very small and does not qualify for exemptions	July 26, 2019
Small businesses—a business employing fewer than 500 persons	July 26, 2020
Very small businesses—a business averaging less than $10,000,000 per year	July 26, 2021

Note: "Businesses" include any subsidiaries and affiliates. All earnings are adjusted for inflation, per year, during the 3-year period preceding the applicable calendar year in sales of human food plus the market value of human food manufactured, processed, packed, or held without sale (e.g., held for a fee).

One important distinction about intentional adulteration pertains to food fraud. While adulteration is an aspect of food authenticity (along with counterfeiting, diversion, mislabeling, overrun, simulation, tampering, and theft), the FDA has stated before audiences on multiple occasions that while food fraud may be an element of intentional adulteration, the agency will not investigate food fraud unless it is part of an investigation related to an incident related to food safety.

Beyond FDA publishing of FSMA rules

Regardless of whether FSMA opens the door to stronger food safety regulations or it limits how far that door can be opened, this Act is the product of the hard work of many stakeholders, including consumers. With some 80% of food being regulated by the FDA and with at least 15% of our food being imported, FSMA offers a new set of science-based regulations. Also important is the proactive nature of these new rules.

The passage of FSMA highlights the differences between the USDA and the FDA. After the landmark 1993 *E. coli* outbreak, the USDA had within their powers the ability to establish a new pathogen reduction program that included shifting to a science-based approach to inspections. The USDA also declared *E. coli* an illegal adulterant. Today industry experts and food safety advocates tend to agree that meat and poultry is much safer as a result. On the other hand, about a decade later, after the pattern of outbreaks and recalls shifted to reflect a larger percentage of culprit foods being regulated by the FDA, an Act of Congress was literally needed to bring about the most significant changes in food safety regulation for foods under their regulatory authority. The FDA's pre-FSMA role was mostly reactive to outbreaks, as it did not involve proactive inspection. The FDA's abilities before FSMA were inadequate, according to former FDA Commissioner of Food and Drugs Scott Gottlieb in his 2017 speech before the NASDA. "… the agency's limited authorities and resources made preventing and handling outbreaks incredibly frustrating and challenging. We just didn't have the necessary tools" (Gottlieb, 2017).

As recent as the 2019 gathering of industry representatives and food safety experts at the annual meeting of the International Association for Food Protection, talk about FSMA included questions about the USDA ever see their own version of FSMA. Some noted specifically how the USDA still does not have mandatory recall authority, unlike that of the FDA.

FSMA not only offered challenges to FDA to do inspections, but the Act made it clear that the FDA needs to work with the states to complete those inspections. FSMA also mandated our federal agencies to better coordinate their efforts with stakeholders. In essence FSMA mandated an integrated food safety system.

This "integrated food safety system" according to Joe Corby, the former Executive Director of the Association of Food and Drug Officials: "... is a change of culture. It's not just the culture at federal agencies. It's the culture at state level. The states have to integrate with the locals that they work with in those particular states as well, of course, with the federal level and with other states and non-profit organizations" (Corby, 2019).

In a world where pathogens do not discriminate, the drawing of lines, whether they are political borders or political divisions of regulatory authority, does not matter to retailers and consumers who demand that the entire food supply is safe.

Ideally, the food industry, itself, will benefit from FSMA's rules. These updated, science-based standards, address gaps in food safety for foods imported to the United States that are transported within the United States, and that are impacted by intentional adulteration. The produce standard rule changes the FDA's role significantly, as evidenced by many outbreaks over the last 15 years tied to produce.

Consumers will gain safer food and stronger confidence in the work between the government and the industry. Though some advocates voiced concern that FSMA passed with the noted purpose of reducing incidents, as opposed to eliminating them, the reality is that there will never be an end to foodborne outbreaks and illnesses. The work ahead is to reduce the risks and reduce the chances of contaminated foods entering commerce and making their way to consumers' plates.

References

Associated Press. (1994). Salmonella Poisoning in 35 States Blamed on Ice Cream. *The Lost Angeles Times*. Available from: https://www.latimes.com/archives/la-xpm-1994-10-15-mn-50399-story.html.

Associated Press. (2017). Man Accused of Grocery Store Poisoning to Get Treatment. *The Detroit News*. Available from: https://www.detroitnews.com/story/news/local/michigan/2017/05/06/man-accused-grocery-store-poisoning-get-treatment/101378586/.

Beach, C. (2019). FDA's Throws new Enforcement Punch; U.S. Importer in the Corner. Food Safety News. Available from: https://www.foodsafetynews.com/2019/08/fdas-throws-new-enforcement-punch-u-s-importer-in-the-corner/.

Burke, M. (2017). Man Accused of Spraying Feces and Urine on Supermarket Salad Bar was Angry Over Money. *The New York Daily News*. Available from: https://www.nydailynews.com/news/crime/man-accused-spraying-feces-urine-supermarket-salad-bar-article-1.3722917.

Bush, L. (2014). Statement from foodborne illness victim Lauren Bush. PEW Charitable Trust. Available from: https://www.pewtrusts.org/en/research-and-analysis/speeches-and-testimony/2014/11/17/statement-from-foodborne-illness-victim-lauren-bush.

CDC. (2006). Multistate Outbreak of *E. coli* O157:H7 Infections Linked to Fresh Spinach (FINAL UPDATE). Available from: https://www.cdc.gov/ecoli/2006/spinach-10-2006.html.

Center for Food Safety v. Hamburg, 954 F.Supp.2d 965 (2013). Available from: https://h2o.law.harvard.edu/cases/4853.

Chrismer, K. (2010). 'How Many More? Consumer Reports. Available from: https://advocacy.consumerreports.org/wp-content/uploads/2010/07/Print-Ad-Rylee-Final1.pdf.

Corby, J. (2019). Comments made opening a panel discussion on Integrated Food Safety System. *Meeting of the International Association for Food Protection*, Louisville, KY.

Dean, L. (2015). FSMA Federalism. Produce Processing. Available from: https://produceprocessing.net/fsma-federalism/.

Dziadul, D. (2014). Statement From Foodborne Illness Victim Dana Dziadul [before the North Carolina Department of Agriculture and Consumer Services]. The PEW Charitable Trusts. Available from: https://www.pewtrusts.org/en/research-and-analysis/speeches-and-testimony/2014/11/20/statement-from-foodborne-illness-victim-dana-dziadul.

FDA. (2016). Report on Regional FSMA Import Safety Meetings. Constituent Update. Available from: https://www.fda.gov/food/cfsan-constituent-updates/report-regional-fsma-import-safety-meetings.

FDA. (2018a). FSMA Final Rule on Sanitary Transportation of Human and Animal Food. Available from: https://www.fda.gov/food/food-safety-modernization-act-fsma/fsma-final-rule-sanitary-transportation-human-and-animal-food.

FDA (2018b). FSMA Final Rule on Accredited Third-Party Certification. Available from: https://www.fda.gov/food/food-safety-modernization-act-fsma/fsma-final-rule-accredited-third-party-certification.

FDA. (2018c). FSMA Final Rule on Foreign Supplier Verification Programs (FSVP) for Importers of Food for Humans and Animals. Available from: https://www.fda.gov/food/food-safety-modernization-act-fsma/fsma-final-rule-foreign-supplier-verification-programs-fsvp-importers-food-humans-and-animals.

Flynn, D. (2017a). States need $100M more for Food Safety Modernization Act. Food Safety News. Available from: https://www.foodsafetynews.com/2017/04/states-need-100m-more-for-food-safety-modernization-act/.

Flynn, D. (2017b). Woman Draws Jail Sentence for Contaminating Chicken in 2016. *Food Safety News*. Available from: https://www.foodsafetynews.com/2017/12/woman-draws-jail-sentence-for-contaminating-chicken-in-2016/#.Wjp5-FQ-fVp.

Gillam, C. (2012). FDA seeks dismissal of lawsuit over delayed food safety rules. Reuters News. Available from: https://www.reuters.com/article/usa-food-lawsuit/fda-seeks-dismissal-of-lawsuit-over-delayed-food-safety-rules-idUSL1E8MUCSC20121203.

Gottlieb, S. (2017). Speech to the 2017 NASDA Annual Meeting. FDA. Available from: https://www.fda.gov/news-events/speeches-fda-officials/speech-2017-nasda-annual-meeting-09122017.

Gustafson, R. (2013). Food Safety Victim Testimony: Rylee Gustafson. The PEW Charitable Trusts. Available from: https://www.pewtrusts.org/en/research-and-analysis/speeches-and-testimony/2013/03/food-safety-victim-testimony-rylee-gustafson.

Hennessy, T., et al. (1996). A national outbreak of *Salmonella enteritidis* infections from ice cream. *NEJM, 334*, 1281–1286 Available from: https://www. nejm. org/doi/full/10. 1056/NEJM199605163342001.

Kingdon, J. (2011). *Agendas, alternatives, and public policies* (2nd ed.). Boston: Longman.

McGuier Woods. (2013). The War Over FSMA.. McGuier Woods. Available from: https://www.mcguirewoods.com/client-resources/Alerts/2013/7/The-War-Over-FSMA.

National Sustainable Agriculture Coalition. (2017). Increased State Funding for FSMA Produce Rule.. National Sustainable Agriculture Coalition. Available from: http://sustainableagriculture.net/blog/produce-rule-implementation/.
Tester, J. (2010). Senate Overwhelmingly Passes Food Safety Bill with Tester's Amendment. Press Release. Available from: https://www.tester.senate.gov/?p=press_release&id=1078.
The New York Times. (2015). Chasing Outbreaks: How Safe is Our Food?. Retro Report. The New York Times. Available from: http://www.nytimes.com/video/us/100000003676533/chasing-outbreaks-how-safe-is-our-food.html. Script, Available from: https://www.retroreport.org/transcript/chasing-outbreaks-how-safe-is-our-food/.
The War Over FSMA: After FDA Ignored Congressional Deadlines, Will Court Order Spur Action? (2013). McGuire Woods. Available from: https://www.mcguirewoods.com/client-resources/Alerts/2013/7/The-War-Over-FSMA.
LGMA. (2015). The WHY behind Food Safety. Video. Available from: https://www.youtube.com/watch?v=AE9G818uJsQ.
Milazzo, D. (2015). Report from Preventive Controls Team for FSMA Implementation. The FDA Food Safety Modernization Act: Focus on Implementation for Prevention-Oriented Food Safety Standards Public Meeting. Presentation for FDA, Washington, DC.
Obama, B. (2009). Weekly Address. The Obama White House. Available from: https://www.youtube.com/watch?v=WjX0iJU3vtY&feature=youtu.be.
O'Hagan, M. (2009). Food-safety lawyer's wish: Put me out of business. The Seattle Times. Available from: https://www.seattletimes.com/seattle-news/food-safety-lawyers-wish-put-me-out-of-business/.
Public Law 107-188—June 12. (2002). The Public Health Security and Bioterrorism Preparedness Response Act of 2002. Available from: https://www.govinfo.gov/content/pkg/PLAW-107publ188/pdf/PLAW-107publ188.pdf.
Rutledge, S. (2016). Spend a Moment with Rylee Gustafson. STOP Foodborne Illness. Available from: https://stopfoodborneillness.org/spend-a-moment-with-rylee_gustafson/.
Schnirring, L. (2013). FDA Finds Field Contamination Links in CANTALOUPES SALMONELLA PROBE. Center for Infectious Disease Research and Policy. Available from: http://www.cidrap.umn.edu/news-perspective/2013/03/fda-finds-field-contamination-links-cantaloupe-salmonella-probe.
US General Accounting Office. (1990). *Truck transport: little is known about hauling garbage and food in the same vehicles: RCED 90-161*. Report to Congressional Requesters, GAO. Available from: http://archive.gao.gov/d23t8/141739.pdf.
WHO. (2002). Terrorist threats to food guidance for establishing and strengthening prevention and response systems. Geneva: World Health Organization, Food Safety Department.
Zhang, J. (2007). FDA food inspections are seen as inadequate. *The Wall Street Journal*. Available from: https://www.wsj.com/articles/SB118463989137768585.
Zuraw, L. (2015). Reid Calls for Full FSMA Funding on Senate Floor. Food Safety News. Available from: https://www.foodsafetynews.com/2015/06/reid-calls-for-full-fsma-funding-on-senate-floor/.

CHAPTER 8

Implementing an integrated food safety system

"For a long time, the FDA would not act on any report from the state regarding problems in a food plant. Instead, the FDA would send its own inspectors in to document those problems before they would initiate an enforcement action."
Mike Taylor, Former FDA Deputy Commissioner of Food Comments made during FDA public meeting on implementation of FSMA, 2015

"... the states that aren't looking for pathogens don't find them."
Joseph Corby, Former Executive Director, Association of Food and Drug Officials (AFDO) Personal Interview, 2019

This chapter focuses not only on an integrated food safety system, but also on the FDA Food Code, the Conference for Food Protection (CFP) (the group that puts forward updates to the Food Code), and where states sit in terms of their ability to prevent and respond to outbreaks, as well as their adopted version of the FDA Food Code. Finally, this chapter presents a set of characteristics and suggested strategies for states to improve their inclusion in such an integrated system while striving to best protect consumers and reduce incidents of food safety failure. The characteristics of focus include states' capacity for regulating food safety, their food regulatory structures, ideal food policies, funding and resources for food safety programs, certifications and universal standards, food safety program collaboration and communication, and food safety program staffing and training.

Integrated food safety system

The FDA's Food Safety Modernization Act (FSMA) includes a strong dependency on state agencies in an "integrated food safety system." More specifically, the Act depends on a mutual reliance between state and federal

Food Safety
http://dx.doi.org/10.1016/B978-0-12-818219-2.00008-9

regulatory and investigatory agencies. While the investigation and reporting of foodborne illnesses by state and county health departments are critical in the prevention of foodborne disease in the United States, one of many concerns is that not all states and counties have the same capacity to carry out the level of food safety regulatory enforcement and inspection specified by the Act.

Prior to FSMA implementation, the FDA invested a considerable amount of work to support not only companies and farms in their developing and understanding of the rules and the various compliance needs, but also with the states. FDA leadership has long had a clear vision of how a healthy partnership between the FDA and the states could benefit food safety. Mike Taylor served as the FDA Deputy Commissioner of Food from the time of FSMA's passage through Congress in 2010 to its implementation in 2016. Prior to FSMA's implementation, Taylor described the relationship between the FDA and the states as such:

> *"In the produce area, the FDA has been doing contract inspections with the states for years and they are able to inspect on our behalf. They have authority to deal with food manufacturing, if they're doing inspections for us. So it's really the produce area [prior to FSMA] where we don't have the history of regulatory program. The FDA needs the states to be playing really even more comprehensive front-line role of being the primary interface with the growers and implementing the produce rule beginning with technical assistance and education and running food inspection compliant, in partnership with the FDA."*
>
> ***(Mike Taylor, Personal Interview, 2015)***

In sharing their vision of states working together with them, one key FDA message has always been the goal of maximizing the food safety benefit that comes from these combined efforts. The nature of America's food safety system is far too complex for a scenario where the FDA could simply be working with just one state (with a strong produce program in place) for facility inspections. "All the states and the federal government, working as a network, is where we would have true sharing of data, whether it's inspection data or analytical results, and the ability to collectively prioritize efforts, understand trends, and share inspection findings" (Mike Taylor, Personal Interview, 2015).

Barbara Cassens, Director of the FDA's Office of Partnership, shared in a 2019 conference panel how she sees standards for food and feed as a "foundation of integration" that helps drive consistency across the different state agencies. Similar to Taylor's view in 2015, Cassens describes this as a "quality management system"—an ideal scenario in which the FDA "can accept this state's work and the state can accept another state's work because we have a common framework that we're operating under" (Cassens, 2019).

While emphasizing the benefits of a National Food Safety Network, Taylor led the FDA's progression toward final FSMA rulemaking and implementation in a changing atmosphere, where the FDA expanded its understanding of states' roles. Further, the FDA embraced the states' needs for both uniformity and diversity, coexisting in federalism and in other contexts, that are inherent in a network like this. Taylor has even referred to uniformity as an ideal view of uniformity as "state empowerment" to be doing food safety work both on their own and in partnership with the FDA. But as FSMA implementation drew closer, the FDA did not lose sight of the states' diversity in terms of how they engage on food safety regulation. According to Taylor, these range from "... diversity of statutory authorities, diversity of institutional arrangement, and diversity of interest—how important is food safety, how important the food system is in a particular state" (Mike Taylor, Personal Interview, 2015).

While most states have a huge stake in the success of their agricultural systems, the FDA recognizes a range based on the level of activity and the level of states' political and resource commitment to food safety regulation. On one end of the spectrum, the FDA—even before implementation of FSMA—has had a strong working with California and Florida on produce safety, through the Leafy Greens Marketing Agreement (LGMA) in California and with state tomato regulations in Florida. In other states, such as Wyoming, the produce sector is vastly different, based in many cases, on geography and land use.

> *"In a state that is getting money from the federal government to do produce work or facility inspections on the FDA's behalf, we've got to have confidence that the states are doing that work at a level that is the same level of food safety ... it's still about protection. It's just that it may be that one of them does that through an agriculture department and one does it through a health department. One has their own statues or the other is through commission to work on our behalf. The goal is the same level of rigor and quality in terms of getting food safety protection."*
>
> ***(Mike Taylor, Personal Interview, 2015)***

So what does this mean in terms of how the FDA responds to the great diversity among the states? Ultimately, the FDA will need to tolerate the fact that there is not necessarily a "one-size-fits-all" state approach. "We have to be working towards a common outcome ....There may be different ways that they choose to play the role and we have to be receptive to that. At the end of the day, if they're going to be doing inspection activity and getting money for us to do it, they have to have adequate authority to do that" (Mike Taylor, Personal Interview, 2015).

The FDA has expressed concern about whether individual states have enough resources, technical staff, lab capacity, and institutional infrastructure to do the work related to the implementation of FSMA. One of the concerns is that resources and staff will have to be diverted from their intended uses, resulting in, for example, decreased restaurant or retail inspections.

> *"If we're going to have a kind of federal-state partnership and engagement of states, we need to look at what their authority is. I think for the FDA, the federal law of FSMA will be the dominant framework, but we have to ask: Do the states have the authority to do the things they need to do from an inspection standpoint? In terms of institutional capacity, do they have the resources? Do they have the technical staff? do they have the laboratory capacities?"*
>
> ***(Mike Taylor, Personal Interview, 2015)***

Another concern is that developing a truly integrated system will be tough because states often vary in the amount of time among a trigger event, the detection of an outbreak, the identification of the source, and the official end of the outbreak. A true integrated system is only as strong as its weakest member and, unfortunately, the states' capacity, in this concern, is nearly impossible to measure. Unfortunately, the states' capacity, in this concern, is nearly impossible to measure.

Beyond governments, one needs to consider the perspective of the industry. Jorge Hernandez is not only the Vice President of Quality Assurance at The Wendy's Company but also has long been a noted expert and industry advocate for food safety. To Jorge:

> *"An integrated food system that includes every actor in the food chain and all regulations and regulators is essential. Consequently, an integrated food safety partnership that communicates across the chain and defines the best practices in each segment, the role of each actor and ensures proper regulatory oversight is critical to any retailer/ restaurant chain who wants to assure 100% food safety, 100% of the time."*
>
> ***(Jorge Hernandez, Personal Communication, 2019)***

While many in the food industry are working hard to develop those partnerships within an integrated system, some, including Jorge, are of the opinion that this idea of a partnership is not complete "until it extends to the customers ..." as "they have a role to ensure the safety of the products they buy too" (Jorge Hernandez, Personal Communication, 2019). This "role" includes critical practices everyone should follow to prevent foodborne illness, such as washing hands, keeping hot foods hot/cold food cold, and not handling foods for others when sick.

Early efforts

Building a national integrated food safety system is not a new idea. The idea of integrating our food safety system has been around for a long time. In 1997, the Association of Food and Drug Officials (AFDO) presented the concept of integrating our food safety system to the FDA and to the USDA's FSIS, in the form of a white paper. The next year, the national food safety system group was formed, consisting of stakeholders (local state and federal agency officials) forming work groups and deciding what needs to be done to integrate our system.

Key questions about what needs to be done to integrate our system arose included those about information technology, protocols for inspections, certification of our laboratories, and how to better share information. A few years after that group was formed, funding was eliminated.

In 2008, a meeting brought together members from every state to talk about how they could improve the food safety system. During that meeting, once again, that idea of integrating our food safety system better coordinating our resources, utilizing resources, where they should be utilized was brought up. Further, at that 50-state meeting, similar to earlier meetings, training took front and center in terms of things that had to happen in order to be successful. One year later, a group called the "Partnership or Food Protection," designated as the group that will draw the blueprint, provided direction of how the food safety system would integrate.

Finally, with the passage of FSMA, not only did that offer challenges to how the FDA to did inspections, but it made it clear that the federal government needed to work with the states to complete those inspections. The Act also mandated that federal agencies had to better coordinate their efforts with stakeholders.

According to Joe Corby, the former Executive Director of the AFDO:

> *"It's not just the culture at federal agencies. It's the culture at state level, too. states have to integrate with the local [stakeholders] that they work with—as well as, of course, the federal stakeholders and non-profit organizations. The culture change taking place is not just to build the integrated food safety system, but to improve the lives of many people because we're able to do our jobs better."*
>
> ***(Joe Corby, Personal Communication, 2019)***

According to Barbara Cassens, Director of the FDA's Office of Partnership, the FDA has been investing a little over $100 million per year into the integration in state programs, local programs, and laboratory accreditation. Further, the FDA's focus on integration is not just getting to an integrated food safety system, but also determining how to measure it. To create this network, the FDA's Office of Partnership builds relationships and, as such, sees a goal of one workforce when it comes to food safety. "It's not a state versus a county versus the feds .... we share commonalities that we oversee for public health" (Cassens, 2019). This work should not be done independently, whereas working together can maximize and leverage many resources. Further, the FDA's work in developing these integrated systems provides industry with efficiency and consistency, including the reality of few duplicate inspections. This also allows the various states' food laboratories the ability to work across the fence with each other, to share resources and data, and to help each other out.

Whereas a safer food system relies on a dependency on that capacity of all state and local resources to do their job through an integrated partnership approach, many could assume that this could have prevented a significant outbreak, such as the 2008–09 *Salmonella* outbreak tied to the Peanut Corporation of America (as previously discussed). Stephen Ostroff, MD, served as acting commissioner of the US Food and Drug Administration from 2015 to 2016 and then as the FDA's Deputy Commissioner for Foods and Veterinary Medicine until December 2018. Dr. Ostroff warns about the limitations of even the best of integrated food safety partnerships.

> *"If there was better oversight of the Peanut Corporation of America, if inspectors went in there, if they had realized how bad the facility was, perhaps all of the problems would have been seen before the outbreaks actually started occurring. However, [PCA executives] were consciously ignoring information that said that they were putting contaminated stuff out in the market. I don't know that you can ever inspect away bad behavior or criminal behavior."*
>
> ***(Stephen Ostroff, Personal Communication, 2019)***

The states' ability to implement federal food policies

In its 2015 report, "All Over the Map: A 10-Year Review of State Outbreak Reporting," the Center for Science in the Public Interest (CSPI) ranked each state on their reporting of outbreaks between 2003 and 2012 and found that 66% earned a "D" or "F" rating. CSPI's 2015 report also identified the number of outbreaks reported to the CDC and solved within each state. Their alarming finding was that only seven states solved 50% or more of their reported, non-multistate outbreaks on their own.

The states considered to be leaders in food safety are those that have strong surveillance programs, can quickly get on top of food illnesses when they occur, and can usually find the source of an outbreak quickly. The FDA has identified the states of Washington, California, Florida, Minnesota, North Carolina, and Georgia as having the strongest food safety programs in the country.

A state with ideal capacity has adequate and appropriate equipment and resources, as well as funding to hire the appropriate technical staff. However, there have been nearly 2000 layoffs in labs and agencies across the country since 2008, which affect the number of restaurant inspectors, laboratory capacity, and surveillance systems available.

With the passing of FSMA, the FDA has expressed concerns over the inconsistencies among the states' regulations. The legislation appears to be Congress's way of acknowledging that there is a need for strengthening regulations across state infrastructure including tribal and territorial governments. However, concern within the FDA still exists over conflicts of interest with various different departments, where one department—such as agriculture—is focused on regulatory insight while another—such as the health department—puts priority focus on public safety.

Many food companies have shared their recent concerns over these new regulations in the context of the lack of guidance from state agencies. Companies with facilities in multiple states express a great deal of uncertainty as to how this will affect them, and when. Even companies with excellent track records for food safety are concerned, as they fear that they will be used as "test cases" for new inspectors and new inspection protocols.

This all leaves consumers highly dependent on their state's capacity. The solution is for each state to focus on building their agency capacity to handle the new responsibilities of inspection and enforcement related to FSMA. And this needs to be done quickly. In the meantime, the food industry is left to pick up the pace of FSMA implementation and, especially for firms with facilities in multiple states, the new political food landscape will include many challenges.

State's capacity for regulating food safety

In their 2015 report, CSPI also ranked states' performance based solely on their reporting of outbreaks, between 2003 and 2012, and adjusted the data for population (Smith DeWaal, Fischer, Glassman, Cororaton, & Martinez, 2015). In this study, CSPI followed up on their similarly titled 2011 study of outbreak data from 1998 to 2007 and removed multistate outbreaks as a variable that might impact the study of a state's capacity without the influence of reporting and investigation conducted by another state (Smith

Table 8.1 CSPI ranking of states (adjusted for population).

Ranking	Outbreaks (per million)	States (based on 1998–2007 outbreak data) (Smith DeWaal et al., 2011)	States (based on 2003–12 outbreak data) (Smith DeWaal et al., 2015)
A	8+	FL, HI, MD, MN, OR, WA, WY	HI, KS, MN, ND, OR, WY
B	6–7	CO, IL, KS, ME, MI, OH, VT	CO, OH, WA
C	4–5	AL, AK, CA, CT, IA, ND, NH, WI	AK, AZ, CA, CT, FL, IL, MD, WI
D	2–3	DE, D.C., GA, ID, MA, MT, NC, NJ, NY, PA, RI, SD, TN, UT, VA	ME, MI, OH, IA, NM, DE, GA, ID, MA, NY, PA, RI, TN, VA, SC
F	1	AZ, AR, IN, KY, LA, MS, MO, NE, NV, NM, OK, SC, TX, WV	AL, AR, IN, KY, LA, MS, MT, MO, NC, NE, NJ, NV, OK, SD, TX, UT, WV, and DC

DeWaal, Klein, Catella, Robets, & Tian, 2011). In both studies, Hawaii, Minnesota, Oregon, and Wyoming remained ranked at the top for reporting while other states rose or fell in the ranking (Table 8.1).

CSPI's 2015 report also identified the number of outbreaks reported to the CDC by each state and the number of outbreaks solved by the state agency, resulting in the ability to identify Alaska, Connecticut, Hawaii, Louisiana, Minnesota, South Carolina, and Washington as the only states to solve 50% or more of their reported, non multistate outbreaks on their own (Fig. 8.1).

One additional finding from CSPI's 2015 report is the number of neighboring states with large differences in outbreak-reporting rates: Maryland (four outbreaks per million) and West Virginia (one outbreak per million); Florida (five outbreaks per million) and Alabama (one outbreak per million); and Wyoming (eight outbreaks per million) and Nebraska (one outbreak per million). The CSPI's 2011 and 2015 analyses include the suggestions that differences in staffing, funding, and infrastructure as potential reasons for the disparity of reporting from the states. These data are not alone in connecting states' capacity to regulate food safety with numerous other factors.

60%–69%	50%–59%	40%–49%	30%–39%	20%–29%	10%–19%	0%–9%
		CA				
		CO	AR			
		FL	DC	MD		
		GA	NE	MA		
		ID	NH	MI	AL	
		IA	NJ	MO	AZ	
	AK	MS	OK	NV	IL	
	CT	NY	OR	NC	IN	
	LA	PA	TN	ND	KS	
	MN	SD	UT	OH	KY	DE
	SC	VA	VT	RI	NM	ME
HI	WA	WI	WY	WV	TX	MT

Figure 8.1 Percentages of foodborne outbreaks reported and solved within that state, 2003–12. *Source: Smith DeWaal et al., 2015.*

FDA food code adoption

The FDA Food Code is not a federally mandated regulation. Rather, it serves as a model guide that state, local, and tribal agencies can copy or amend to keep food retail and restaurant establishments safe from biological, chemical, or physical hazards. The FDA Food Code represents the FDA's best advice for a uniform system of regulation in order to protect public health and ensure the safety of food at retail and foodservice operations (Eisenbeiser, 2018). The first version of the Food Code was published in 1993, with later versions in 1995, 1997, 1999, 2001, 2005, 2009, 2013, and 2017. The vehicle through which changes are proposed is the CFP.

In a meeting sponsored jointly by FDA and the American Public Health Association, CFP first met in Denver in 1971. Representatives focused primarily on microbiological aspects of food safety. The group met again in Washington, DC, in 1984, focusing on both the microbiological and toxicological contributors to foodborne illness. CFP incorporated in 1985 and met for the third time in Ann Arbor, Michigan, in 1986, making the decision to focus on retail food safety, establishing a constitution and bylaws, agreeing to meet every other year, and receiving nonprofit status.

The current version of the CFP focuses primarily on identifying emerging problems related to retail food safety and seeking viable solutions through collaboration and consensus building among its members—

representing the food industry, government, academia, and consumer organizations. In his 2019 presentation at the International Association for Food Protection, David McSwane, PhD, CFP Executive Director, identified the goal of the biennial meetings:

> *"We find solutions that we think are acceptable to both the regulators and industry. Now that's not always a panacea. There may be some groups that will be more pleased with what we recommend than others, but at least we want to make sure that all of these groups are actively involved in the process so that hopefully they're going to be more attuned and receptive to the outcomes of that process."*
>
> ***(McSwane, 2019)***

Though the Conference has no formal regulatory authority, the overall body of council members works with the FDA, CDC, USDA, and the AFDO through memoranda of understanding to influence the FDA Food Code model laws and minimize disparate interpretations and implementation. Though all states can play a role in revising the FDA Food Code, not all have adopted the most recent versions in part or in whole.

In its 2018 report "Adoption of the FDA Food Code by State and Territorial Agencies Responsible for the Oversight of Restaurants and Retail Food Stores," the FDA's National Retail Food Team looked at all 50 states, plus the District of Columbia's Department of Health/Health, Regulation and Licensing, along with the territories. All told, the report recognizes 65 "State agencies" responsible for providing regulatory oversight of either restaurants, or retail food stores, or both. One important note is that 19 states regulate food safety through their state's Department of Agriculture, whereas 26 do this through their department of Public Health. Further, five states use some other agency (Table 8.4).

Some states delegate regulatory oversight to multiple agencies within that state, some even assigned to regulate different segments of the retail food industry. Most states (38) and Washington, DC, have one agency regulating both restaurants and retail. However, 13 states have multiple agencies, with 12 states using two agencies. These 13 states also have variations. Georgia, Maine, New York, Oregon, Tennessee, Utah, and Virginia all have two agencies, but one is responsible for restaurants, while the other is responsible for retail food stores. Connecticut, Mississippi, Ohio, and Vermont also have two agencies, but one is responsible for both restaurants and retail food stores and the other is responsible for retail food stores. Minnesota has two agencies, both responsible for both restaurants and retail food stores. Finally, one state (Florida) uses three agencies, with two agencies responsible

Table 8.2 List of FDA Food Code adoption by states—as of 2016.

Version adopted (as of February 2016)	Abbreviations of states that use them
1995 Food Code	SD
1997 Food Code	MN
1999 Food Code	AZ, LA, MA
2001 Food Code	CT, ID, IN, NJ, NY, VT
2005 Food Code	AL, AK, CA, GA, IL, KY, RI, VA, WV
2009 Food Code	AR, CO, FL, HI, IA, KS, MD, ME, MI, MO, NC, NE, NH, NV, ND, OH, OK, OR, TN, UT, WA, WI, WY
2013 Food Code	DE, MS, MT, NM, PA, SC, TX

Source: AFDO, 2016.

for both restaurants and retail food stores and a third agency responsible for restaurants.

In 2016, at the time of FSMA's implementation, states adopted versions of the FDA Food Code ranged from the 1995 to 2013 versions, with most states having the 2009 version as the most recent adopted (Table 8.2).

Many states, in the wake of FSMA's implementation, have started, if not completed the political processes of adopting new versions of the FDA Food Code. Though this is not the same as FSMA, the use of the FDA Food Code as a guidance and the adoption of new versions signal great strength in a state's willingness and regulatory alignment to support federal food policies. According to the FDA's National Retail Food Team (2018), the most recent adoption statistics for each state are as such (Table 8.3).

With such variations in adoption throughout the 3000 US regulatory jurisdictions, wide-ranging and inconsistent regulatory requirements provide significant challenges for multistate food retailers and restaurants that operate in numerous jurisdictions because they must comply with each iteration of the Food Code (Weeda, 2017). As a result, multistate retailers and restaurant chains must overcome inconsistent health inspection standards, inconsistent training requirements, and inconsistent jurisdictional authority. Each of these inconsistencies creates tremendous barriers for retailers and restaurants to protect public health to the best of their abilities. Ideally, by harmonizing one single version of the Food Code, consumers will not have to worry whether the zip code they are eating food in will place them at a higher risk of contracting foodborne illness.

Table 8.3 List of FDA Food Code adoption by states—as of 2018.

Version adopted (as of February 2016)	Abbreviations of states that use them
1995 Food Code	**SD**
1999 Food Code	**AZ**
2001 Food Code	**IN**, LA, **NY** (one of two agencies), **VT** (one of two agencies)
2005 Food Code	**AK, KY**, NJ, **WV**
2009 Food Code	**AR, MD, ME, MI, NC, NE, NH, NV, OR, TN, WI**, WY, and DC
2013 Food Code	AL, CO, CT, **DE**, FL (one of three agencies), GA, HI, ID, IA, MA, MN, MO, **MT**, ND, OH, OK, RI, **SC, TX**, UT, VA
2017 Food Code	IL, MS, NM, PA *(KS and WA started 2017 Food Code adoption in 2018 and are still in progress)*

Note: **Bold**, did not change since 2016.
Source: National Retail Food Team, 2018.

Ideal state characteristics for an integrated food safety system

A focus on six key characteristics of states' capacity (for regulating food safety as well as preventing and responding to foodborne illness incidents) includes (1) states' food regulatory structures, (2) ideal food policies, (3) funding and resources for food safety programs, (4) certifications and universal standards, (5) food safety program collaboration and communication, and (6) food safety program staffing and training.

States' capacity for regulating food safety

State policymakers should focus on strengthening county and state capacity beyond simply regulating FDA FSMA rules compliance so as to include outbreak prevention, detection, and response, as well as for more efficient collaboration with other county, state, and federal agencies.

A state that has the ideal capacity to not only perform its duties, but to be able to pivot and respond to crises as they arise is characterized as one that can detect, report, and solve outbreaks within its borders, has adequate and appropriate resources as well as sufficient quantities of technical staff to use these resources, food laboratory capability, appropriate institutional infrastructure, and adequate funding for FSMA implementation at capacity and beyond.

State and local food regulatory capacity for outbreak prevention, detection, and response, as well as for regulatory inspections for FSMA compliance is tied to a variety of characteristics: state regulatory infrastructure, food regulatory policies, funding and resources, certification and universal standards, collaboration and communication, as well as staffing and training.

According to Mike Taylor, former FDA Deputy Commissioner of Food "... it is all about resources when it comes to capacity—basically staffing, training, and how you have those basic ingredients" (Mike Taylor, Personal Communication, 2016). Capacity is characterized as a complex characteristic, perhaps one that combines many characteristics to assess the agency's ability to not only perform its duties, but also to be able to pivot and respond to crises as they arise. A state agency's capacity to implement the FSMA is also tied to funding, with the concern for resources and staff being diverted from how they are intended to be used.

In his 2018 article "Unfinished Business: Keeping the Focus on Food Safety," Mike Taylor expressed his concern that leaders in Washington have "lost their focus on food safety" (Taylor, 2018). As evidence of this, Taylor points to the lack of follow through to fully fund implementation of FSMA. President Trump's 2019 budget request for the FDA was essentially flat for food safety, translating to a decrease in actual purchasing power due to rising costs for delivering services.

> *"... success requires continued investment to build the capacity of states to provide the education and technical support to farmers, coupled with the high-quality inspection and enforcement, needed to prevent illness outbreaks in this crucial sector of our food system."*
>
> ***(Taylor, 2018)***

Stronger states, ones that are considered to be leaders in food safety, are those that are seen as having better surveillance programs, they are able to get on top of food illnesses when they occur the fastest, and they are usually the ones that also find the source the quickest. Essentially, Joe Corby, former Executive Director of the AFDO, explains that "... the states that aren't looking [for pathogens] don't find them" (Joe Corby, Personal Communication, 2016).

According to Robin Stombler, President of Auburn Health Strategies, LLC, "If we are going to build and maintain proper lab capacity—we need equipment and resources funding, not to mention funding to hire the appropriate people." When looking at time lags between a trigger event, detection of outbreak, identification of source, and the official "end" of the outbreak, some suggest that one way that a state's capacity has been assessed is by asking: "Why did this take a week or ten days? Was this the only guy doing this? Was he on vacation and all work stopped during that period?" Ultimately, capacity is one of the key differences between states' agencies. (Robin Stombler, Personal Communication, 2019)

Another view of capacity can be seen in the essential role of trained and qualified staff. The right people play critical roles in driving a state's response and success rates with solving outbreaks. Industry experts still talk about how much capacity was lost when Dr. William Keene, Oregon State's senior epidemiologist, died in 2013. His legacy is found not only in the International Outbreak Museum he started in Portland, Oregon, but also in how his peers revered him.

"Bill was one of the best, and an extraordinarily able voice for public health," said Robert Tauxe, MD, MPH, Director of the Division of Foodborne, Waterborne and Environmental Diseases at the CDC (Weise, 2013). In a statement made for his publication *Food Safety News*, Seattle lawyer Bill Marler noted how the two states that almost always solve their foodborne illness outbreaks are Minnesota and Oregon. He then went on to describe that "Minnesota has Team Diarrhea. Oregon just had Bill, and that was enough" (Flynn, 2013).

Capacity can also be defined by the nature of the state and local food testing laboratories used for investigation. Robin Stombler is the Director of the Food Laboratory Alliance. She asserts that laboratory testing is a "foundational element of food safety validation and verification" and that the "accuracy and quality of those test results is essential" (Robin Stombler, Personal Communication, 2019). Robin holds that we have much to achieve in order to support these labs and their critical role in food safety.

> *"At the present time, we do not know how many or where food laboratories exist in the United States. If we cannot answer this basic question, it is difficult to determine if all food testing laboratories follow recognized standards, methods and practices. Accountability is needed through accreditation and the use of quality controls, proficiency testing and appropriately trained personnel."*
>
> ***(Robin Stombler, Personal Communication, 2019)***

State food testing laboratories importantly monitor, detect, and investigate foodborne disease outbreaks throughout the country. Adequate, dedicated funding is needed to ensure that state public health laboratories are accredited and continue to perform this critical testing. Some states' contracted, private labs can be slower than others, more difficult to communicate with, and more detached from the area of the problem. As a result, having a lab that is owned by the state is important. To build a food safety partnership, laboratories—public and private—must be included. Effective communication networks that include laboratories will help support the health of the public.

> *"It is now eight years after the FSMA was signed, and one important section of the law remains outstanding. Section 202 would recognize food testing laboratory accreditation, develop model standards by which those laboratories must operate, and account for these laboratories through a publicly available registry. As of this writing, this section has not been promulgated."*
>
> ***(Robin Stombler, Personal Communication, 2019)***

Capacity is also clearly tied to funding. According to Joseph Corby, former Executive Director of the AFDO, "Some states are more able to spot and identify [sources of foodborne pathogen outbreaks] because they have put more state money into it. They haven't been as severe with staffing cuts" (Joseph Corby, Personal Communication, 2016). Corby points to how AFDO has followed the staff reductions that have occurred throughout the 2700 state and local health districts across the country. "... there's something like 2000 layoffs that occurred ... since [2008]—a lot of those are the restaurant inspectors and the laboratory capacity and all the other parts of just having a good surveillance system" (Joseph Corby, Personal Communication, 2016). Corby also described staff needed for capacity as a "pretty easy area for states to cut," as policymakers at the city, county, and district health organizations are the ones whose decisions form that capacity. Some states tend to make staffing capacity a better area of funding priority than others.

State- and county-level regulators interviewed defined capacity as a growing concern under the Act. One participant described his job as being impacted by "real time, complaint increased pressure and accountability ... we expect accountability as a nation." The reality, however, is that all interview participants at the state level expressed capacity as being a purely ideal or theoretical concept. "At capacity, we want to hire more staff. We cannot do that because the need was not anticipated." If new needs or concerns arise, local agencies cannot simply request for an increase in staffing. Any budget requests for increasing capacity. Annual budgets are fixed and "based 100% on last year ...." We "cannot grow." One possible result, as predicted by one participant from the state level, is that "inspections at retail food establishments will suffer." This comment echoes that of one federal-level participant who worried about resources and staff not being supplied adequately.

The CDC reports that, as new money recently became available to support better surveillance for antimicrobial resistance, they started building the data infrastructure in the states and expanding the state laboratory and epidemiologic capacity. They now have trained and certified staff in all states partnering closely with the FDA genome tracker labs, the FSIS labs, and NIH (Tauxe, 2019).

Ultimately, state policymakers need to evaluate other states' food regulatory programs, those with highly rated capacities, and consider a variety of measures to assess their state's current capacity and anticipated growth under FSMA. New policy should not be driven solely by industry or agency economic burdens, but also by the true burden of disease experienced by the very constituents elected officials represent.

Characteristics of states with ideal food regulatory structures

A state that has an ideal regulatory structure for food inspection and outbreak response is one that does not place all regulatory and inspection authority in a state agency that also carries the conflict of interest of promoting the food industry. During a 2015 FDA public meeting on implementation of FSMA, Mike Taylor, then, the FDA's Deputy Commissioner of Food, stated that, in passing FSMA, "Congress was acknowledging the need ... for strengthening state infrastructure around these areas" (Mike Taylor, Personal Communication, 2015).

According to data collected by the Institute of Medicine, 26 states use a State Department of Public Health while 19 other states use a State Department of Agriculture. At the same time, some divide the authority and responsibilities between two agencies. Finally, some states use other forms of regulatory agencies, such as Department of Consumer Protection, Department of Environmental Conservation, and Department of Inspections and Appeals. This report included an analysis which asserted that the use of one regulatory agency over another can impact not only the resources available, but also the priorities and goals of states' programs (Wallace & Oria, 2010) (see Table 8.4 for a list of states and their food regulatory agencies).

The FDA, and thus the American consumer, must have confidence that all states are doing food safety work at the same—highest level of protection. One must look at the missions or priorities of a state's agriculture department and compare them to that of a states' health department. According to the FDA: "Congress enacted FSMA in response to dramatic changes in the global food system and in our understanding of foodborne illness and its consequences, including the realization that preventable foodborne illness is both a significant public health problem and a threat to the economic well-being of the food system" (FSMA, 2019). Thus, the FDA would theo-

Table 8.4 List of food regulatory agency types and the states that use them.

Type	Abbreviations of states that use them
Department of Agriculture (19)	AL, FL, GA, ME, MI, MN, NE, NY, NC, OH, OR, PA, SC, TN, UT, VA, WA, WI, WY
Department of Public Health (26)	AZ, AR, CA, CO, DE, HI, IL, IN, KS, KY, LA, MD, MA, MS, MO, MT, NV, NH, NJ, NM, ND, OK, RI, TX, VT, WV
Split between Health and Agriculture	ID
Split between Commerce and Agriculture	SD
Department of Environmental Conservation	AK
Department of Consumer Protection	CT
Department of Inspections and Appeals	IA

Source: Wallace & Oria, 2010.

retically prefer the scenario of a state's food program aligned under public health—as opposed to under state agriculture.

Great differences already exist between the states in terms of the quantity and characteristics of challenges their food regulatory agencies face, as well as their performance, such as ranking and percentage of in-state outbreaks solved. Variations in the priorities and policies of different agencies (such as that of agriculture vs. public health) may play a significant role in the overall effectiveness of an integrated food safety system.

With different types of state agencies involved in one way or another—state health departments, state agriculture departments, or some other state agency—each one of them can be doing something entirely different in terms of resourcing their public health agencies. They may choose to regulate through a board or through a department that is primarily assigned to promote safe products, such as an Agriculture Department. They may choose to regulate through their public health activities, such as in public health departments.

For states making the transition to a single food regulation agency, such as Michigan did a few years ago, communications can become easier, but they may have challenges when it comes to large-scale investigation of a plant as this may cause a resource issue. Single agencies can worsen the load on inspectors, epidemiologists, and on labs.

State policymakers need to consider similar arguments made at the federal level to create an independent food inspection agency, one that has as protecting consumers as its sole mission. Keeping budget issues in check while maximizing staff support and training would benefit from one agency with this one mission. Further, with the variety of types of inspections, the different types of commodity expertise needed, and the types of farm, food production, retail, restaurant, school, institution, and other facilities to inspect, this strategy could best support the state's efficient, effective, and sustainable implementation of FSMA regulation.

Characteristics of states with ideal food policies

States must adopt legislation that aligns with FSMA rules or agree to allow the FDA to control the regulation of the food industry within that state through contracted agents. A state that allows the federal government to take over local control of policy will weaken their relationship with farmers, local business owners, and large businesses with facilities in their state. Industries in states that turn over regulatory control to the FDA will encounter challenges to federalism and their power to regulate at the local level. Adopting legislation quickly will help bring needed funds to the agencies that are trying to redesign or start new programs and put resources and staff into place for implementation.

To avoid complications from lack of funding and resources needed to implement the Act, states should adopt legislation that aligns with FSMA rules. They should also do so with great speed, so as not to weaken the safety of produce and food products from their state, but also to support the economy of their farms and food industry. Further, states may decide to increase the level of strictness with exemptions as a measure to better support small farms and businesses that might otherwise elude inspection under current FDA exemption definitions. These states will also lose the ability to manage the funds related to regulating the food under FSMA rules.

A 2000 report from the US Department of Health and Human Services' Inspector General highlighted the agency's concern over states' food regulatory agency standards, programs, and practices, whereas they are not all equivalent (Brown, 2000). The US Government Account Office (GAO) has criticized the FDA for their "underutilized" interagency agreements and memorandums of understanding (MOU) with states (GAO, 2004, 2005). These reports, along with the concerns expressed by former FDA Deputy Commissioner of Food Michael Taylor, in his recommendations for strengthening state and local roles make clear the need for improvement with food policy enforcement across the nation (Taylor & David, 2009).

In a study that explored the differences between the established food safety regulatory systems in the United States, Canada, and in the United Kingdom (Martinez, Fearne, Caswell, & Henson, 2007), the authors recommended that government agencies need to take a more prescriptive and proactive in their regulation of the food industry. The authors also acknowledged potential barriers to change in regulatory structure, concluding that state disparities exist and, based on their study of EU and Canadian systems, could be resolved. Some reports indicate that policy variations could stem from differences in the states themselves.

Significant differences can be seen between the states when it comes to the full scope of the food industry from farm to table. A recent CDC analysis of infectious diseases, specifically *Escherichia coli*, highlights the geographic distribution of outbreaks. The CDC classified more than one in six foodborne outbreaks reported between 2003 and 2012 as multistate and having affected more people than single state outbreaks. CDC data also revealed a median rate of outbreaks in northern states being more than twice that of southern states. Of particular note in this CDC analysis is its data pertaining to foodborne illness related to a variety of settings that fall outside federal regulation and depend of a wide range of state and even smaller government resources (Heiman, Mody, Johnson, Griffin, & Gould, 2015). State-level outbreak characteristics need to be looked at in a different light than the reporting of outbreaks.

This same study revealed some patterns but great differences from state to state in terms of the number of reported incidents (per 100,000 people), and breaking down the illnesses by mode of transfer (foodborne, waterborne, person-to-person, and animal contact) researchers noted significant variation in regions and by state (Heiman et al., 2015). Another notable observation from the study pertains to person-to-person infections of *E. coli*. Specifically, the authors noted that the vast majority of cases reported came from daycare or similar facilities. However, the authors noted that a problem with their findings lies in the fact that not all states report such illnesses from daycare or school settings. Another, more significant problem exists with differences in states' food regulatory policies that might affect how or when FSMA is implemented in each state.

For states that have a big stake in respect to their produce sectors, for example, taking ownership of the regulation carries political and economic importance, both of which should carry a great deal of motivation. As states are assessing their regulatory foundations, their law, their regulations, to see if they need to go through their legislative process, adopt the produce safety rule, it is not enough for them to just adopt the rule, they have to see if they have authority to go onto farm and do surveillance work. They also need to have authority to collect samples. As a result, some states will take longer than others to move forward with FSMA adoption and implementation.

In theory, though based on descriptions from FDA leadership at public meetings on FSMA implementation, states will choose to progress with FSMA adoption in one of three ways:

1. A small number of states will automatically adopt federal regulations as written.
2. Most states will adopt FSMA through their legislative process, and they may actually amend and change and modify. A state may even make their legislation more stringent than the federal regulation. Sometimes, they will just take certain provisions out that they just do not want to adopt. Ultimately, however, the federal regulation overrides the state regulation.
3. Other states may never adopt federal regulations. The FDA will contract with state regulators who will be inspecting under the FDA's authority.

Reflecting on the multiple outbreaks tied to romaine lettuce in 2018, taking place near or after the 2-year anniversary of FSMA's implementation, one cannot overlook the fact that several FSMA rules should have aligned to increase the safety of leafy greens, and, thus, preventing the incidents. Applicable FSMA rules include Rule #1—Preventive Controls for Human Food, Rule #3—The Produce Safety Rule, and Rule #6—Sanitary Transportation of Human and Animal Food. In his November 1, 2018, press statement on the romaine lettuce outbreaks, (then) FDA Commissioner Scott Gottlieb, MD, stated:

> *"Fully implementing the Food Safety Modernization Act (FSMA) is critical to these efforts. We must continue to advance FSMA's Produce Safety Rule in collaboration with our state regulatory partners and ensure that we craft agricultural water standards that work across the incredible diversity of commodities and growing conditions."*
>
> ***(Gottlieb, 2018)***

State policymakers need to avoid turning over regulatory control to the FDA. State policymakers also need to avoid picking and choosing which parts of the rules to adopt as this will result in two negative consequences. First, picking and choosing random elements of the Act to adopt will increase the length of time for policymakers to complete the process. FDA estimates that this direction could take as long as 7 years for a state to complete. Second, this will ultimately weaken any definition of a set of universal standards and of an integrated food safety system. The foods we eat do not come solely from within the state in which we live. Weakening the safety of food will have an impact on the lives of consumers in other states.

State policymakers should adopt legislation that essentially adopts FSMA rules by reference. This strategy is not without precedence. Some states adopted the FDA Food Code by reference and are among those states that, according to the study, work with the most current version of the FDA Food Code. During the 2016 Biennial meeting of the CFP, a state regulator, supported by some of these states, proposed an amendment to the FDA Food Code that labels adoption of the codes by reference as a "best practice." This strategy would be efficient and would allow for timely implementation at the state level.

Characteristics of states with ideal funding and resources for food safety programs

A state should have the needed funding and resources to conduct food programs for public education, industry education, illness prevention, outbreak detection, and outbreak response at the regulatory and investigatory agencies and laboratories. Like public education and public health, these programs should not be limited by budget constraints and decision-making processes that are distant and untimely.

Great differences exist between the stated in terms of the amount spent (adjusted for population) per foodborne illness event and in the ways in which states fund their programs. State budget cuts hurt staffing and training, thus impacting the capacity and effectiveness of state and local regulators. Other concerns for funding include roadblocks to county agency access to funding, as well as a state's public health program funds being redirected by their governor to unrelated needs or being denied due to a funding formula that does not take into consideration unanticipated emergency needs—often the case with large outbreaks.

Not all states fund food safety regulation, prevention, and response similarly. The AFDO conducted a survey of state health agencies in 2008 in which they collected data on several items, including sources of funding for food safety programs. The study found, from responding states, that two states, Kansas and Ohio, use fees to fund 100% of their food safety programs, while four other states use fees to fund 80% or more of their programs. In all, 28 states use fees as one if not the only means of funding food safety programs. The study also found that Iowa, Maine, Pennsylvania, and Wyoming use general fund appropriations to fund 100% of their food safety programs (with Rhode Island using it to fund 99.9%). Three other states use general fund appropriations to fund 80% or more of their programs. Well more than half—38 states use general fund appropriations as one if not the only means of funding food safety programs. Eight states apply for and use federal grants as one of means of funding food safety programs, while 23 states use direct federal dollars as one source of funding their programs (AFDO, 2009).

Another difference between the states can be found in how much each state spends in the investigation and aftermath of an event. In a 2015 study, researchers analyzed foodborne illness incidents per 10,000 residents, with a focus on the estimated annual expenditures of each state for total illness incidence, cost per resident, and cost per case for a long list of bacterial, parasitic, viral, and even unknown foodborne pathogens. The study uncovered a large range of incident costs between states from as low as $537 per 10,000 residents in West Virginia to a high of $5,134 per 10,000 residents in Maryland (Scharff, 2015).

At a meeting with a state's regional environmental health association members, a discussion of funding allowed county-level inspectors an opportunity to offer specific recommendations regarding the use of federal food safety funds.

1. Some of the federal dollars should be to help state inspectors become well rounded and cross-trained.
2. Increase local access to and control of funds.
3. Change budget structure. The local levels could be funded more by doing what some agencies do: charge a fee for service.
4. Help county offices apply for grants from the federal government.
5. Allow inspectors to increase efficient use of funds, such as double-dipping with two inspection sites or types in one trip.
6. Allow anticipated costs. At capacity, local agencies want to hire more staff. Budgets and funding are most often based on data the previous year.

State policymakers need to consider the overall impact of increased investments in county agencies. Further, they need to reevaluate the processes through which county agencies request budgets and additional funding for capacity growth. Policies can include steps for empowering county agency leadership, such as training or other support for federal grant writing, thus local control of funding for some programs.

Characteristics of states with ideal certifications and universal standards

States with highly certified inspectors and laboratories are highly regarded by the FDA and NGOs for their efficiency, their novel approaches to food programs, and their track record with in-state and multistate outbreaks. These states invest in training and even create their own training programs. Ideally, all states would share the same high level of certifications for state food laboratories. This scenario would allow the CDC to accept and believe in valid data without the need to retest or decline to use the data.

Ultimately, a truly integrated food safety system demands that all states are performing at an acceptable standard. Consumer advocacy groups have expressed concern about the lack of uniform standards, even for states' food labs, as they will all have to be accredited to best participate in an integrated food safety system. While most states' labs are working toward accreditation, this will require funding and may take several years. The FDA has been audited by GAO, resulting in criticism that the FDA has not been showing competency of state labs but giving them money for contracts anyway. In addressing this criticism, prior to FSMA implementation, Mike Taylor stated that "there has to be criteria and standards that ensure that we are putting money into a state that is doing a good job with the same level of protection from state to state" (Mike Taylor, Personal Communication, 2015).

Significant holes exist in state and county agencies staffing, due to the loss or lack of retention of highly qualified staff and, thus, the loss of a significant level of expertise in complex, commodity-specific policies. The lack of adequate funding for professional development has resulted in deficiencies at the state and county levels. Some states higher employees with only a bachelor's degree level of education while others can attract and retain those with doctorates. The lack of universal standards would undermine the intent of an integrated food safety system and create weak areas in industry.

State policymakers can attach funding mandates to policies that provide for and require minimum levels of qualification for inspectors and laboratories. Further, this level of minimum certification needs to include standards and certification standards that go beyond that needed for implementation of FSMA. Many other standards, such as ISO, GFSI, HACCP, and Food Safety System Certification 22000 (FSSC 22000) will help inspectors and auditors maneuver through commodity-specific and complex industry policies. Further, state policymakers need to adopt FSMA in its entirety, not select elements, into state legislation. Any policies that are less restrictive than federal policy would, again, weaken the safety of the nation's food supply.

Characteristics of states with ideal food safety program collaboration and communication

A state that has ideal collaboration and communication with other agencies is one that shares data, is trusted by other state and federal agencies, and pools resources and expertise if needed. These states have minimal confusion between multiple state agencies that share outbreak or inspection responsibilities. County agencies should not bypass consulting with their own state agencies because they will find better support from counties in other states. However, many county inspectors characterize collaboration and communication as needing "hands-on support from the state level, like the state agencies are doing with the federal level" (from feedback at a regional training event, 2019). According to some county-level inspectors who participated in investigating a multistate outbreak (but wish to remain anonymous):

> *"The state helped us, but our state is more of a coach than a team player. They more often sat on the sidelines than provide technical information when we need it. And that's a shame in a way. Other health departments in neighboring communities helped us more. In fact, we got more information from the CDC than from the state department of health."*
>
> ***(Anonymous state-level inspector, 2019)***

Inadequate collaboration or communication has been observed from time to time between multiple agencies, between states, and between state and federal regulators. Food safety experts and even the FDA have tied gaps in outbreak investigations to deficiencies in collaboration and communication. As the frequency of outbreaks has increased, along with the quantity and size of multistate outbreaks, state- and local-level inspectors and regulatory staff rely on outside resources and support when they are at capacity.

In addition to the FDA providing IT support for FSMA implementation and documentation, state policymakers should direct state agencies to collaborate with the FDA on ways to better communicate between county and state agencies during implementation. States and NGOs can work with academia to conduct studies of communication and collaboration patterns to identify and resolve problem areas.

Characteristics of states with ideal food safety program staffing and training

According to Steve Moris, Program Manager for the Kansas Department of Agriculture, "The states perform over 65% of the inspections in the U.S. at food processors, and almost all of the produce inspections that are starting now. And that requires a lot of training … that requires a lot of time on the state's part, sending their inspectors and their managers to train" (Moris, 2019).

Early on, the Partnership for Food Protection's training and certification work group established a goal of creating national curriculum standards as a way to have a defensible, valid way to measure that the workforce (state, local, federal, tribal, etc.) meet certain standards. According to Gerald Wojtala, Executive Director of the International Food Protection Training Institute (IFPTI), "We need to have assurance that we can count on each other and have this mutual reliance that we have to have some assurance that, foundationally, the workers are trained in the same way" (Wojtala, 2019).

A state with adequate staffing for food safety programs is one that can easily expand its capacity as needed and can anticipate areas of growth with changes in industry, detection science, and even population. A state staffing and training support for regulators, laboratory, and investigatory staff is one that not only demands a high level of certification, but also provides funding and programs, such as partnerships for professional development of staff. The quality of inspections and outbreak response should not be a characteristic that varies from state to state, therefore, neither should the certification and training level of staff.

Whereas great differences from state to state in their ability to solve in-state outbreaks that they reported to the CDC, timelines for investigation completion are often impacted by the lack of staff or their inadequate expertise. Hiring freezes and staff budgets are being cut at a time when more outbreaks are being found on a regular basis. As a result, staffing and resources are top concern for FSMA funding.

Robin Stombler adds that building and maintaining strong state labs and inspection programs is critical and demands adequate funding for hiring the appropriate people and for training them.

> *"At the Federal level, you see inspectors who are usually well-trained and sometimes they are very accomplished in their field—they'll have masters' degrees and they will have been on the job for some time, but at state level you might not see that. At the state and county levels, you might see people with a high school education, who got into this as a job that they applied for and got—not as a job where they can see themselves in a career field or they are seeing themselves as having wanted to be in public health or public safety type roles and then the state may not fund adequate training, and that means that the scope of their inspections is going to suffer, thus hindering the possibility that they will catch things."*
>
> ***(Robin Strombler, Personal Communication, 2016)***

While the produce safety alliance and other alliances have training programs, more is needed from state and federal levels. Many experts call for more regulator training, particularly on produce safety. As the states do not have a high level of expertise in regulating farms for food safety, this will require comprehensive training. That specific need aside, training cannot be a one-size-fit-all scenario for the states, as too many differences exist among the states on farming scale, harvesting period, water (surface well water drought irrigation) soil fertilize, as well as with different commodities.

State and county participants expressed similar concerns over staffing issues. They suggest that the changes brought about by FSMA have triggered new obstacles related to staffing and training. "Obstacles for this may be people's familiarity. Are they uncomfortable to change or prone to change, how will this impact available resources?" They want states to start investing more time and funds into training. However, these new responsibilities will "challenge administrative needs, cultural issues, training, availability of resources, and this is all at a time when there is a hiring freeze within state government." And, as one state-level participant pointed out, "agriculture has an older workforce than public health."

Similar to communication, state and county regulators see training as creating significant challenge. Ideally, local-level agents need a successful, engaging, ongoing, training to provide consistent, timely messaging across the state for new regulations and foodborne illness surveillance. Marcia Lee served as a Senior Food and Drug Inspector for the Massachusetts Department of Public Health. She offered blunt advice to deal with this obstacle:

> *"Don't impose a rule then expect local departments to train afterword. Training at the local level is very difficult. Training can require a health department to close so agents to participate—doing this for several days in a row is not feasible for many departments. We cannot bring 45-50 people into a classroom one or two days a year and give them everything they need to know."*
>
> **(Marcia Lee, Personal Communication, 2019)**

Marcia offered a look at how this impacts the Commonwealth of Massachusetts, with 351 towns and cities that operate autonomously from the state's Department of Public Health.

> *"One or two FDA Standardizing Officers per state is insufficient to properly standardized heath agents in Massachusetts. The problem with trickle down standardization where the FDA standardizing Officer train some agents and then they are expected to train others is that it is largely ineffective—like playing telephone, inter-*

CHAPTER 9
Predicting the future of food safety

"Pick any day of the week and you will find stories of
train derailments, plane crashes,
funds used inappropriately at a nonprofit organization,
explosions in a manufacturing facility,
workers shot or injured on the job,
or E. coli-*tainted beef, turkey, chicken, or even bean sprouts."*
William T. Coombs, Author—
"Information and Compassion in Crisis Response"
in* Journal of Public Relations Research, *1999

"... the tools we use really do define what we can see."
CDC's Robert Tauxe, MD, MPH,
***in his* Silliker Lecture at the**
International Association for
Food Protection Meeting, *2019*

From "poke and sniff" to artificial intelligence (AI)

After Upton Sinclair's novel *The Jungle* triggered consumers' criticism and the government's investigation into meat industry practices, the 1906 Federal Meat Inspection Act brought USDA inspectors into the slaughter houses with the authority to physically monitor all carcasses and cuts of meat as they moved down the slaughter line by literally touching, smelling, and prodding the meat to test its wholesomeness, a practice of organoleptic inspection referred to as "poke and sniff."

While the "poke and sniff" system of inspection was intended to prevent rotten, damaged, or otherwise deleterious meat from being sold and consumed, its very nature prevented it from detecting invisible pathogens such as *E. coli*. Worse, this method was actually responsible for transmitting pathogens from infected meat to clean meat, thus making consumers less safe.

Generations of consumers were raised to base their faith in the safety for USDA inspected meat in "poke-and-sniff" inspections from 1906 until the 1990s. After the landmark 1993 *E. coli* outbreak tied to contaminated beef, the USDA's Pathogen Reduction; hazard analysis and critical control point

Food Safety
http://dx.doi.org/10.1016/B978-0-12-818219-2.00009-0

systems (9 CFR Parts 304, 308, 310, 320, 327, 381, 416, and 417) included a shift to a science-based inspection system.

> *"The Food Safety and Inspection Service (FSIS) is establishing requirements applicable to meat and poultry establishments designed to reduce the occurrence and numbers of pathogenic microorganisms on meat and poultry products, reduce the incidence of foodborne illness associated with the consumption of those products and provide a new framework for modernization of the current system of meat and poultry inspection."*
>
> ***(Pathogen Reduction, 1996).***

Robert Tauxe, MD, MPH, is the CDC's Director, Division of Foodborne, Waterborne, and Environmental Diseases. During his 2019 John H. Silliker Lecture at the annual meeting of the International Association for Food Protection (IAFP), Tauxe shared how, during the 1970s, 1980s, and 1990s, the CDC detected or received reports of an average of two to four multistate outbreaks per year. In total, 3 years after the landmark 1993 *E. coli* O157 outbreak, along with many other changes taking place in our food safety system, the CDC began its national laboratory network "PulseNet" connecting foodborne illness cases to detect outbreaks. As PulseNet expanded to include other pathogens beyond *E. coli*, the number of identified multistate outbreaks increase to 25 or 30 a year (Tauxe, 2019). The CDC hails Pulsed-field gel electrophoresis (PFGE)—a laboratory technique used to produce a DNA fingerprint for a bacterial isolate, such as *E. coli* or *Salmonella*—as the current "gold standard" fingerprinting method.

> *"... the tools we use really do define what we can see. So with PulseNet using [PFGE], the subtype* E. coli *O157 first and then others, in a network of state health departments, we began looking for clusters we couldn't see before. We later expanded them to* Listeria *Monocytogenes,* Salmonella *and all the other STEC. And the central premise of this was that if we saw a cluster of strains that were very similar, indistinguishable by the PFGE method, they might very likely share a source."*
>
> ***(Tauxe, 2019).***

Tanya Roberts, Ph.D., author of *Food safety economics: Incentives for a safer food supply* (2018) is a retired Senior Economist with over 30 years of experience at the USDA's Economic Research Service. Her published economic research is some of the most respected in the industry. Roberts points to some facts about her career that highlight just how much pathogen monitoring has changed over the past 45 years. When she started working during the Carter administration, she started investigating data from the McDonald's outbreak in 1982. Until that time, *E. coli* O157:H7 was not even identified as a human illness pathogen tied to consumption of food.

"I talked to some microbiologists a little older than me and they said that they only learned about five foodborne pathogens in college. Today, there are some 250 pathogens that the CDC is monitoring. It's just that for 80% of illnesses we can't really identify link with a specific pathogen."

(Tanya Roberts, Personal Communication, 2019).

As a result, Roberts believes the future of food safety surveillance will see industry and regulators embracing data collection and analysis technology as a tool "try and get more depth and get more specific and more accuracy" (Tanya Roberts, Personal Communication, 2019).

While PFGE offers many advantages, it has some limitations, such as how it is described by users as time consuming and that it cannot type all strains. Today, the CDC is transitioning toward using whole genome sequencing (WGS)—a method that "reveals the complete DNA make-up of an organism" and, according to the FDA, is used to "perform basic foodborne pathogen identification during foodborne illness outbreaks," thus helping to "reduce foodborne illnesses and deaths" (FDA, 2018).

"... with new technology ... you have a Pulse Field Gel Electrophoresis and Whole Genome Sequencing ... comes new sources of data and more opportunity for more widespread and clearer data. And with this new technology and data comes opportunity for updated and more refined economic evaluations."

(Tanya Roberts, Personal Communication, 2019).

A recent Northeastern University graduate with a master's degree in Regulatory Affairs of Food, Adam Friedlander is a Manager of Food Safety and Technical Services at Food Marketing Institute. Friedlander envisions a future in which food safety is more data-driven at the consumer level.

"In the future, if I were to eat a cell-cultured hamburger, I foresee, as a consumer, having access to the data that's in that hamburger and it's going to go through my body and I see myself having access to the data that's in my stool because it's going to end up being all crowd-sourced. So if I feel sick, and I believe it must've been something that I ate, I see us collecting that data and I see being able to report out that this sample from this food has this specific pathogen."

(Adam Friedlander, Personal Communication, 2019).

Friedlander is not alone in his predictions of immediate results and availability to data from foodborne pathogen detection. Experts at the CDC are hopeful regarding future solutions for challenges associated with improving the speed of detection for foodborne pathogens. Robert Tauxe stated, in his 2019 presentation at the IAFP, that he sees a bridge between the current WGS database and having, what he calls, "the post-isolate future" (Tauxe, 2019).

"Public health needs more advanced molecular diagnostic tools for direct use on the clinical specimens to get the sequence information in a matter of hours. We know a number of diagnostic companies are working on solutions to this and we're beginning to explore meta genomic strategies as well. And I'm expecting … that 5 to 10 years from now, we may have diagnosis and pathogen sequencing using meta genomic methods even as close to the patient as the bedside."

(Tauxe, 2019).

New technologies

The "food safety culture" that emerged after the landmark 1993 *E. coli* outbreak has not only impacted the industry, but consumers as well. Consumers are more aware of the many safety risks inherent with their meals. Today, consumers want the ability to see clearly the many links between the creation of a food product all the way to its final placement in a customer's hands or onto their plates. Shoppers want to trust brand names and the certifications and claims on labels. Food reputation concerns are key elements in consumers' decision-making process.

Whereas the primary questions surrounding food were once simply:

1. Will this taste good?
2. Will this fill me up?
3. Can I afford it?

Modern questions for food decisions now include:

1. Does this food's taste, appearance, smell meet my standards? (food quality)
2. Will this food be safe from contaminants? (food safety)
3. Was this food impacted by sabotage, terrorism, or intentional adulteration? (food defense)
4. Will this food satisfy my nutritional needs and be sustainable? (food security)
5. Is this food what the label claims it is? (food authenticity)

Innovation and even industry disruption are no longer seen solely in consumers' perception of the look and taste of a food product. Valerie Madamba is Senior Counsel, Regulatory Compliance and Government Affairs at Blue Apron. Blue Apron (an "ingredient-and-recipe meal kit service" company launched in 2012) is future minded in terms of how food is manufactured, prepared, and delivered and offers clients convenience while still connected to current food manufacturing and food safety practices. Madamba describes Blue Apron as being a draw for consumers who like forward thinking and innovation. "Logistically there's incredible innovation … in terms of how we do cater to the kind of convenience that our consumers are looking for" (Valerie Madamba, Personal Communication, 2019).

One of the hottest topics at food industry events is technology. Any discussion of the food industry and technology will inevitably include a focus on data collection and analysis related to compliance and reputation. Some new technology, or "RegTech" are promised as a key optimization tools not only for the future of the industry, but also for consumers as they "can now expect to see the entire histories of the products they buy, and hence make more informed decisions" (Rivers, 2019). Exhibitor halls at conferences are full of booths displaying everything from sanitation devices to sensors to software. But the most talked about and written about of all technologies today is Blockchain. Some in the food industry describe Blockchain using words such as transparency, traceability, network, partnership, and big data. Some retail giants use words such as required.

Walmart describes itself as "... the world's largest retailer" due to having become "the masters of supply chain management." The retail giant has "endeavored to become a leader in the area of implementing supply chain technologies to achieve the kind of operational efficiency that make these cost savings possible" (West, n.d.). In a September 24, 2018 press release, Walmart and Sam's Club (a chain of membership-only retail warehouse clubs owned and operated by Walmart Inc.) announced that they will require real time, end-to-end food traceability from their suppliers of leafy green vegetables by September of 2019. Specifically, their suppliers must use IBM Blockchain technology (Walmart, 2018).

Blockchain, as a form of regulatory technology, offers a decentralized eLedger; a collection of blocks of information for each step, farm to fork. It lives in multiple locations at once, making it extremely difficult to edit, change, or forge. Being immutable, Blockchain creates a permanent record, which can be referenced quickly and with greater confidence than traditional records in the event of an emergency.

According to Walmart:

> *"Blockchain is a way to digitize data and share information in a complex network in secure and trusted way. For food safety, this helps to more accurately pinpoint issues in the food chain and further protect customers against foodborne illnesses .... For more than a year, Walmart, working with IBM and 11 other food companies, has successfully developed a Blockchain-enabled food traceability network built on open-source technology. In an initial pilot conducted by Walmart and IBM, the amount of time it took the retailer to trace an item from store to farm was reduced from seven days to just 2.2 seconds."*
>
> ***(Walmart, 2018).***

According to IBM:

"Blockchain offers complete visibility of the data behind the many stages of product creation. Manufacturers, farmers, wholesalers, suppliers, delivery services and stores each input information that details and verifies their roles in the process—creating a log that provides irrefutable evidence of a product's provenance."

(Rivers, 2019)

Before digging deeper into Blockchain, an important note is that this imperative from Walmart is not the first time that retailers, including Walmart itself, served as the driving force for technology change in the food industry. This first step toward the types of today's "cutting edge" technologies can be found over 50 years ago in the development of barcodes found commonly on today's food packaging and labels.

The Kroger Company, which runs the largest supermarket chain (by revenue) in North America, published a wish for a better future in a 1966 booklet, stating: "Just dreaming a little … could an optical scanner read the price and total the sale …. Faster service, more productive service is needed desperately" (Weightman, 2015). A few years later, grocery industry advisers searched for a solution to standardize the storing of a product's pricing information. Their work came to fruition on June 26, 1974, when, at a Marsh supermarket in Troy, Ohio, a worker swiped a 10-pack of Wrigley Juicy Fruit gum—the first item scanned for its Universal Product Code (Hirst, 2014). Today, visitors to the Smithsonian National Museum of American History in Washington, DC, can see one of the first barcode scanners used at that Ohio supermarket.

From that point on, information in the hands of the giant retailers became as valuable as the products on their shelves. Their "control over information" is described by UCLA Sociology Professor Edna Bonacich as the start of the "shift in Wal-Mart's power" (Lewallen, 2004).

The goal of standardizing is not only to scale its common language on a barcode on an item that can be scanned anywhere in the world, but also to boost efficiency and profit at that retailer. To do this, the food industry, as well as health, transport, and logistics sectors, have relied on GS1 US to manage the barcode standard used by retailers, manufacturers, and suppliers.

Kevin Otto is the Senior Director of Community Engagement at GS1 US. He leads their cross-industry Blockchain efforts bringing together stakeholders from various industries to discuss how Blockchain can support supply chain imperatives, what needs industries currently must address to enable widespread adoption, and the critical role of GS1 Standards to effectively leverage this technology.

From Otto's perspective, he thinks that the challenge for barcodes faced by food service industry and retail food has been further upstream. Large major retailers helped push the development of the barcode. "It's really a matter of how those [companies] far upstream in the supply chain are getting support from their trading partners." The challenge, then, is to engage more of the small to midsize farmers "who don't have the technology background and think that maybe the application of a barcode is something incredibly technical, when it's not." Specifically, Otto states that these farmers need to:

> *"... understand the value of coding information and then be able to track it through the supply chain. So, when you get to distributor and then ultimately to a retailer or food service operator level, many of them, if not all of them, have the capability of scanning and storing this information."*
>
> ***(Kevin Otto, Personal Communication, 2019).***

While barcodes are still used today, their format and how they are read has changed. In 2004 Walmart announced that it was taking barcode technology a step further, requiring its suppliers to provide radio frequency identification (RFID) microchips identifying the item to which it is attached. This provides for more detailed inventory and supplier information than a bar code and increasing speed and efficiency of stocking and at checkout lines. Walmart looked at shifting over to RFID technology by the end of 2006 (Lewallen, 2004).

The reality of Walmart's experience with RFID technology, which should sound an alarm for any future technology, is that, according to Bill Hardgrave, former Walmart RFID technology consultant, "RFID technology was relatively new" for Walmart at that time, "and didn't work that well. Despite the hype around Walmart's pilot project, the tags were not giving suppliers useful data" (Kaplan, 2018).

Newer formats, such as those seen with the longer barcodes came out of the work associated with the Produce Traceability Initiative (PTI)—a voluntary program for companies in the produce industries to maximize tracking and tracing efforts. With PTI, companies label cases with GS1-128 barcodes to significantly expedite outbreak investigations and recalls through globally unique identification of the brand owner of the product and other information, such as the batch/lot information. As of 2018, industry estimates of produce cases with PTI labels were at 60% (Nickel, 2018), but these changes did not happen overnight. In 2010 the Produce Marketing Association and the United Fresh Produce Association conducted an industry survey about attitudes and implementation of traceability measures in which they polled more than 260 industry members selling in the United States. While nearly 75% of produce companies polled indicated that they were working to implement the PTI at that time, the survey revealed a number of reasons preventing implementation. Similar to what is seen with Blockchain today, the top three obstacles to implementation of PTI at that time were the perception of high costs, lack of awareness of the initiative, and waiting on government regulation (Karst, 2010).

Another change to barcodes is the use of quick response codes—those square, matrix (or two-dimensional) machine-readable barcode labels that contain information about the item to which it is attached. Consistent in these changes are the increased amount of data that can be accessed from these codes and how it helps understand the products, in this case, food.

All of these changes are part of the continuous improvement process seen in any industry. However, while the food industry has been quick to adopt new technologies in their efforts to gain a competitive advantage, regulators have struggled to keep up with advancements.

When the food industry agreed to adopt bar codes (creating to digitally identify and track data) and supported the launch of the first GS1 barcode in the 1970s, federal and international regulators only had a paper-based requirement for proof of production, sales, and distribution.

After the introduction of barcodes, the GS1-128 code and the PTI moved the industry forward to relay more information from the farm to retailers and even to consumers. However, according to Nathan Libbey, Sales Director CERTUS Food Safety (an innovative leader in food safety, through revolutionary technologies and strategic partnerships), "regulators still remained static in their requirement and suggestion of a paper standard for one-up-one down traceability and accountability" (Libbey, 2018) (Fig. 9.1).

Even with the 2011 FDA Food Safety Modernization Act (FSMA) that had effective implementation dates of 2016–18, paper was the standard for records. Only recently has the industry seen a change in the government's stance on digitization of records.

FDA Commissioner Scott Gottlieb, after multiple outbreaks tied to Romaine lettuce and other leafy-green vegetables in 2018, issued a statement in which he declared that "Complicating this already large-scale investigation,

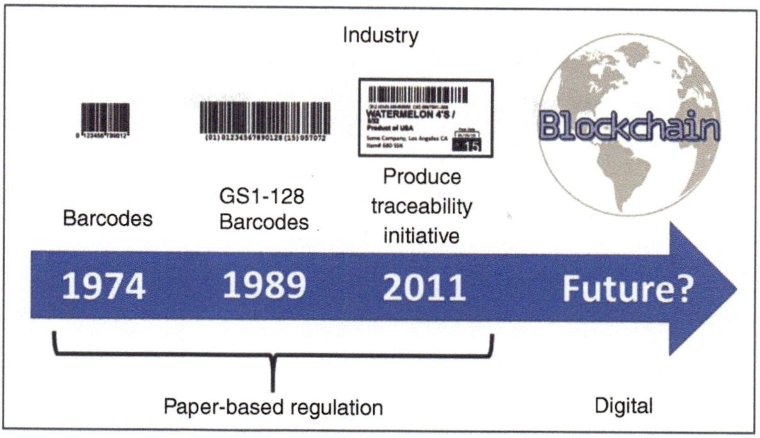

Figure 9.1 ***Timeline of barcode evolution to Blockchain and from paper-based to digital.*** *(Based on presentation by Libbey, 2018).*

the majority of the records collected in this investigation were either paper or handwritten" (Gottlieb, 2018). Thus the FDA's emphasis on industry work to standardize record keeping and adopt traceability best practices now includes the use of state-of-the-art technologies. But this was only a suggestion from the US government.

In Canada, the Safe Food for Canadians Act (S.C. 2012, c. 24) (SFCA) and the Safe Food for Canadians Regulations (SOR /2018-108) (SFCR) came into effect in January 2019. SFCA and SFCR cover imported, exported, inter-provincially and, in some cases, intra-provincially traded food products.

> *"As risks to food, animal health and plants have changed considerably and continue to change rapidly, the Agency must continue to adapt and be more efficient and responsive while supporting Canada's ability to compete in the global market."*
>
> ***(Canadian Food Inspection Agency, 2018).***

What makes Canada's SFCA stand out is that it was the first widespread regulation in North America to suggest that "standard commercial software" is acceptable for recordkeeping (Canadian Food Inspection Agency, 2019).

So where does the United States' FDA stand on digitization?

In the opening session for the 2017 Dubai International Food Safety Conference, Frank Yiannas, then Walmart's Vice President in charge of food safety delivered his thoughts on "Why should technology trend in food safety: exploring Blockchain." Yiannas shared his observation of weaknesses in the food industry when it comes to traceability and how he was once a major skeptic of blockchain. Having become a believer that Blockchain can be a digital solution, he showed the international audience a video in which he highlighted his work at Walmart with IBM and nine other major food brands including Dole, Nestle, Tyson, and Unilever to pilot a blockchain technology. Today, Frank Yiannas is the FDA's Deputy Commissioner for Food Policy and Response.

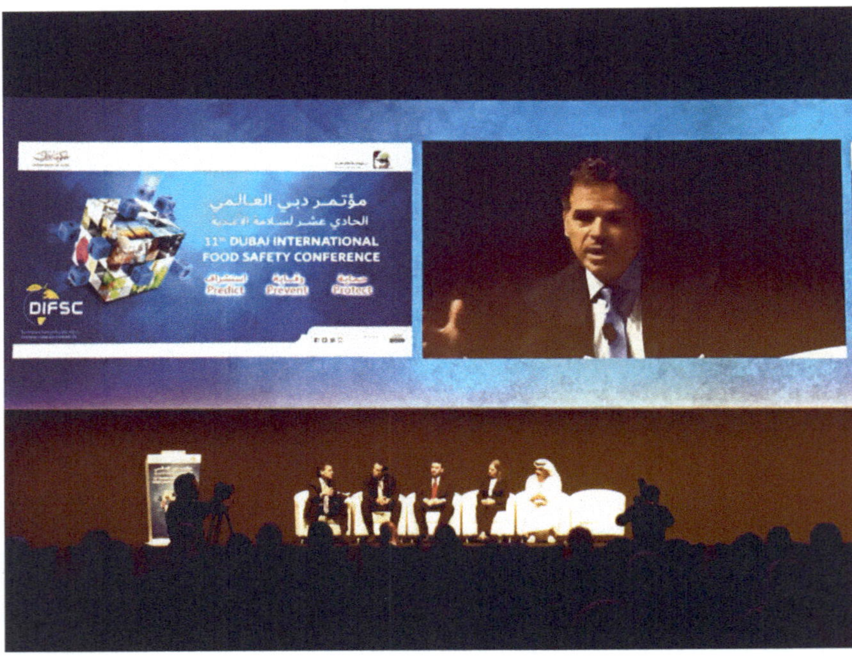

Photo by Author of Frank Yiannas November 19, 2017, delivering his opening remarks at the 2017 Dubai International Food Safety Conference.

As of June 2019, the FDA, authorized under the US Drug Supply Chain Security Act (DSCSA), has embarked on a pilot program with Walmart, IBM, and Merck that will explore using Blockchain. The goals of this real-time monitoring test of the pharmaceutical supply chain include improving the security of prescription drug supply and distribution as well as increasing regulatory oversight of counterfeit, stolen, contaminated, or otherwise harmful drugs (Mathias, 2019). While the role of large retailers over the past 50 years in increasing the use of digital solutions within the food industry, one can see how success with this pilot will impact the FDA's initial steps toward a more proactive position on digital solutions for food industry's future.

From bar codes to Blockchain

The industry perceives that Blockchain, or some other form of accessible, cloud-based method of storing and tracking data from transaction to transaction throughout the entire chain, is the next step in the evolution of regulatory compliance and traceability technology. One of the first large-scale projects of this nature is taking place in Dubai, UAE. In the United States, and around the world, the food industry is following Dubai's findings to help provide a blueprint for future Blockchain implementation.

Dubai is filled with people who look to the future. They can be found in the city's stunning skyscrapers, malls, and highways. This can also be found in their determination to explore ways to use Blockchain and big data to protect their food. According to municipality statistics, Dubai imports about $200 billion of food annually from nearly 200 countries (Saseendran, 2017). In 2017 government leaders there took a step to digitize food data to ensure better food safety and to help consumers with their nutritional needs and preferences.

During the opening ceremonies for the 11th Dubai International Food Safety Conference in 2017, Hussain Nasser Lootah, Director General of Dubai Municipality, launched "Food Watch," a digital platform that aims to completely digitize the food safety and nutritional information of all edible items served through more than 20,000 food establishments operating in the emirate. The Food Safety Department of Dubai Municipality developed the Food Watch platform to facilitate data exchange between authorities, food businesses, service providers, and consumers. According to the Dubai Municipality's website:

> *"By utilizing digital monitoring techniques, data analytics and customized applications, the platform will offer full tractability of foods with validated ingredient and nutritional information. Smart contracts, services, and customized applications will deliver every user a unique experience based on their requirements. Digitized exchange of data will enable the delivery of real-time assurance based on predictive insight, from what went wrong to what is likely to go wrong."*
>
> ***(Dubai Municipality, 2019).***

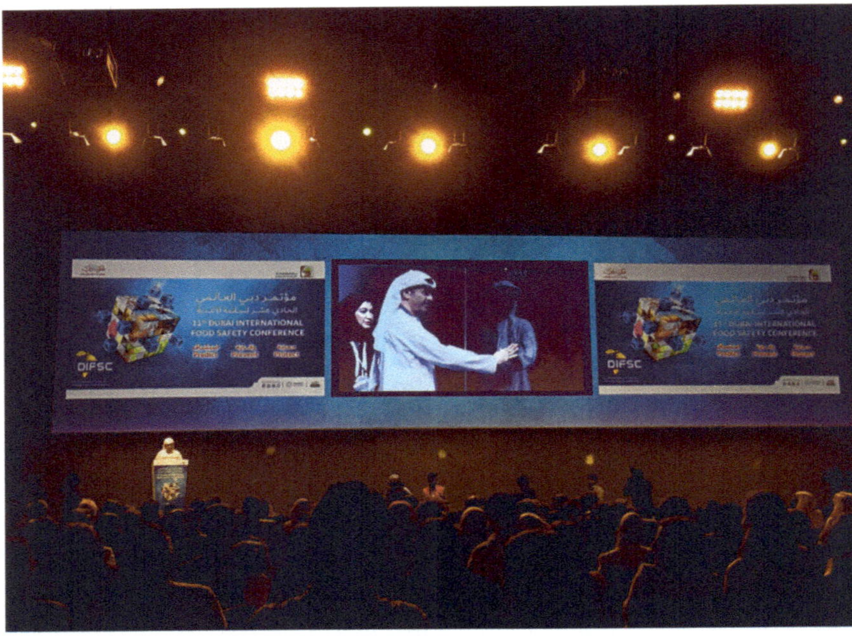

Photo by Author of the Dubai Municipality's November 19, 2017 launch of "Food Watch" program at the Dubai International Food Safety Conference.

According to leaders at the conference, the initial phase of data compiling focused on food establishments that are handling high-risk foods. Eventually, all other food establishments will be required to update the platform with information about their food items, including health and nutritional claims, details about their premises and food handlers, and even certifications. These pieces of data will give inspectors and consumers unprecedented access to critical information.

More important than the information being gathered about food is how having that data can facilitate action. Future phases of Dubai's new food monitoring system will focus on incorporating Blockchain and Internet of Things to quickly and accurately track food products from farm to fork and everywhere in between. Making this data easily accessible can enhance the ability of officials and consumers to take action before and after a health violation or food poisoning incident takes place, thus underscoring the municipality's larger outcomes of predicting foodborne issues, preventing illnesses and protecting consumers proactively through blockchain and big data. The stated goal is for the system to be in place before Dubai hosts the World Expo in 2020.

In the United States, outside of a dozen or so companies working directly with Walmart, most of the food industry sits somewhere on a learning curve in the early stages of Blockchain. During his opening keynote for the 2019 Blockchain for Food and Beverage event in San Francisco, Bob Wolpert, Golden State Foods' Corporate Senior Vice President, stated that "Nobody is going to trust Blockchain in the beginning .... If you cannot define how the customer will benefit, then you cannot identify the business value" (Wolpert, 2019).

Consumers will ultimately pay higher prices for food from a company that uses Blockchain. The industry promises for improved food safety are easy for consumers to buy into—especially when they have no idea how complicated the initial implementation is perceived at this time. This mountain to climb, in order to have Blockchain up and running smoothly throughout the entire industry as intended, is not lost on industry leaders.

One way of looking at the challenge of Blockchain is that this will require a fundamental shift in how companies deal with their data and what their competition, as well as their customers. Otto describes this as a "visibility" dilemma.

> *"Ultimately what we're talking about is persistent supply chain visibility. So, it's not just knowing where product is within your four walls—it requires a partnership upstream and downstream in a supply chain that hasn't historically existed, because the way that most people have built their visibility programs is one up, one down. I know where it came from, I know where it went when it left my four walls."*
>
> ***(Kevin Otto, Personal Communication, 2019).***

While Jorge Hernandez, Vice President of Quality at the Wendy's Company, views Blockchain technology as "amazing" and that the possibility of using it to improve the traceability in food is real, he has some hesitations.

> *"My hesitations are around the practicality and cost to implement, what some consider a 'rigid' technology, across the different segment of the entire food industry. To make the traceability goal tangible we are not only talking about U.S. implementation, but global implementation. The plan to get implementation appears to be having big players buy it and mandate it for the rest of the industry as a 'cost of doing business.' This thinking, in my opinion, is a significant challenge. Especially without a clear and demonstrated business 'value' to all players (something very real for small and medium size companies)."*
>
> ***(Jorge Hernandez, Personal Communication, 2019).***

In 2018 when Walmart announced their Blockchain requirement for suppliers (Walmart, 2018), they started with leafy green vegetable suppliers. Leafy greens provides not only a good example of a commodity that has had its food safety failures make world news headlines over the past few years, but is also a good example of a food in which the consumer does not necessarily always know the difference between the big name and the small supplier. Those small suppliers or smaller company labels want to be seen by shoppers at the grocery store as being on the same shelf (both literally and figuratively) as the trusted, large brand labels. But if these smaller suppliers not buying in to traceability technology, they are not investing in it or even prioritizing it, this ultimately puts them—and consumers—at a disadvantage. Otto points to how major retailers are dealing with this difference in suppliers.

> *"When you're talking about a food safety journey, major retailers aren't going to be willing to take the hits for these safety issues. If it's just the bigger suppliers that are willing to get on board, you may see a shift in that direction. I do think that people like Walmart obviously have a say over these smaller suppliers."*
>
> ***(Kevin Otto, Personal Communication, 2019).***

For the smaller supplier, successful implementation of new technologies related to traceability and regulatory compliance can be a clear differentiator in the market. This involves being able to demonstrate their investment into and development of a strong, efficient, and successful a differentiator for them. This differentiator element can also be seen as a disruptor in the industry.

A small company's failure to embrace new technology related to compliance technology and traceability may result in a loss of sales or even to a barrier to market. Major retailers will start to move away from engaging in business with small suppliers. "If it's just the bigger suppliers that are willing to get on board, you may see a shift in that direction. Major retailers aren't going to be willing to take the hits for these safety issues" (Kevin Otto, Personal Communication, 2019).

Thus, the use of newer technologies, such as Blockchain, becomes a differentiator for the small suppliers and for new companies or products. "If [smaller suppliers] are doing a better job than the large supplier, it can mean sales for them. This can help set you apart from your competitive set … because ultimately the information is going to be digitized ... there's going to be a way of coding this across the entire supply chain. If you're not setting herself up for that today, then you put yourself behind the eight ball, as this isn't going away" (Kevin Otto, Personal Communication, 2019).

One of those specific challenges with Blockchain is the need for a company to put the entirely of data across a supply chain of a specific product out into the open for transactions down the line. That requires a partnership well beyond the "one-up-one-down" model that the food industry has observed in the past. Blockchain is only going to be successful "if companies are willing to partner and can coalesce around what information it is that they need to share" (Kevin Otto, Personal Communication, 2019).

Seafood offers a current glimpse into this relationship between access to information and a company, large or small, differentiating itself with Blockchain or some version of it. In a scenario where a restaurant operator (in order to protect the restaurant's reputation) wants to know that they are purchasing authentic seafood for his customers, this is where Blockchain becomes a disruptor that benefits smaller suppliers who leverage this technology in order to compete with the larger suppliers.

Understanding a new technology's value is one thing, not all stakeholders can see Blockchain as anything beyond theoretical. Valerie Madamba of Blue Apron believes that some in the food industry will view drones as being more tangible than Blockchain.

> *"I could see how, at a large, perhaps multinational company it could be more challenging to grapple with adoption of new technology. There are more resources, but getting it up the chain or showing that acceptance, for certain people within an organization like that can, be challenging."*
>
> ***(Valerie Madamba, Personal Communication, 2019).***

Change, itself, is not always an easy decision. Jill Hollingsworth, DVM, the Vice President of Food Safety and Regulatory Affairs at CHEMSTAR, worked at the USDA from 1978 to 1996, ultimately serving as their Assistant Deputy Administrator of the Food Safety Inspection Service. Hollingsworth has witnessed many industry discussions around technologies viewed as the next "Silver Bullet," but has also heard how executives see timing for change.

> *"I remember once talking to a whole big room of industry people, these happened to be meat guys … I remember them saying, 'Here's the new technology …' 'We hear so much about this…' 'Here's a new thing that's going to change it, make everything better…' 'The investment is worth it,' and 'We've been down this road so many times.' And this one guy said: 'everybody in this room wants to be the second person to try it.' It's a brilliant comment because it is true. Everyone wants to be the second one because they want to see if it worked for the first guy."*
>
> ***(Jill Hollingsworth, Personal Communication, 2019)***

As recent as early 2019, the journey to Blockchain becoming a successful, industry-wide reality was projected as a 5-year process. By the middle of 2019, at an industry meeting on Blockchain updates, most representatives in attendance agreed that they now see it as taking 20–25 years to achieve.

Some in the food industry also view a timeline for technology change in terms of what problems can be solved now, not years down the road. Jorge Hernandez is the Vice President of Quality Assurance at The Wendy's Company. Long an advocate for food safety, Jorge thinks about "new and disruptive technologies and products that modify the issue/problem themselves" as being impacted by "the world ... moving faster and picking up speed" (Jorge Hernandez, Personal Communication, 2019).

> *"When thinking ahead I used 3, 5 and 10 years increments as markers. I no longer do that because What I thought was 5 years away is now 2 or 3. What I thought was 3 years away is now 1 or 2 months. My approach now to just look at an issue/problem and consider what will I need to do/find/get/solve as if it was here next month. That helps me keep my mind open and looking constantly at my environment for ideas, tools, fluctuations, technologies and disruptions that can help ME adapt and evolve to deal with new situations."*
>
> ***(Jorge Hernandez, Personal Communication, 2019).***

When asked during a 2019 food industry event on technology, some food company representatives talk about Blockchain as being "Interesting, but we are not prioritizing it now." They add that transparency and traceability are two major elements of food safety regulatory compliance that "... you don't need Blockchain for." A representative from one fast food chain stated that Blockchain "is a tool—it will not be the solution." A representative from another fast food chain, (one that has had multiple food safety failures that captured the media's attention) stated how Blockchain is a "wait and see technology. We have many other issues to fix before we can invest in it." Perhaps the most startling comment came from a major meat company's representative who stated that Blockchain as a system would not be only expensive, but "if we have that system in place" we could be "crucified faster." In a similar comment, one company talked about future work with Blockchain involving the need to "rely on sensors" in such a way as to "protect you from lawyers." Three companies admitted that they "put the brakes on pilots with Blockchain" (All comments from 2019 event attended by the author, but intentionally kept anonymous.)

Based on his direct interactions with industry partnerships, GS1 US's Kevin Otto sees this trend in companies that were once racing toward Blockchain as a solution, but are now slowing down or even deciding to place its adoption on hold.

> *"I think initially people were latching on for Blockchain to help drive greater partnerships and what we're hearing, in the meetings that we have sat in [is that] they're starting to take a step back from Blockchain and realize- 'Hey, we still have even*

more work to do before we can really make this project work' .... you're seeing a lot of companies step back and say- 'We're not ready for Blockchain yet because we haven't had the initial partnerships in our supply chains to actually make sure that the information that you need to feed to a Blockchain even exists"

(Kevin Otto, Personal Communication, 2019).

Though Blockchain will not solve all the industry's quality assurance and food safety concerns overnight, many leaders in food policy view this as being a part of the modern, digital toolkit in the future. They also anticipate that the industry will use Blockchain to meet the demands that consumers are placing on retailers in terms of trust: label information, origins, temperature control, and more. However, leaders must balance the talks of strengths and opportunities with that of weaknesses and threats. Strengths include its format as a digital record database, put together with information pertinent to multiple stakeholders. There must be consensus of all stakeholders for the blocks of data in the chain tied to a product. The ease of access to the multitude of documents (thousands of transactions within the supply chain for a product on the retail shelf), now made digital, is seen as one of Blockchain's greatest strengths.

Smart contracts are also the strength of Blockchain. Attaching terms and conditions to transactions that are automated, so a computer (artificial intelligence) can execute the terms (such as transportation temperature sampling data specifications), thus preventing a shipment from being finalized and sent out by a supplier if it did not meet buyer requirements. Blockchain also offers democratization of information with real-time visibility of the chain to all parties in a transaction at the same time. This is what can enable quick recalls. However, recalls and traceability alone may not be enough to make consumers safer.

Stephen Ostroff, former FDA Deputy Commissioner of Food, sees the link between Blockchain and traceability, but adds a cautionary note.

"When I think about blockchain—traceability is really important for a whole variety of reasons. But the main reason that right now traceability is important is when there's a disease outbreak, we can get stuff off the market more quickly. But that's after the fact. So, I understand that enhanced traceability through blockchain is likely also preventative. But, Blockchain, in and of itself, doesn't make food inherently safer'

(Stephen Ostroff, Personal Communication, 2019)

Weaknesses of Blockchain include the fact that the inclusion of multiple parties opens the door to potential issues in how it is configured, who authors the blocks of information, and who controls (public vs. private) the blocks of data. As the size of the eLedger gets larger over time, it gets harder to manage and secure. This assumes 100% buy-in and participation. True recall traceback requires complete—and authentic—participation and accurate data from all participants. Furthermore, all participants must be using platforms that can communicate with each other. As competitors might tend to use conflicting technology providers, then the ultimate goals of Blockchain become weakened by a different set of principles, or commercial-driven decisions, as opposed to strengthened by cooperation.

Another weakness is the shift in supplier and customer culture, as we will see a much different, nonlinear supply chain than currently exists. This will force changes in industry job roles as trust providers. Similarly, a weakness can be found in current certifications as this culture continues to shift. How do mangers or directors verify and validate information governance?

Strengths and weaknesses aside, much progress can be found in building the understanding of Blockchain's use and potential. While significant food industry coalition tests have already produced some great results, many experts continue to discuss the changes needed in the workforce to support Blockchain. In addition to a focus on ethics, data management, and data security, organizations and universities are now developing training programs and certifications for Blockchain leadership. Beyond data entry, many industry skill sets related to regulatory compliance can be blended with analytics and even project management.

Also, Blockchain is all about data, which has value, but for data to become actionable information, people (not just artificial intelligence) need to ask the right questions. To overcome this potential weakness, those who use Blockchain for food safety and authenticity must understand the true burden of disease, not just the various aspects of the commodity. All stakeholders must develop a stronger understanding of this culture shift with the relationship between the supplier and the consumer. A third party or digital tool alone cannot achieve the goals associated with brand trust and public health.

Beyond data and technology

The hype around Blockchain or any other data collection and analysis technology, in terms of being able to improve food safety, typically includes how it would improve traceability and speed up a recall. It is important to note that while this increased reactive focus on data collection has a definite place in response to failures in food safety, the timing comes after incidents or crises have occurred, when real people have been harmed, and consumers have become victims, hospital patients, and worse.

Much like a car's airbag, Blockchain has the opportunity to be part of the solution, but deployment after an incident has already happened, regardless of its efficiency, forces us to accept that harm already has occurred. Over time, after-the-fact responses reduce a company's options to identify, stop, and correct a failure while the liabilities of that company continue to increase. This is where hindsight and insight usually include lawsuits, court trials, and sometimes even changes in legislation. This is where, according to the 2012 economic study discussed earlier in chapter six, many companies will experience a sharp drop in their NYSE stock value over an entire quarter of trading, then may only return to pre-incident values after at least three additional quarters of stock trading.

Consumers are aware that new technologies and food safety practices come with a price tag that increases the grocery bill. But what are we paying for if these steps fall short of protecting us? Consider, also, that while companies frequently recover (or at least survive) after these incidents, those consumers and their families most impacted by a foodborne illness or food allergen crisis never fully recover.

Industry use of Blockchain must include a parallel focus on its use to predict and prevent failures before they become crises that harm consumers. This approach brings an increase of options while minimizing (if not eliminating) liabilities. The impact on consumer safety adds great value to technology used in the most proactive sense. (Fig. 9.2)

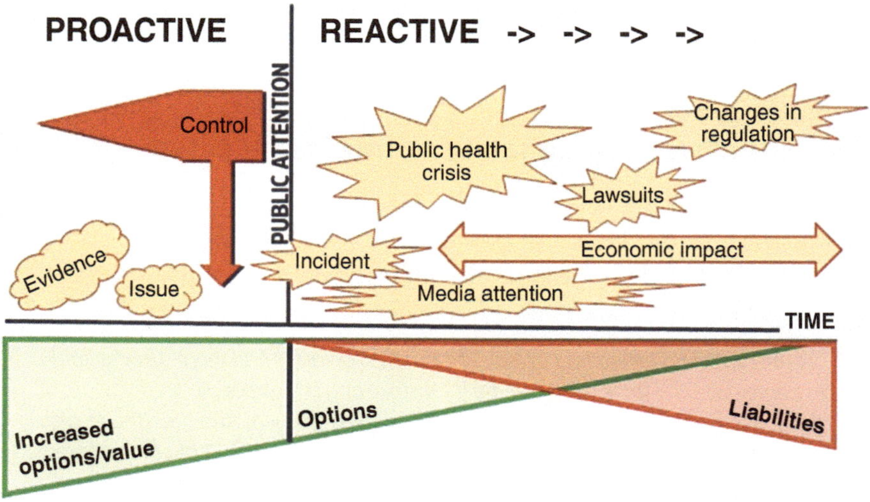

Figure 9.2 ***Proactive versus reactive approach to food regulatory compliance technology.*** *(Modified by Author. Proactive vs. Reactive approach to Food Regulatory Compliance technology).*

Not all failures can be identified and stopped before it is too late. However, if industry leaders fail to develop practices and even a culture that embraces predictive analytics driven by a balance of data/technology literacy and human literacy (understanding the true burden of disease, asking the right questions, prioritizing consumers' safety), then families will ultimately pay for the newest technology that protects industry more than it protects consumers. Though Blockchain and other advancements offer promises in reducing the numbers of recalls, outbreaks, and victims, how data and technology are used is not enough to solve all the problems inherent in food safety.

Future generations of food industry leaders and regulators will need data literacy to manage the flow of big data, and technological literacy to know how their machines work, but these understandings will only succeed if partnered with human literacy (the humanities, communication, and design related to how human beings function) to adapt to change (Aoun, 2017).

This "human literacy" includes an understanding of the true burden of disease. It is an essential element behind the "Herculean effort" (an incredible amount of work, strength, and courage) and behind the mitigation of food safety failures. As no single person can protect food alone, it will take a strong culture of understanding and prevention in order to make progress. As such, predictions for the future of food safety culture cannot ignore the role that the many consumer advocacy groups and victim advocates will continue to play in bringing about changes in industry board rooms and on Capitol Hill.

The outlook for a "food safety culture" of the future

Alan Baumfalk is the recipient of the 2018 SQF Auditor of the year award. His perspective on the future is shaped by years of auditing the good, the bad, and the ugly. He sees significant improvement in how many in the food industry view compliance and a food safety culture today.

> *"You're still going to find bad actors. Somebody is going to find them. They're going to come out. But I think there's so much at stake and I think people are so aware of the damage that can happen to children and to consumers. And then there's also an awareness that this could cost a company their reputation, impact their brand, and ruin it. The idea of a food safety culture is prevalent. In fact, people are really aware now that failures affect everybody in the food industry."*
>
> ***(Baumfalk, Personal Communication, 2019)***

Baumfalk still has an optimistic view of the future of food safety.

> *"I think the future is brighter. There are more professional people, more ethics, and more caring. While I believe that there is always going to be mistakes that happen, I see a lot of resources being put in to trying and preventing failures in food safety as much as possible. I only see better things for the future."*
>
> **(Baumfalk, Personal Communication, 2019).**

As opposed to the notion that future food safety progress will only happen because of "bodies in the street" ("Chasing Outbreaks: How Safe is Our Food?", 2015), the politicization of "victim advocates" is still recognized as having immeasurable impact and will likely remain so in the future.

When Jill Hollingsworth, DVM, served as the Assistant Deputy Administrator of the USDA's Food Safety Inspection Service at the time of the 1993 *E. coli* outbreak, she encountered victim advocates for the first time. "When so many people were pointing fingers, being angry, and blaming everybody, although they had every right to do that, [very few people] really had much more of a 'what are we going to do? what can we do? What are we going to do?' approach" (Jill Hollingsworth, Personal Communication, 2019). To her, this approach taken by some parents, who lost children during that landmark outbreak was really one of the big influences on making change, as this attitude kept them sane and provided greater motivation for forward thinking.

The role of consumer advocates can also be seen in the Herculean efforts behind FSMA. According to Sandra Eskin: "I think whether it would have passed without Pew, that's sort of beside the point. We were able to infuse all these resources and fly people in and use all the tools of the advocacy tool chest. I think that victim advocates were a huge part of our effectiveness" (Sandra Eskin, Personal Communication, 2019).

The Pew Charitable Trusts and STOP Foodborne Illness honored young food safety advocates, such as Rylee, Dana, and Lauren, for their advocacy and efforts to improve our nation's food safety. These advocates gained much more than simply the ears and support of legislators.

Rylee is now studying Japanese language and culture at university. She believes that her advocacy became instrumental in her on-going recovery.

> *"Talking with legislators helped me recover emotionally because I was talking to them about my foodborne illness story and participating in a process that could prevent other people from becoming ill as well. Sharing a voice made me believe that I was doing something right."*
>
> **(Rylee Gustafson, Personal Communication, 2019).**

In 2014, at the age of 16, Dana Dziadul wrote *Food Safety Superstar*, a children's book teaching kids about food safety practices. Her book gained the attention of FDA, resulting in support for its release at the US Capitol. Today, Dana is also a college student, studying human development and family studies.

Lauren Bush completed her studies and earned an MPA in public policy analysis. Working in government and community affairs in New York, Lauren continues to advocate for food safety and serves as the co-leader of the Board for STOP Foodborne Illness.

Another example of the contributions from consumer advocates can be found in the aftermath of the Peanut Corporation of America (PCA) *Salmonella* outbreak. "The Parnell brothers" (PCA's owners) "created perhaps, though, not intentionally, some of the most articulate and passionate advocates I've ever worked with … who were close to my age, if not older" (Sandra Eskin, Personal Communication, 2019). One of these advocates is Jeff Almer who, after the death of his mother from this outbreak, collaborated with the prosecution team in advance and throughout the PCA trial and testified at the sentencing. He also worked with Pew to support their work (Detwiler, 2015).

People all the way through the highest levels of federal, state, and county agencies hold the utmost of respect for consumer advocacy organizations and for advocates. Government and industry representatives who once sat isolated from consumers now share panels and stages with them. Rarely is an industry conference or training planned anymore without inclusion of those whose presence is to bring to the conversation the true burden of disease. Consumer perspectives are present in editorial advisory boards and now featured regularly in industry magazines such as *Quality Assurance and Food Safety Magazine*.

At the same time, no food safety advocate, who was an outbreak victim or whose work stems from the loss of a loved one to foodborne illness, wishes to be in that role in the first place. While not every young survivor or grieving parent has the ability or interest to advocate for others' safety, most assume that they should never have needed to do so in the first place.

According to Mitzi Baum, CEO of Stop Foodborne Illness, "Consumer advocacy is an essential part of the system of checks and balances when food industry, regulatory policy and the public interest intersect" (Mitzi Baum, Personal Communication, 2019). Over the last 25 years, Stop Foodborne Illness has earned the trust of a growing constituency by organizing and amplifying the voices of people who have been impacted by foodborne illness. Together, these victim advocates and consumer advocates initiate change through the sharing of stories of survival and death due to foodborne pathogens.

This organization also works with food industry executive leadership through their "Alliance to Stop Foodborne Illness" program. Their goal is to harness the power of individual stories to create awareness that behind every statistic for illnesses, hospitalizations, and deaths related to food is an individual. This is critical, as it puts the humanity in the data. Embedding these stories within companies' internal food safety training programs would then serve as a constant reminder of the "why" of food safety.

> *"As we look toward the future, it is imperative that consumer advocates raise their voices and participate in organizations such as Stop to initiate real change. They must lead and continue to call upon industry executive leadership and regulators to rely on scientific research to initiate regulatory and process change that institutes meaningful improvements and continual monitoring of the country's food supply chain to protect the nation's population from preventable deaths."*
>
> ***(Mitzi Baum, Personal Communication, 2019)***

Just as the technologies of today and tomorrow will bring us closer to a global food supply that truly is safe, so, too, will the next great voice from a victim advocate. Unfortunately, new voices will only come about after yet, again, some future food safety failure that could have been prevented.

Future case studies

Today, over 25 years after the 1993 "Jack in the Box" *E. coli* outbreak, this landmark event in food safety culture and history is still taught in academic programs, discussed at conferences, and referred to in journal articles. Most experts interviewed for this book, when asked about what outbreaks or recalls from the past will still be used as case studies for new students and food safety leaders 25 years from now, their answers are nearly the same.

1. The 1993 "Jack in the Box" *E. coli* outbreak
2. The 2006 Dole baby spinach *E. coli* outbreak
3. The 2011 Jensen Farms Cantaloupe *Listeria* outbreak
4. The various (2018 and earlier) leafy green/Romaine lettuce outbreaks
5. The 2016 and beyond Chipotle outbreaks of various pathogens

Each one of these events offered a different lesson for those who are willing to listen and learn as a person, as a company, or as an industry. They offer many lessons on the importance of food safety, importance of documentation, need for the evolution of regulations, importance of a food safety culture, as well as liability and accountability for the failures.

Not all experts agree on two cases as still being taught 25 years from now—the 2008–09 Peanut PCA outbreak and resulting trial and sentencing, and the DeCosters' eggs incidents and resulting trial and sentencing.

Stephen Ostroff, former FDA Deputy Commissioner for Foods and Veterinary Medicine, offered a reason for why these two cases might not be taught as much as the others.

> *"There weren't many lessons from either of them, other than the fact that these were really, really, really heinously bad people. That's not a failure of food safety, that's just bad people who shouldn't be making food. And there's no way sort of up front that you're going to be able to put in place something to prevent people from doing really bad things. When they do stuff criminally, okay: throw the book at them, but I don't know that there's a lot of lessons to be learned there."*
>
> ***(Stephen Ostroff, Personal Communication, 2019).***

References

Aoun, J. (2017). *Robot-proof: Higher education in the age of artificial intelligence.* Cambridge: MIT Press.

Canadian Food Inspection Agency. (2018). *Understanding the safe food for Canadians regulations a handbook for food businesses.* (CFIA Publication No. P0965E-18 Catalogue No.: A104-142/2018E-PDF ISBN: 978-0-660-26985-6). Available from: https://www.inspection.gc.ca/DAM/DAM-aboutcfia-sujetacia/STAGING/text-texte/regs_safe_food_regulations_handbook_business_1531429195095_eng.pdf.

Canadian Food Inspection Agency. (2019). Safe Food for Canadians Regulations Tool Kit for Food Businesses Fact sheet: Traceability. Available from: https://www.inspection.gc.ca/food/toolkit-for-food-businesses/traceability/eng/1427310329573/1427310330167.

Detwiler, D. (2015). Holding Food Companies Accountable. *Food Quality and Safety Magazine.* Available from: http://www.foodqualityandsafety.com/article/holding-food-companies-accountable/.

Dubai Municipality. (2019). Food Watch System. Dubai Municipality. Available from: https://www.dm.gov.ae/en/Business/FoodSafetyDepartment/Pages/Food-Watch-System.aspx.

FDA. (2018). Whole Genome Sequencing (WGS) Program. FDA. Available from: https://www.fda.gov/food/science-research-food/whole-genome-sequencing-wgs-program.

Gottlieb, S. (2018). Statement from FDA Commissioner Scott Gottlieb, M.D., on Findings from the Romaine Lettuce E. coli O157:H7 Outbreak Investigation and FDA's Efforts to Prevent Future Outbreaks. FDA. Available from: https://www.fda.gov/news-events/press-announcements/statement-fda-commissioner-scott-gottlieb-md-findings-romaine-lettuce-e-coli-o157h7-outbreak.

Hirst, E. (2014). 40 Years Ago Today: Wrigley Gum the First Product to Have Its Bar Code Scanned. *The Chicago Tribune.* Available from: https://www.chicagotribune.com/business/chi-bar-code40-years-old-wrigley-gum-20140626-story.html.

Kaplan, D. (2018). The Rise, Fall and Return of RFID. Supply Chain Dive. Available from: https://www.supplychaindive.com/news/RFID-rise-fall-and-return-retail/530608/.

Karst, T. (2010). Produce Traceability Initiative Releases Survey Results. The California Fresh Fruit Association. Available from: https://www.cafreshfruit.org/news/230.
Lewallen, B. (2004). Wal-Mart and the Bar Code. PBS Frontline. Available from: https://www.pbs.org/wgbh/pages/frontline/shows/walmart/secrets/barcode.html.
Libbey, N. (2018). Presentation on Evolution of Food Traceability. Food Safety Consortium, Schaumburg, IL.
Mathias, T. (2019). IBM, Walmart, Merck in blockchain collaboration with FDA. *Reuters New Service*. Available from: https://www.reuters.com/article/us-fda-blockchain/ibm-walmart-merck-in-blockchain-collaboration-with-fda-idUSKCN1TE1SA.
Nickel, A. (2018). Walmart reaffirms Produce Traceability Initiative effectiveness. Produce Retailer. Available from: https://www.produceretailer.com/article/news-article/walmart-reaffirms-produce-traceability-initiative-effectiveness.
U.S. Department of Agriculture. (1996). Pathogen reduction; hazard analysis and critical control point (HACCP) systems. *Federal Register, 61*(144). Available from: https://www.govinfo.gov/content/pkg/FR-1996-07-25/html/96-17837.htm.
Rivers, S. (2019). Win Customers' Hearts with a Transparent Supply Chain. IBM Food Trust's Blockchain Pulse: IBM Blockchain Blog. Available from: https://www.ibm.com/blogs/Blockchain/2019/04/win-customers-hearts-with-a-transparent-supply-chain/.
Saseendran, S. (2017). Dubai Launches High-tech Food Watch Programme. *Gulf News*. Available from: https://gulfnews.com/uae/health/dubai-launches-high-tech-food-watch-programme-1.2126769.
Tauxe, R. (2019). From Outbreak Catastrophes to Clades of Concern, How Whole Genome Sequencing Can Change the Food Safety Landscape. John H. Silliker Lecture presented at the annual meeting of the International Association for Food Protection, Louisville, KY.
Walmart. (2018). Walmart and Sam's Club to Require Real-Time, End-to-End Food Traceability with Blockchain [Press release]. Available from: https://corporate.walmart.com/media-library/document/leafy-greens-on-Blockchain-press-release/_proxyDocument?id=00000166-0c4c-d96e-a3ff-8f7c09b50001.
Weightman, G. (2015). The History of the Bar Code. *The Smithsonian Magazine*. Available from: https://www.smithsonianmag.com/innovation/history-bar-code-180956704/#7SjtIpUFxC14Ztyk.99.
West. C. et al. (n.d.). RFID Technology. Walmart Supply Chain. Available from: https://walmartsupplychain.weebly.com/rfid-technology.html.
Wolpert, B. (2019). Unlocking the Potential of Blockchain to Transform the F&B Supply Chain. Presented at the Blockchain for Food and Beverage event, San Francisco, CA.

CHAPTER 10

Beyond food safety

"One thing that not everybody thinks about when they think about climate and food sustainability, is the scale of that challenge. Food is the biggest and most widespread human undertaking."
Joseph Robertson, Global Strategy Director, Citizens' Climate Lobby, 2019

"The things described by Mr. Sinclair happened yesterday, are happening today, and will happen tomorrow and the next day, until some Hercules comes to cleanse the filthy stable."
From literature Review of* The Jungle *in* The London Times*, 1906

"With this ever-changing landscape, we know we must continue preparing to take advantage of new opportunities and address potential risks."
From FDA Press Release, 2019

Beyond the obvious topics related to food safety, this book concludes with a series of topics related to change—either changes we cannot avoid or ignore any longer, changes in the evolution of the food industry over time, or changes that we need to consider making. This chapter will also align changes with a look at the four industrial revolutions.

First, let's define the four Industrial Revolutions.

The First Industrial Revolution

The First Industrial Revolution (18th–19th centuries in Europe and America) included the progression from hand production methods to machines and new processes for manufacturing and production. At the same time, along with a population increase, America and Europe experienced a shift from mostly agrarian/rural to industrial/urban societies. This period is also noted for the steam engine making possible the rise of the mechanized factory system and centralized food operations.

Food Safety
http://dx.doi.org/10.1016/B978-0-12-818219-2.00010-7

The Second Industrial Revolution

With the Second Industrial Revolution (between 1870 and 1914, pre-World War I), development of the internal combustion engine, along with production of steel, oil, and electricity, all resulted in urbanization and, in terms of food, an increase in the distribution distance of food as well as the consumption of international foods. This industrial revolution included many events and transitions that impacted economic, political, geographic, and social elements of America.

This was a period of American Imperialism—purchases and annexations beyond the continent. In 1867, the United States purchased Alaska from Russia and annexed the Midway Islands. In 1898, the United States, motivated by economic interests, annexed the Hawaiian Islands—which, only a decade later, became one of America's greatest sources of sugar.

America had now become an "Industrial Power," with advanced ways of manufacturing (especially with electricity), new industries (including steel, oil, and canned foods), growing labor force in expanding urban cities, and growing economic forces and needs. By this time, the growth of these new industries demanded greater and more reliable sources of products, while new territories meant new markets. Also, America's continued population increase expanded domestic markets for food. Railroads and ships moved people and products to markets across the nation and beyond. One great engineering feat during this period was the completion of the Panama Canal in 1914, eliminating the need to navigate around tip of South America, becoming a significant benefit for the American military—and America's import/export economy.

America also became "The Land of Immigrants." Chinese immigrants made a huge impact in the Transcontinental Railroad and brought about major advances in the growth of agriculture in the West. Similarly, those who emigrated from Japan made a large impact in agriculture, on West Coast fishing, and in the canning industry. Filipinos freely migrated to the United States, mainly in response to the need for agricultural workers following the exclusion of Chinese and Japanese laborers. Mexican immigrants dominated California's agricultural labor force after 1900. Also, during this period, small numbers of immigrants from India also came to America as farmers. Obviously, with more people, the demand for food increased. New markets opened and with the influx of laborers came new ideas and techniques.

However, immigration—and how we react to immigrants—divided the nation, divided the labor force, and even divided the food industry. We can see the repetition today in our agricultural industry with exclusions and deportations impacting immigrant laborers. Many states' food industries have long depended on immigrants as migratory farm labor. Immigrant settlement helped to distinguish the American geography between urban and rural areas. Finally, immigration can be seen as a driving force in differentiating the two coasts, as the East Coast became more industrial, while the West Coast became more agricultural.

Finally, a novel written during this time focused on a man from Lithuania who had immigrated to Chicago and worked at a fictional Chicago meatpacking firm. Upton Sinclair's 1906 novel, *The Jungle*, as noted earlier in this book, changed consumers' perspectives of food quality and safety and triggered new regulations for purity and inspections. Sinclair was one of many writers and investigative reporters referred to as "Muckrakers" and "Progressives." Around the turn of the century, they pushed social activism and political reform to eliminate problems caused by industrialization, urbanization, immigration, and political corruption.

Before the Third Industrial Revolution started, the food industry would experience radical changes in how consumers get food, namely frozen foods, microwaveable meals, ready-to-eat foods, and fast-food restaurants. Children would want a new lunch box, with images from the latest TV show or movie, to take lunch to school. Supermarkets would become the central gathering place for shoppers. Malls would offer fashion and food courts for American teens.

The Third Industrial Revolution

The Third Industrial Revolution (The Digital Revolution) began in the 1980s and still can be seen now. This era includes the advancement of technology from analog electronic and mechanical devices to digital technology, the acceptance and growth of the personal computer, as well as the birth of the internet. Now, consumers have access to food and brand information and can even order meals online.

The technological changes that came about during this period allowed for the agriculture industry could keep up with two conflicting pressures: rapidly decreasing land available for farming and rapid population growth. This was a time when farmers began using new tools—including biotechnology in the forms of weed- and insect-resistant crops, genetically engineered crops and satellites for precision farming.

This was also the time (as pointed out in Chapter 2) when new concerns about food reputations (safety, security, defense, and authenticity) came about due to failures and to economically motivated crimes.

Food safety failures gained national and even global headlines as consumers' illnesses and deaths due to foodborne pathogens prompted demand for new regulations at a level not seen since Sinclair's book from almost 90 years earlier.

Food defense became priorities after the 1984 Rajneeshee bioterror attack through food poisoning in Oregon, the 2008 melamine scandal in China (when adulterated milk and infant formula caused over 300,000 illnesses, some 54,000 infants hospitalizations, and the deaths of 6 babies (Macartney, 2008)), and after the attacks on September 11, 2001.

Food authenticity grew slowly as a concern in the United States, when fraud within certain commodities (honey, seafood, etc.) began capturing headlines. Internationally, the 2013 horsemeat scandal in Europe prompted new laws and new agencies to investigate and prevent.

Finally, food security, which includes sustainability, has grown as a major international concern. The United Nations General Assembly passed a resolution in 2015 on Sustainable Development Goals (SDGs)—a set of 17 global ambitious, yet critical, goals for the year 2030 (see list of all 17 SDGs later). Though all the 17 goals have a connection to food (Rockström, 2016), some SDGs have names that provide a clearer connection to food, such as zero hunger, good health and well-being, clean water and sanitation, sustainable cities and communities, responsible consumption and production, climate action, life below water, and life on land. These SDGs reflect the challenges that technological advances in the Fourth Industrial Revolution (4IR) are geared to solve.

The 17 United Nations Sustainable Development Goals (SDGs):

1. No poverty
2. Zero hunger
3. Good health and well-being
4. Quality education
5. Gender equality
6. Clean water and sanitation
7. Affordable and clean energy
8. Decent work and economic growth
9. Industry, innovation, and infrastructure
10. Reduced inequality
11. Sustainable cities and communities
12. Responsible consumption and production
13. Climate action
14. Life below water
15. Life on land
16. Peace and justice strong institutions
17. Partnerships to achieve the goal

List of UN Sustainable Development Goals. Available from https://sustainabledevelopment.un.org/sdgs

Joseph Robertson is the Global Strategy Director at Citizens' Climate Lobby, an international grassroots environmental group that trains and supports volunteers to build relationships with their elected representatives in order to influence climate policy. In terms of the United Nations' SDGs, Robertson holds that:

> *"The more appropriate view of the SDGs is that they are a map of the challenges that determine whether human society will succeed or fail. The better we do, in terms of all of the SDGs, the easier everything is that we're trying to do. Food is of the things that is affected by all of this. If people are too poor, it's going to be harder to get food to people in traditional ways."*
>
> ***(Joseph Robertson, Personal Communication, 2019)***

Robertson stresses that these goals that came about near the end of the Third Industrial Revolution are a driving force for how we conceptualize the importance of the 4IR. To make his point, he uses a direct product of the Second Industrial Revolution as an example of the domino effect for us to consider:

> *"The 1930's Dust Bowl situation shows what happens if people [responsible for] producing food are too poor. They don't produce [as needed] and you have further difficulties such as the lack of education, gender equality, the ability to access energy affordably, decent work, sustainable cities, all of this determines whether or not we're able to produce food efficiently, reliably and sustainably, and affordably. When any of them are not working well enough, we find that it creates difficulties. So... the SDGs are not 'idealist aspirations'—they are ways of measuring whether we are succeeding or failing as a civilization."*
>
> ***(Joseph Robertson, Personal Communication, 2019)***

Gina McCarthy holds that this responsibility for the successes of civilization should reinforce the mission of the federal government to protect the people. As Professor of Public Health at Harvard University who previously served as the EPA Administrator during the Obama administration, McCarthy describes where this role of the federal government comes from.

> *"The federal government's role is to ensure that the public's rights to clean air, water and food are protected. When these public health necessities are compromised, the government's job is to step up and step in. For example, if air or water pollution is harming people' health then federal laws require that people's health be protected through the local, state and/or federal rules and regulations. Those regulations must be based on sound, independent, peer-reviewed science. They should be tailored to intervene in ways that are informed by history and analysis to ensure they will be effective at addressing the risk in the most cost-effective way. And they must be strongly enforced. Rules without compliance, and poorly designed rules are worse than doing nothing all. Why? Because they give the public a false sense of security. They make people believe that the government has done its job and their health is protected when in truth, people's ability to live health lives is still at risk."*
>
> ***(Gina McCarthy, Personal Communication, 2019)***

While the products of the Third Industrial Revolution opened new markets and created new job markets, this increasing sense of need to improve society and the environment shaped the next step in industry.

The Fourth Industrial Revolution

The 4IR (Industry 4.0) builds on the "Digital Revolution" with technology becoming embedded within societies and even the human body. We see the rise of robotics, Artificial Intelligence (AI), nanotechnology, quantum computing, blockchain, biotech, the Internet of Things (IOT), and autonomous vehicles. Many examples of using existing technologies to improve the food industry and benefit consumers include how blockchain pilot testing for use in food transparency and traceability is a key topic in the industry today. Additionally, automation is being explored in food manufacturing while companies are field-testing drones for food delivery.

Klaus Schwab, the founder and executive chairman of the World Economic Forum, describes how this 4IR is fundamentally different from the previous three, which were characterized mainly by advances in technology. The underlying basis for 4IR lies in advances in communication and connectivity rather than technology. These technologies have great potential to connect billions of more people to the web, improve business and organization efficiency, and help the environment and future generations. Schwab also describes this revolution as "... disrupting almost every industry in every country" as "the breadth and depth of these changes herald the transformation of entire systems of production, management, and governance" (Schwab, 2017). Thus, this 4IR is not so much about new technologies as it is about what we can do with existing technologies.

This concept can already be seen in early 2019; the FDA addressed these advancements and the agency's expectations for the future of food safety and technology. According to a joint statement from Norman Sharpless, MD, the FDA's Acting Commissioner of Food and Drugs, and Frank Yiannas, the FDA's Deputy Commissioner for Food Policy and Response:

> *"We expect to see more innovation in the agriculture, food production, and food distribution systems in the next 10 years than we've seen in the past 20, which will continue to provide an even greater variety of food options and delivery conveniences to American consumers. With this ever-changing landscape, we know we must continue preparing to take advantage of new opportunities and address potential risks."*
>
> ***(FDA, 2019a)***

Specifically, the FDA announced what they are calling a "New Era of Smarter Food Safety" to augment food safety compliance by leveraging "the use of new and emerging technologies" with a goal to develop a "Blueprint" to "address several areas, including traceability, digital technologies and evolving food business models" (FDA, 2019a). The FDA held a public meeting on October 21, 2019, in which the focus for this "Blueprint" included four key areas:

1. **Tech-Enabled Traceability and Foodborne Outbreak Response**: Looking at technologies, data streams, and processes that will greatly reduce the time it takes to track and trace the origin of a contaminated food and respond to public health risks.
2. **Smarter Tools and Approaches for Prevention**: Enhancing the use of new knowledge from traceback, data streams and tools for rapidly analyzing data. The ability to use new data analysis tools and predictive analytics will help FDA and stakeholders better identify and mitigate potential food safety risks and advance the preventive controls framework that FSMA established.
3. **Adapting to New Business Models and Retail Food Safety Modernization:** Advancing the safety of both new business models, such as e-commerce and home delivery of foods, and traditional business models, such as retail food establishments.
4. **Food Safety Culture:** Promoting and recognizing the role of food safety culture on farms and in facilities. This involves doing more to influence what employees and companies think about food safety and how they demonstrate a commitment to this work. Strengthening food safety cultures also extends to the home and FDA is working to educate consumers on safe food handling practices. (FDA, 2019b).

Industry provides many examples of innovation along these lines. Sean O'Leary is the CEO of FoodLogiQ, a company that provides traceability, food safety compliance, and supply chain transparency software solutions that companies can integrate with their existing systems. Before a large meeting of platform users from a variety of major brands in food manufacturing, retail, and restaurants, O'Leary pointed to an image of the CDC's annual estimates for foodborne illness, hospitalizations, and deaths. After a pause, he introduced a call-to-action as he stated: "If the food industry could use technology with the goal of reducing these numbers by just 1%, imagine the impact that would have on thousands of American families each year" (O'Leary, 2019). This is exactly the kind of solutions-based use of technology that embodies the 4IR.

Another company, Relevant Systems, Inc., based in Boston, has developed FoodCode-Pro, "an innovative, intuitive software platform for food safety inspectors. According to Michael Hicks, the company's President and a cofounder, "We are staking the future of the company on the adoption of digital, mobile tools that will drive the efficient and effective operationalization of the FDA Food Code" (Michael Hicks, Personal Communication, 2019). Thus, this company's model of helping inspectors uniformly collect data is not so much new technology, but a way of using existing technology to enable data-driven assessment of food establishments and, thus, better protect consumers from foodborne pathogens.

For consumers, this current revolution has allowed new gains in access to information about foodborne illness symptoms and precautions, recalls and outbreaks, restaurant inspection results, and other information critical for making decisions. Another addition is the ability of consumers to contribute to crowdsourced data related to foodborne illness. Patrick Quade's website "IWasPoisoned.com" is one of a new collection of online platforms that provide opportunities for stakeholder voice and impact for the industry. The website sees 600,000 page views per month, but these are not all from consumers.

> *"It's not just restaurants but, grocery chains... the food industry, in general, corporate through industry, and public health agencies. And then we also have had a decent amount of interest from the insurance and investment fund sectors. They want to understand the risks inside their portfolio. Some companies are riskier on food safety than others and there's not really a good way to look at that. So, we provide insights into what we're seeing from a consumer reporting perspective."*
>
> ***(Patrick Quade, Personal Communication, 2019)***

I attended the FDA's October 21, 2019, public meeting on the New Era of Smarter Food Safety and provided insight from my multiple perspectives. Here is the statement I provided in an attempt to frame these 'eras' with how they relate to those who impact and are impacted by them.

> *"As a professor of food policy, I now teach graduate students who were born after the landmark, 1993 "Jack in the Box"* E. coli *outbreak. In the era since then, the food industry has embraced a "food safety culture"-described by some as a change in farm-to-fork beliefs, practices, and values behind combating foodborne illness. Food safety regulations are still being modernized while new technologies offer promises for enhanced traceability and transparency. During this same time, however, consumers have been continuously bombarded with evidence of the seemingly uninterrupted cycle of crisis-and-reform. They - we - witness the growing variety of contaminated foods, new ways in which foods became contaminated, unpredicted causes for failures in food safety mitigation, and the addition of thousands of*

families each year who will live with a chair forever empty at their dinner tables. Unlike most of us, my graduate students grew up with words and phrases such as "E. coli," "foodborne pathogen," "multi-state outbreak," and "recall" as part of their social media feeds, Instagram posts, viral videos, and even memes. They developed skillsets and confidence with digital tools and technology platforms that we are only now exploring for use in the food industry. What should we call these future food industry workers and leaders? The most useful designation I have found for them is Food Safety Culture's Next Generation, *as they are native speakers of the culture, having been born into the modern era of legal, economic, political, technological, and social aspects of food safety. So what does that make the rest of us... who were not born into this culture of food safety, as it came about at some later point in our lives and careers? Perhaps we are* Food Safety Culture's Founders. *The importance of the distinction is this: The* Food Safety Culture's Founders *may not share the fluency of digital tools like artificial intelligence, Blockchain, and predictive analytics that this* Next Generation *has acquired through their years of interaction and practice. However, in an industry bursting with big data,* members of this Next Generation *stand to benefit from the* Founders' *knowledge and experience of the true burden of disease as well as compliance challenges before and throughout the previous era of change in food safety. With all the discussion of artificial intelligence in this new FDA blueprint, failure to incorporate ethics and a better understanding of the human condition will not support the effective and sustained efforts to Promote Food Safety Culture Throughout the Food System. As a father who lost his son to* E. coli *in that landmark, 1993 outbreak, I have high expectations for any and all Eras of Smarter Food Safety. My son and too many others are part of* Food Safety's 'Lost' Generation" *(Detwiler, 2019).*

Detwiler, D. (2019, October 21). "Personal Statement at FDA Public Meeting." Rockville, MD.

With an understanding of this current period of the 4IR and how we got here, one can now explore a number of changes—beyond the obvious ones related to food safety—that can be connected clearly to the increase in population (Fig. 10.1). These changes will ultimately have an impact on consumers' confidence and on their lives.

Climate change

Food reputation reaches beyond food safety as consumers have become increasingly more at-risk due to failures or attacks related to food defense, food security, and food authenticity. "One thing that not everybody thinks about when they think about climate and food sustainability, is the scale of that challenge. Food is the biggest and most widespread human undertaking" (Joseph Robertson, Personal Communication, 2019). Protecting consumers in today's global food supply is, thus, a complex issue as it involves fundamental changes in science, technology, policy, and industry

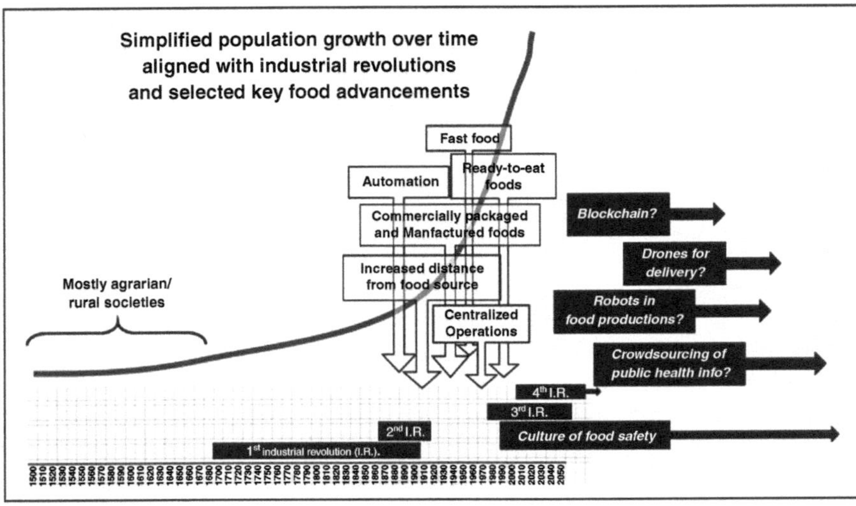

Figure 10.1 Simplified population growth over time aligned with industrial revolutions and selected key food advancements. *(Author from Lecture Material).*

considerations from the farm to the fork. Further, this challenge is one on the international stage.

Climate change impacts food safety hazards at various stages of the food chain. One 2010 multinational study found a series of climate-related factors to include: changes in temperature and precipitation patterns (which also impact the transmission of parasites and foodborne pathogens); increased frequency and intensity of extreme weather events; ocean warming and acidification; changes in contaminants' transport pathways; and socio-economic aspects related to food systems such as agriculture, animal production, global trade, demographics, and human behavior (Tirado, Clarke, Jaykus, McQuatters-Gollop, & Frank, 2010). In the future, part of that human behavior concern is the expected increase in the frequency of pesticide applications.

Gina McCarthy speaks before audiences and her students about climate change's impact on air pollution and water supply, and the displacement of agriculture and of people as a result of climate change's damage to land. Her call to action for audiences: "People need to reframe the narrative around climate change as an issue about people" (McCarthy, 2019).

Though climate change and food may seem like a new concern today, it is anything but new. "Throughout history, much of the instability in the world is a result of a fight over arable land and over clean water. We just think we're well beyond that, but we're not—fundamentally. Those two staples are what life is all about and the world will fight over them and climate change will make those fights more frequent, more intense, and much more difficult to manage over time" (Gina McCarthy, Personal Communication, 2019).

For consumers, climate change can be seen as a threat to two of the lower "Needs" pertaining to "Physiological Needs" (air, water, food, shelter, sleep, survival) followed by those needs pertaining to "Safety and Security" (personal and financial, health and well-being) in Abraham Maslow's "Hierarchy of Needs" from his theory in psychology proposed in his 1943 paper "A Theory of Human Motivation" (Maslow, 1943, as cited in Healy, 2018). Higher needs include "Social Needs" (friends and family), "Esteem" (self-esteem, confidence, achievement), and "Self-Actualization" (creativity, realization of potential).

Clearly, when consumers are unable to achieve either of the first two of Maslow's "Needs," then they are unable to even approach the higher "Needs" in life.

Placing Maslow's Hierarchy alongside Archie Carroll's 1991 "Pyramid of Corporate Social Responsibility" relative to the "Moral Management of Organizational Stakeholders," one can see why corporations may not prioritize food and climate and the environment in the same way as consumers.

According to Carroll, corporations' first "Responsibility" is that of simple economics: be profitable. Next, a corporation can start focusing on legal responsibilities: obey the law. Only after meeting these two responsibilities can most corporations start to shift their key focus on to ethical responsibilities and philanthropic responsibilities—both of which are where the alignment with consumers' basic needs can be found (Fig. 10.2).

Granted, many companies do not need to be legally required to do the right thing, as they will do this as part of their own ethos. But erosion of legal and economic consequences has and will continue to allow some corporations to maximize profit at the expense of the climate, the environment, their consumers, and of future generations. Joseph Robertson cautions that environmental concerns, much like all the UN's SDGs, must be taken more seriously than as seen in how they are often prioritized in industry.

> *"People think of [SDGs] like 'nice ideas' that you might achieve in an 'ideal world' and that we think about and work towards only for charitable reasons. That way of thinking is self-defeating on all sides. If you're the cynic who thinks that way, it is self-defeating to think that is ideal and that they will never affect you . . . one can just choose not to care. And if you are the idealist that you think that [these goals] are only nice or idea, then it is also self-defeating, because you're narrowing your team to those who think like you and you're kind of giving a pass to those who are not."*
>
> **(Joseph Robertson, Personal Communication, 2019)**

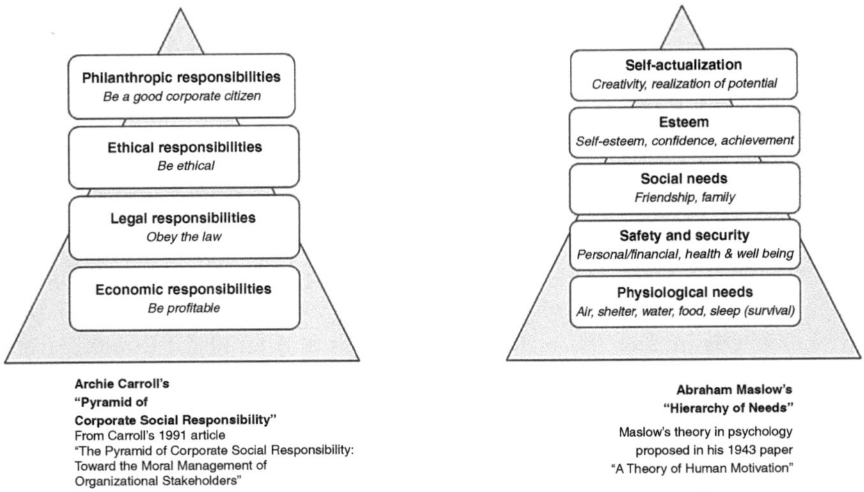

Figure 10.2 "Alignment of Maslow's Hierarchy of Needs" with Carroll's "Pyramid of Corporate Social Responsibility." *(Based on the work of Maslow, 1942, cited in Healy, 2018 and Carroll, 1991).*

Climate change, thus, becomes equally a focus on the transition of the environment, and what we consume from it, as well as the transition of how we, as a society, as consumers, and as voters prioritize it. During a 2019 public event "The Climate Is Changing, Are We?" held by Gina McCarthy, former EPA Administrator, and John Kerry former Secretary of State, neither were not shy about her dismay at the Trump administration's political inaction. McCarthy and Kerry reframed the issue of climate change as one concerning national security, the economy, public health, and listed food safety and other food concerns as one of the top five benefits of reducing carbon emissions.

McCarthy asserts that "When an administration [looks towards] goals of smaller government … they neglect to understand the implications from a health and safety perspective." To combat this way of thinking, she stresses that we, as a society, need to stop ignoring history, which tells us that "no company and no person is fit to be the best judge of their own work" (Gina McCarthy, Personal Communication, 2019).

Beyond the United States, geopolitical factors also need to be considered. Kerry reminded the audience of our nation's achievements in World War II. He recalls his trips to Normandy and the lessons written by Yale historian Paul Kennedy in his book "The Engineers ofVictory" (2013) about four or five key decisions made in order to win the war. Bringing this point to climate change, Kerry added that:

> *"We are at an equal level of critical choosing right now. We ought to be on a war-time footing with respect to this issue because it's going to take nothing less than that, to orchestrate the size of the transformation that has to take place with respect to transportation, with respect to industry … with respect to agriculture … all of which are the key parts of what is causing climate change."*
>
> ***(Kerry, 2019)***

Specifically, Kerry described how the numbers of "climate refugees" exist and are going to increase. He also offered a warning about the fight over water that is already taking place and how, "when the great rivers [of the world] start drying up and changing their capacity to provide food to people, we're going to have a huge food dislocation" (Kerry, 2019). McCarthy also ties climate change to how, in many parts of the world, food instability forces migration:

> *"After significant floods in Syria and years of drought in Honduras and Guatemala and other places (that are likely very consistent with climate change that we're seeing) it's literally forcing people to leave, not because they want to or they are looking for a better life, but because they have no life there, they can't put food on the table."*
>
> ***(Gina McCarthy, Personal Communication, 2019)***

Every part of the food system is, in one way or another, impacted by climate change: how we store food and transport that food effectively, how we keep it fresh and keep it refrigerated and at the temperature that it needs to be with increased heat and all the flooding that's happening. At the same time, climate experts warn that food manufacturing impacts the environment and climate change itself, as a source of significant greenhouse gas emissions. Change can come through finding disruptive technologies and shaping consumer demand for companies to "refrigerate without the use of high global warming chemicals," to stop "using excess amount of pesticides," and to "prevent spoilage or to reduce the food waste from farm to table" (Gina McCarthy, Personal Communication, 2019).

For the food industry, entire economic models still depend on one critical element—the demand of consumers. As such, their business is impacted by the same basic threats faced by human beings. Several major food companies can already be characterized as prioritizing, investing, and training with a look to the future and how climate change impacts not only their brand's success, but also their sustainability.

One might not think of climate change while eating a burger, but Jorge Hernandez, Vice President of Quality at the Wendy's Company, has often shared with audiences how he sees disruptive technologies and changes in consumer preference impacting food safety. Another issue he brings up is how global warming impacts food safety here in the United States—not just in more obvious places like Dubai. To Hernandez, climate-based technologies in the food industry "bring economic opportunities to regions that previously have been unable to support year-round agriculture production due to geography and climate" (Jorge Hernandez, Personal Communication, 2019).

Founded in 1987, Amy's Kitchen is a family-owned, privately held company in California that manufactures organic and non-GMO convenience and frozen foods. Anna Jesus, their Vice President, Quality and Food Safety, describes how Amy's Kitchen views responding to climate change not only as part of sustainability and social responsibility, but also as "integral foundations for food safety."

> *"We believe that without the basic human needs being met (safety, security, food, and shelter), it's not possible for individuals to make higher level food safety decisions for other people. Amy's was built on the principles of respect for Earth. Organic practices such as those espoused in* Silent Spring *[Rachel Carson's landmark 1962 environmental science book] were part of our founding principles. Additionally, climate change threatens vegetables crops as much as anything, so that's our bread and butter."*
>
> ***(Anna Jesus, Personal Communication, 2019)***

Changes in farming

A look at just one of the leafy-greens outbreaks from early 2018 highlights the need to think about food safety solutions that are not, on their face, food safety solutions. The *E.coli* outbreak tied to farms in Yuma, AZ, responsible for 210 reported illnesses across 36 states, 96 hospitalizations, 27 patients developing HUS, and 5 deaths (and which drew criticism after the CDC warned the public to avoid lettuce grown in that region).

Investigators who went to the farms in Yuma, AZ, to determine the source of the *E. coli*, found that it came from canal water used to irrigate the region. On November 1, 2018, the FDA released a statement from FDA Commissioner Scott Gottlieb, MD, on findings from the outbreak investigation and FDA's efforts to prevent future outbreaks. In the statement, Gottlieb discussed how federal and state officials tested the irrigation water, looked at other factors, including "soil amendments, growing and harvesting practices, animal intrusion, adjacent land use, and employee health and hygiene practices" (Gottlieb, 2018). They also examined potential contamination sources at manufacturing and processing operations.

"When and how the irrigation canal became contaminated with the outbreak strain of E. coli *O157:H7 is also uncertain. We know that a large concentrated animal feeding operation (CAFO) is located adjacent to this stretch of the irrigation canal where the samples were collected. This is one potential source. However, the investigation did not identify an obvious route for contamination of the irrigation canal from this facility. In addition, samples collected at the CAFO did not yield* E. coli *O157:H7. The investigation did not exclude other ways the irrigation canal could have become contaminated with this outbreak strain."*

(Gottlieb, 2018)

The FDA Commissioner recommended that leafy-greens producers take steps to prevent future, similar outbreaks, including assuring that agricultural water is safe for its intended use and assessing potential direct or indirect contamination risks (such as CAFOs) near growing fields. One way to do this, though not mentioned in Gottlieb's statement, is the use of alternative farming operations, such as hydroponics, container farming, and other similar practices.

Whereas this may seem like a way of farming that is not currently visible, hydroponics and container farming (sometimes both in the same operation) has gained considerable support from industry experts and in the government sector.

Former FDA Deputy Commissioner for Foods and Veterinary Medicine, Stephen Ostroff, MD, has thought about these operations as a solution for many food concerns, including food safety, for some time. He agrees that there would never be any guarantee of "zero risk," but, at the same time, recognizes that this is a way we can lower the risk:

"There's just something inherently problematic about things like leafy-greens. And even with all of the research ... trying to figure out how you can make them safer, there are still going to be risks associated with those types of products. I try to remain an optimist about this, but, either they've been ignoring the last 10 years or so of repeated problems, or they haven't quite figured out what the right basket of changes is.

What would really be a game changer for something like leafy-greens: grow them hydroponically or grow them indoors. You know, such as taking big office buildings in New York City and turning them into greenhouses ... some call it vertical farming or indoor vertical farming. I'm sure that there's probably enough data these days to show that hydroponically-grown products, aquaponically-grown products, and products that are grown indoors will not have the same risk profile for foodborne pathogens as the stuff grown outside. In fact, I'm not aware of outbreaks associated with hydroponically-grown products."

(Stephen Ostroff, Personal Communication, 2019)

Brad McNamara is the CEO and cofounder of Freight Farms, the world's leading manufacturer of container farming technology, in Boston, MA. McNamara's journey into the future of produce farming included a shift in how the next generation of technology for food sustainability impacts food safety and even food defense. Hydroponic vegetable production through container farming, also known as vertical farming and by other variations, fits the very definition of 4IR (Fig. 10.3).

> *"We have officially been a company since 2012. At the time, we were a complete outlier. Indoor or controlled environment agriculture was a greenhouse and there were some people who are talking about maybe you should do that in warehouse. When we started, our view of the industry was that we can use technology and design to create more efficiencies that allows you to go smaller, not bigger and go to more places, not less. I think we were officially the first to put a commercial type farm into a modular set up. Now, you've got all the indoor agriculture conferences, controlled environment conferences, the greenhouse track, and container track."*
>
> ***(Brad McNamara, Personal Communication, 2019)***

> *"When we first envisioned what we were trying to build, we had come off with the urban rooftop greenhouse development and it seemed like an obvious fit. What*

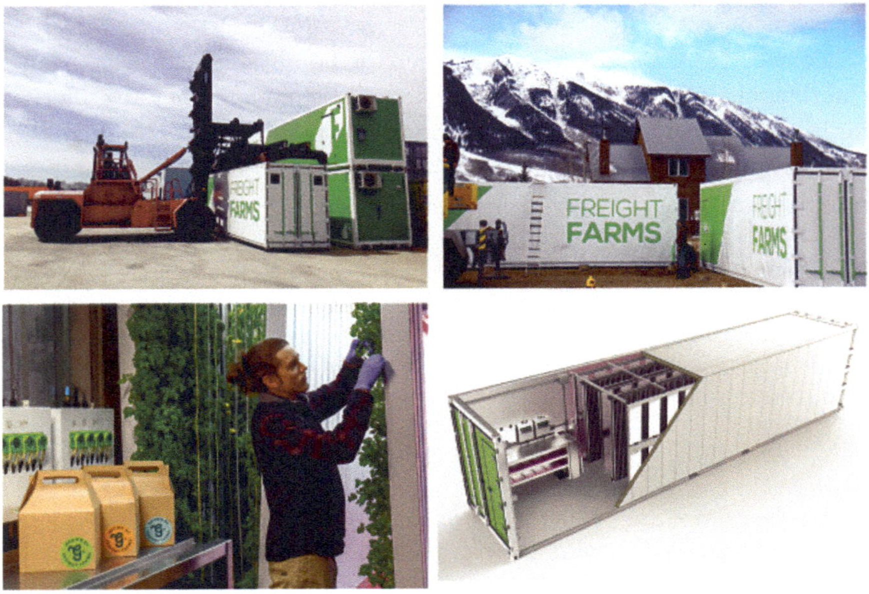

Figure 10.3 Container farms being stacked (top left), container farms in operation through winter (top right), inside a leafy-green vegetable container farm (bottom left), and computer rendering of cut-away view of container farm (bottom right). *(Photos from Freight Farms (used by permission).)*

was really fascinating, and I think something that we underestimated, was the kind of the market and the demand for it was when we put together a really nice solution that anybody could access, anybody could use and they could put it anywhere and grow food. And what's been the most fascinating part of the journey has been seeing what the different use cases have been."

(Brad McNamara, Personal Communication, 2019)

Before Freight Farms could sell a food technology solution for concerns such as sustainability, a characteristic most of their clients think of first, the company had to satisfy food safety compliance aspects of the concept.

"When we started to grow ... we had to think about food safety very differently, because some of our partners are going to be at the big foods, institutional food service companies. They would walk into the room and drop a 400-page book and one would think 'Whoa, all right, they must be safe.' When we were looking at food safety, so much of it just didn't apply: not manure handling, not the chemicals, not runoff, etc."

(Brad McNamara, Personal Communication, 2019)

Another aspect of container farming is how much, or little, opportunity for alignment with blockchain it offers. Blockchain, as an optimization tool for complicated food supply systems, is intended to document all the various transactions in harvesting, holding facilities, processing facilities, and distribution centers. Using a container farm to do this for a school, an assisted living center, a restaurant, even for a prison or a military base (all examples of where Freight Farms' containers can be found), the "chain" of transactions becomes extremely short. What increases for the users, then, includes accountability, protection from outside attacks (food defense), and isolation from potential recalls and outbreaks out in the market.

"Actually, it was almost like a rethinking or reimagining of food safety in terms of new risk factors by doing things the way we're doing them. And what we realized was that it came down to the human element. In any food safety protocol, humans tend to be the weak link."

(Brad McNamara, Personal Communication, 2019)

Many companies agree with this notion, adding that we have all the technology that we need to radically reduce foodborne risks, but what it comes down to is humans either who are unaware of safe practices or who do not care about them. Whereas the human factor inside the operations may be categorized as a risk, the human factor in the market, however, is seen as an asset.

"For us, the first wave is moving the farm right to where people are, and we already have this generation of 'Millennials' that's aware, and then you have 'Gen Z,' which is in reality going to be bigger than 'Millennials,' going to have more buying power

and all the things that move the needle economically in this world and this country, and who are going to have exposure to how food could be grown, what food safety really means, and how to simplify things."

(Brad McNamara, Personal Communication, 2019)

Large fast-food chains are starting to explore and even use indoor and hydroponic farming operations for their ingredients. Jorge Hernandez believes we should "explore any technology that can improve food safety, provide business value and a better product for the customers. In fact, growing romaine lettuce in greenhouses and hydroponic farms is not a far-fetched reality" (Jorge Hernandez, Personal Communication, 2019). Hernandez not only agrees with the use of indoor and hydroponic farming, but also points to examples at The Wendy's Company.

"Here at Wendy's we've been working to get all our tomatoes for US and Canada grown in greenhouses and hydroponic farms. This source allows us to control and improve not only their food safety and quality but also their flavor/taste. In addition, greenhouse farms provide supply predictability, protection of crops from harsh weather, a safe, indoor growing conditions and a significant reduction of pesticides use. Greenhouses also support local economies by sustaining the agricultural workforce with fresh produce that can be grown year-round in comfortable, indoor environments."

(Jorge Hernandez, Personal Communication, 2019)

Changes in protein production

The previous examples of new farming processes are nowhere near as controversial as new processes for protein production. Consumer trends in lifestyle and diet have become a driving force in the food industry. However, Stephen Ostroff's experience at the FDA left him with the insight that the food supply is going to change whether consumers want it to or not.

"You have a large swath of the population that is very much traditionalist: they like the food supply that they knew and they loved. They want animal-slaughtered meat, they want traditional produce, they want stuff that they've known and are comfortable with. And those folks may never gravitate to some of the newer innovations going on in the food supply. But some part of the population will."

(Stephen Ostroff, Personal Communication, 2019)

Soy burgers, veggie burgers, quinoa burgers, and pea protein-based burgers, such as "Beyond Burger" and "The Impossible Burger" offer vegetarian- and vegan-friendly options for protein. Impossible Foods, Inc., the company behind "The Impossible Burger," differentiates itself in stating that, "compared to cattle production" they use "95 percent less land,

74 percent less water, and create 87 percent less greenhouse gas emissions" (Migala, 2019). Opponents of plant-based hamburger patties argue that these products are made of over 20 ingredients and that some of them may not be that healthy for consumers. Some also point out that the impossible meat "uses genetically modified soy protein, drawing criticism from anti-GMO groups" (Atkin, 2019).

Opponents of "clean-meat," also called cell-cultured or lab-cultured meat, argue that these new, disruptive company products that will try to compete with traditional meats cannot call themselves "meat." In February 2019, the US Cattlemen's Association (USCA) filed a petition with USDA's Food Safety and Inspection Service (FSIS) requested that the agency officially limit the labeling of "beef" and "meat" to products that meet their common dictionary definitions. Specifically, the association requested that "products that are labeled as 'meat' should be limited to those that are derived from the tissue or flesh of an animal harvested in the traditional manner" (USCA, 2019). Those who support these new products argue that people know that "plant-based meat" and "lab-cultured meat" do not actually come from animals, just as almond milk does not come from a cow. Further, they argue that prohibiting the use of the word "meat" on the label is a violation of the First Amendment (Selyukh, 2019).

In terms of regulation, the USDA's FSIS and the FDA announced a formal agreement in March 2019 to collaborate their resources to regulate the development and oversee the production of human food using new technologies "to derive cell-cultured products derived from the cell lines of livestock and poultry." This shared regulatory approach is intended to ensure that these foods are produced safely and accurately labeled before entry into commerce (USDA, 2019).

In terms of food safety, experts assert that these alternatives to meat offer consumers a way to reduce their chances of becoming sick from foodborne pathogens. Stephen Ostroff very much agrees.

> *"One of the things that I think is an overlooked aspect of this is that … these new products can potentially really make a dent in the incidence of foodborne disease. I truly believe that lab-grown meat is not going to have* Salmonella *in it. It's not going to have campylobacter in it. It's not going to have* E. coli *O157 in it. At least when this stuff comes into your home, it's not contaminated. The fact that you're bringing less [pathogens] into your kitchen, I think probably would be beneficial."*
>
> ***(Stephen Ostroff, Personal Communication, 2019)***

In August 2019, Stefan Palzer, Nestlé's Chief Technology Officer, spoke before an audience in Switzerland about the many trends in food that Nestlé sees. Palzer described how "plant-based nutrition is exploding" while listing a number of other formats as part of an "explosion of different dietary patterns" that are "causing a lot of challenges but also opportunities in the food space." These new, growing trends in food formats include vegetarian, paleo, pagan, pescatarian, ketogenic, low carb diets, lactose-free, and dairy-free (Morrison, 2019).

Whereas consumer trends may gain traction in the industry and attention on social media, the creation of new food market opportunities comes at a time when new definitions of these products and manufacturing technologies challenge the regulations meant to protect consumers. In 2015, prior to publishing the seven rules under the Food Safety Modernization Act, the FDA found the need to update some seemingly common definitions from regulatory statutes that dated back over 100 years. The new regulations came with a more broadened definition of "farm" and with specific differentiation for "raw agricultural products" (from the simple definition of produce) as a means to ensure that the implementation of the Act would reflect and encompass the modern food production landscape. Future food trends, including where it comes from, the ingredients used, and the manufacturing process, will continue to challenge regulations and the authority of state and federal agencies.

Changes in food retail

Another challenge to regulating food safety can be found in the ways in which food is sold to consumers. The US Department Commerce reported in 2015 that sales at restaurants and bars overtook spending at grocery stores for the first time in American history (Jamrisko, 2015). At the same time, the line between retail and restaurant became blurred by what the National Restaurant Association calls "retail-host restaurants"—"one of the fastest growing segments for restaurant food" (Flynn, 2016). These types of hybrid establishments actually existed earlier in the 20th century, such as seen with the Woolworth Department Store's lunch counters made famous by the 1960s Civil Rights sit-ins.

That trend had died off until now. Modern examples include major supermarkets with restaurants/self-serve options that offer hot meals, as well as beer and wine service—including full-service pubs, as well as many convenience stores offering sit-down food services. Even movie theaters have joined this trend and have gone beyond retail of drinks, popcorn, and candy to include full-service dining options. The National Restaurant Association's definition of retail/restaurant hybrids now includes health and personal care store restaurants, general merchandise/variety store restaurants, food store and grocery store restaurants—including a portion of deli and salad bars, and gasoline service station restaurants. This trend is growing at surprising rates. Sales by these in-store restaurants in 2015 topped $40 billion. Hybrids took in about $3 out of every $4 in revenue generated by the retailer. Further, hybrid establishments are growing at a rate of nearly 6% per year (Flynn, 2016). With this trend, perhaps, comes an explanation for why the CDC reports that 40% of foodborne illness cases are related to retail food consumption (Jones, Pavlin, & LaFluer, 2004).

Regulations pertinent to restaurants and retail stores (see Chapter 8) are perceived by consumers as being uniform, when, in fact, FDA Food Code guidance as interpreted and adopted by local jurisdictions are anything but uniform from state to state and, in some cases, county to county. Another consumer trend is the growth of farmers' markets, Community Supported Agricultures (CSAs), "on-farm markets," home or community food gardens, and cottage foods. Jurisdictional differences aside, one must also consider the impact on food safety for these operations.

Farmers' markets/CSAs/on-farm markets

The Foods Safety Modernization Act (FSMA) (see Chapter 7) targets foods that are usually consumed raw, such as apples and grapes. For food that is not usually consumed raw, like grains, rhubarb, and potatoes, the rule does not apply. Further, FSMA is only for food intended for sale in the United States—thus, the rules do not apply to a family that grows food solely for themselves.

In terms of businesses that averaged less than $25,000 in sales over the last three years, some operations are exempt from the FSMA rules. Some other exemptions do apply. However, a number of other regulations, such as those under the Pure Food and Drug Act and local commercial or other laws, still apply.

The popular CSA operations would only need to meet modified requirements of FSMA, as long as their annual sales are less than $500,000 a year and sales are all to qualified end users. Seasonal, weekly farmers markets, with annual sales less than $25,000, are not covered under FSMA. On-farm markets, such as ones with large-scale produce operations and, on Fall weekends open to the public for activities such as apple picking, hayrides, petting zoos, sandwich counters, packaged foods, etc., are not likely exempt from FSMA rules if their total food sales exceed $500,000.

Home/community food gardens

Whereas FSMA does not apply to these types of farming operations, local regulations—even some that have nothing to do with food safety—often apply and become prohibitive. Michigan State, along with other states, banned backyard farming, thus limiting, if not preventing altogether the ability for Americans to grow their own food and feed themselves. Michigan also removed protection for small home farmers from the Right to Farm Act (RTFA). Again, other states have their version of RTFAs as well. Some interpret these laws as protecting large producers who do not want individuals to provide for themselves or their families, thus ensuring that American consumers depend on grocers and major brands for their food. This is not simply a city problem, however. "The new changes affect residents of rural Michigan too. It is not simply an urban or suburban concern" (Papple, 2014).

In some locations, zoning codes ban front-yard vegetable gardens. In one case, a family, fighting for the right to replant their garden, after being fined and forced to dig it up, was declined having their case heard by the Florida Supreme Court (Leibrock, 2018). Some states and counties have revised or removed these preventative laws, but not all.

Local laws aside, a 2014 report by the National Gardening Association found that the number of home food gardens increased by 29% from 2008 to 2013 with some 9 million urban households growing their own food. Similarly, the National Gardening Association found that the participation of households in community gardens increased 200% during the same period (National Gardening Association, 2014). A 2012 *New York Times* report noted that the rise in home food gardens is a byproduct of water shortages and the "growing interest in sustainability" (Kurutzdec, 2012).

Cottage foods

According to guidance documentation from the Association for Food and Drug Officials (AFDO), a "cottage food operation" is one in which a person produces cottage food products only in the home kitchen of that person's primary domestic residence and only for sale directly to the consumer. A cottage food operation shall not operate as a food service establishment, retail food store, or wholesale food manufacturer (AFDO, 2012).

Important to the interpretation of this definition are a few more of AFDO's guidance definitions. "Cottage food products" are defined as "non-potentially hazardous baked goods, jams, jellies, and other non-potentially hazardous foods produced at a cottage food operation." "Domestic residence" is defined as a single-family dwelling or an area within a rental unit where a single person or family actually resides. A domestic residence does not include any group or communal residential setting within any type of structure, or outbuilding, shed, barn, or other similar structure. A "Home kitchen" is defined as "a kitchen designed and intended for use by the residents of a home but that is also used by a resident for the production of cottage food products. It may contain one or more stoves or ovens, which may be a double oven, designed for residential use. It shall not include commercial types of equipment typically used for large wholesale manufacturing." And finally, "Potentially hazardous food (time/temperature control for safety food)" is defined as "a food that requires time/temperature control for safety to limit pathogenic microorganism growth or toxin formation" (AFDO, 2012).

Joe Corby, former Executive Director of AFDO, warns about cottage food businesses and food safety. "We [AFDO] deal with cottage foods, which concerns us. Some of those people don't have any insurance on those food products and when they're involved in an outbreak ... they're definitely out of business. There's no question" (Joe Corby, Personal Communication, 2019).

At the 2019 International Association for Food Protection (IAFP), David McSwane, Executive Director at Conference for Food Protection, shared his worries about why food safety regulations pertaining to cottage foods are prioritized (or not).

> *"We know there's some social values and value-related aspects to that are going to drive some of the decisions that people make. A lot of discussion going on, even this conference, when it comes to some food freedom laws and cottage food laws. If you dig down deep and you see what's happening in the state level, there's a lot of conversations, a lot of them are far from a science-based conversation."*
>
> ***(McSwane, 2019)***

With changes in how and where consumers are buying food, their assumptions that they are making better, healthier choices are not always supported by regulatory oversight—at least not on oversight that is consistent across jurisdictions. Future considerations for food safety regulation must be based on science and not allow for gaps due to consumers' zip codes or the type of retail establishment they frequent.

Changes in food delivery

Valerie Madamba, Senior Counsel, Regulatory Compliance and Government Affairs at Blue Apron, envisions the food industry using greater automation to remove human error when interacting with food: "I predict new models in the future—driver-less delivery cars or unattended delivery drones .... the continued course of greater automation, delivery, production .... different ways in interacting with our food and maybe taking a lot of the human element and human error out of food handling and food production" (Valerie Madamba, Personal Communication, 2019).

Madamba's predictions are not too far off. In addition to the start of "Food Watch" in Dubai (as discussed in Chapter 9), advances in technologies related to food delivery in that region are also being embraced to answer the impacts of population density, climate, and the amount of food imported to the region. Delivery from restaurants to homes has long been handled by motorcycle delivery. But this increases food costs to consumers while failing to solve some access problems caused by traffic and high-rise building. Consumers in Dubai took part in trials of food delivery by drones last year (Lewis, 2018).

New Zealand has already tested drones—also known as "unmanned aerial vehicles" for food delivery service. Domino's Pizza completed a 2016 trial in New Zealand after the government reviewed laws for driverless vehicles and initiated new aviation rules applicable to commercial use of drones (*Khaleej Times*, 2016). This year, trials of food delivery by drone are being conducted in North Carolina and Virginia (Kelso, 2019).

Changes in food production technology use

While unmanned aerial and ground vehicles offer solutions for delivery to consumers, robotic technologies inside the food manufacturing plant offer new solutions for issues related to labor, safety, and sanitation. Early adopters of this kind of technology brought in robots for palletizing operations with heavy loads to prevent injury. Other actions currently being handled by robots include cutting, handling, sorting, and sensing—including X-rays and CT scans along the food production line. But even these technologies in the food industry are often criticized for not having been adopted earlier.

At the 2019 meeting of the IAFP in Louisville, KY, a panel of experts convened to discuss the "Impact of Robotics and Artificial Intelligence on Food Safety." One panelist, Mike Harper, representing Soft Robotics in Massachusetts, shared his views on the "Impact of Robotics on Food Manufacturing." He pointed out how the 1915 Ford Motor Company "Model T" assembly line used people, while the 2019 Tesla "Model S" assembly line uses robots. At the same points in time, produce operations in 1915 used people where today these same fields look no different (Harper, 2019).

Another panelist, Ian Jenson, representing meat and livestock in Australia, presented on the "Potential for Robotic Processing of Red Meat: Food Safety Implications." Jenson (2019) highlighted how the early 20th-century Ford Motor Company assembly line was derived from the meat slaughter lines after the implementation of USDA inspection in 1906. Using robots may be one way of thinking outside the box for solutions in food production, but others are thinking inside the box.

Change in how consumers align food with values

Aside from the Culture of Food Safety talked about earlier in this book, the food industry has come to better understand significant changes in consumers' behaviors and decision-making. Beyond food safety, blockchain is hyped as "the" tool to make the supply chain more transparent and to assure consumers that they are supporting brands that align with their personal ethics. Consumers vote with their food dollars and often make purchase decisions on issues unrelated to food safety. Call it the Millennial Effect or just a sign of the times for all of us, but today's consumers bring a set of values and beliefs that include issues related to animal treatment, the environment, global warming, fair labor practices, and human rights (Smith, 2015), and on very specific issues, as seen by Americans boycotting food companies and retailers based on owners' stance on supporting LGBTQ rights (Fiorilla, 2019), gun regulations (Holson, 2018), and even breastfeeding in public (Morran, 2010).

More and more, consumers making ethical choices on how they eat have become one of the most significant impacts on customer loyalty for retail and restaurant, as well as for brand loyalty for ready-to-eat and packaged consumer goods. According to Ali Berlow, publisher of *Edible Vineyard Magazine* and author of The Food Activist Handbook: Big & Small Things You Can Do to Help Provide Fresh, Healthy Food for Your Community (2015), "I feel like with the imperative of climate activism and building up local and regional food systems in a safe way … there's just a heightened awareness now. I think this next generation and the younger generations are going to be demanding it" (Ali Berlow, Personal Communication, 2019).

Climate change, the environment, and the ethical treatment of animals are some of the chief concerns of consumers in a new era of "Food Ethics"—moral principles about "the rights, duties, and harms associated with the ways in which we produce, process, and consume our food" (Berlow, 2019). Consumers' values around labor conditions are a relatively new element that impacts their decisions.

> *"Consumers are acutely aware of how the CAFOs [concentrated animal feeding operations] are placed in the marginalized communities in North Carolina and the amount of environmental injustice that happens in those communities because of that type of growing system to meet the supposed demand and feeding the world. They are learning how growers in Florida [earn a] penny a pound for their worker. And workers in Vermont who are milking cows at some of these mega dairies can never really leave the property for fear of deportation. People working in dangerous working conditions for fear of retribution if they complain."*
>
> ***(Ali Berlow, Personal Communication, 2019)***

Once perceived only as conditions of long ago or in developing nations, these dangerous conditions for food workers are found here in the United States. Back in 1991, a fire engulfed a Hamlet, North Carolina chicken processing plant. Workers were trapped by blocked or locked doors. Worse, according to authorities, 25 people were killed and 40 were injured (Associated Press, 1991). Authorities at the California Division of Occupational Safety and Health reported in 2012 how an employee was cooked to death in a steamer machine at Bumble Bee Food's seafood plant in California (Colgrass, 2015).

These examples are not alone. In 2015, the National Safety Council published results from an Emory University study of 2008–10 data from the Bureau of Labor Statistics. The researchers found that food industry workers (in areas of food production, processing, distribution, storage, and retail) "have a 60 percent higher rate of occupational injury or illness than workers in other industries" (National Safety Council, 2015). The National Safety Council also highlighted three additional facts about food industry jobs:

1. They made up about 15% of US private-industry jobs during that time period;
2. As opposed to workers from other industries, these workers' "severe injuries that required time off work" were "more than twice as frequent"; and
3. These food industry workers' risk of occupational death was 9.5 times higher than in nonfood jobs (National Safety Council, 2015).

This is not the same type of food safety as intended by the title of this book, nor are they similar to the many cases and advancements discussed in earlier chapters. Even if these conditions reflect the doings only a minute percentage of food companies and, similar to how Stephen Ostroff described the unsanitary conditions at the Peanut Corporation of America (PCA) being caused by "bad people who shouldn't be making food" (Stephen Ostroff, Personal Communication, 2019), consumers buy products on retailers' shelves with the assumption that all stages of production are compliant to a range of standards under the jurisdiction of multiple authorities.

These examples of modern—yet horrific—conditions and casualties of industry resemble the same eye-opening descriptions in Upton Sinclair's pivotal novel *The Jungle*. The real images that Sinclair wrote, and special agent from the Roosevelt administration verified, triggered not only worldwide shock, but, perhaps more importantly, consumer demand for changes in regulatory oversight of the meat industry.

Sadly, these headlines are more likely to capture readers' attention today than CDC's estimated 48 million people who get sick, 128,000 who are hospitalized, and 3,000 who die from foodborne diseases each year in the United States.

Change in how media covers outbreaks

Perhaps even in this age of social media and viral videos, one should consider the importance of a newspaper headline. Much discussion on social media related to the news of the day still originates from original reporting in traditional news outlets. Newspaper headlines are still one of the most powerful contributors to readers' opinions and actions related to public health or consumer behavior. However, as pointed out in the 2014 media study "The Personal News Cycle," only about 4 of 10 Americans surveyed delve deeper into a particular news subject beyond the headlines (Rosenstiel et al., 2014). Thus, in a non-read article, the headline is the only contributor to such action. As a result, "headlines have become almost like articles in and of themselves" (DeMers, 2016). Additionally, in the 2016 study "Social Clicks: What and Who Gets Read on Twitter?" scientists discussed how news is influenced and how it becomes influential, supporting the idea that public opinion related to politics, and even natural disasters, is influenced by editorial decisions and the source of the information (Gabielkov, Ramachandran, Chaintreau, & Legout, 2016).

A look at newspaper headlines from the landmark 1993 Jack in the Box *E. coli* outbreak exposes a clear pattern. An analysis of the headlines from articles covering the 1993 outbreak reveals differences in the words used and, thus, the message communicated. An important note here is that the reporters and investigative journalists at that time faced the same challenges as consumers in that *E. coli* and outbreaks such as this were a relatively new phenomenon (Fig. 10.4).

The words in the images represent the key nouns and verbs, while the size of the font indicates the number of times the word appeared in headlines. The word cloud on the left reflects key words found in the headlines from *The New York Times*, *Los Angeles Times*, and *Washington Post* from

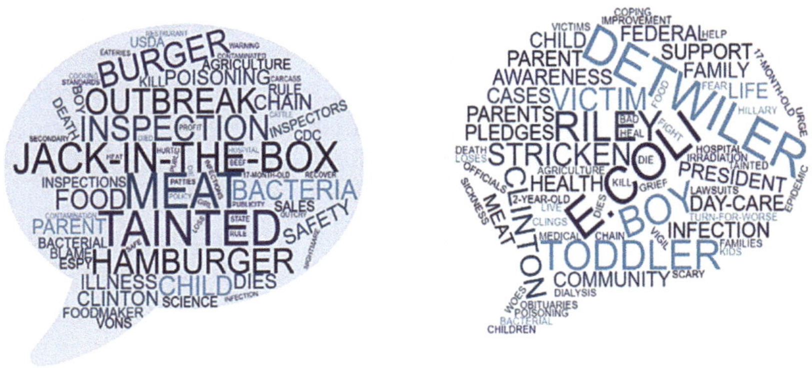

Keywords in 1993 headlines from **National Newspapers** (NY Times, LA Times, Washington Post)

Keywords in 1993 headlines from **State / Local Newspapers** (Seattle Times, Seattle Post Intelligencer, Bellingham Herald)

Figure 10.4 Comparing national newspaper headlines and local newspaper headlines from the 1993 *E. coli* outbreak. *(Graphics by Author).*

January to April 1993. While these papers originated a great distance from the actual outbreak, they have long been regarded as leading and influential papers from which other papers derive content.

In contrast, the word cloud on the right reflects key words found in the headlines from papers at or close to the outbreak, including *The Seattle Times*, *The Seattle Post-Intelligencer*, and *The Bellingham* (WA) *Herald* from January to April 1993. The national papers never mentioned *E. coli*, focused on the names of the companies involved, and, perhaps more concerning, sent messages that focused more on the problem of the product and less on the public health concern. In contrast, local papers' headlines focused on the victims, community, public health, and the true burden of disease. Ultimately, the local papers' headlines seen in 1993 would have impacted consumer opinion and behavior more than those in national papers.

The way in which this kind of public health event is covered by the media can make an impact on the public, as well as on the industry and lawmakers if journalists go beyond data and sound bites. However, a great amount effort and consideration, not to ignore the sets of circumstances, are needed for national news coverage to have the same level of public health impact as the state and local news outlets. According to her research on journalism at The Ohio State University, Catherine Gynn, PhD, revealed that "It was only through the interaction of Riley Detwiler's parents with President Clinton that the national news coverage developed a human face for the events" (Gynn, 1995).

Today, Linda Byron teaches investigative reporting at the University of Washington. In 1993, however, she was an Investigative Reporter on criminal justice and special projects, ultimately becoming a producer and local TV news anchor in Seattle. She earned more than a dozen Emmy Awards and a National Edward R. Murrow award during her career. One of the topics she talks about to this day is the 1993 outbreak.

> *"It was a story that was really important on a local level .... I think that happened with the Jack in the box and the* E. coli *outbreak—there was a sense of outrage and then it snowballed and that reinforced the outrage ... when you have children dying, that strikes at our collective sense of wrong and of caring. And so, I'm not surprised that it was a big story on a national level."*
>
> ***(Linda Byron, Personal Communication, 2019)***

A former staff writer at *The New York Times*, Christine Haughney Dare-Bryan's career in reporting on food includes Senior Investigations Reporter and Editor for the series "Food Crimes" at Zero Point Zero Production, and Agriculture Reporter for POLITICO. She sees how the divisions of reporting specialties at newspapers impact the coverage of topics at the intersection of business, public health, food, and crime: "that has a lot to do with the structure of media, because these ideas would come out of the food section versus the national or foreign pages. It's like a territory issue. And so that's why a lot of these stories were falling through the cracks" (Christine Haughney Dare-Bryan, Personal Communication, 2019).

To Linda Byron, journalists' coverage of these stories is extremely important for "how food safety warnings got out and how people understood what some of the threats were in their communities." However, she also believes that these messages became critically important at a time when she saw "corporate pressure from lawyers, arguing that the public doesn't need to know the details about *E. coli* outbreaks even if dozens of people are sick" (Linda Byron, Personal Communication, 2019).

> *"And that argument, wouldn't go anywhere now because with social media, people would put the information out so quickly and it would go viral. So, there was a higher burden on journalists and on local news and national news to protect the public and to provide information under the belief that the public has a right to know about safety threats. And that includes food safety. We talk all the time about threats from guns and violence and infrastructure failures and all these other things. But the idea that something you do every day—consuming food—could be that level of threat is, wasn't really understood before this big story broke in 1993 and the fact that I remember distinctly that Jack in the Box said they were fixing the problem and then they would test and it showed that they were still weren't cooking a hamburger enough. So, then there's that sense of outrage double because*

wait a minute, like everyone can make a mistake, but you know, this is unsafe and you're still not fixing it. And oh, by the way, where are these federal regulatory agencies that are supposed to be protecting us and what are they doing?"

Again, one cannot fault the national papers for this observation of difference in message. The overall culture change related to food safety since that 1993 outbreak has impacted national news and the words used to describe outbreaks and recalls. Events as recent as the Chipotle Mexican Grill outbreaks and the incidents with 2018 romaine lettuce highlight the fact that the media covers these food concerns more and with greater accuracy.

At the time of the PCA incidents and investigation, she observed that "in the TV world, there seem to be a fascination with crime shows and a fascination with food shows. There were two cases before PCA that were pretty egregious: the DeCosters' case, and the Jack-in the-Box case. I wondered why audiences weren't getting extensive coverage of these topics?" (Christine Haughney Dare-Bryan, Personal Communication, 2019). With seemingly limitless cable TV channels and new internet-based platforms for investigative reporting, Christine Haughney Dare-Bryan found an opportunity to conceive and develop the "Food Crimes" web series that ran on the website foodrepublic.com.

Industry journals have also become a platform that invests an enormous amount of research and advisory input to their articles. Lisa Lupo is the Editor of *Quality Assurance and Food Safety Magazine.* She sees the role of industry journals as being a partnership with industry, a place where companies and food experts in general can talk with each other about information important to the future of the industry. This magazine has become a place where company leaders have talked about their recalls and how they overcame them. *Quality Assurance and Food Safety Magazine* has become a platform where it is safe for a company to be open about how they're making changes and to engage in these conversations that are being seen by others. Lupo points to her magazine's coverage of the 2006 spinach recall:

"Even back then, when we did that article, you know, [the company's executives] were very open. 'Yep, we have this issue. Everybody knew about it and here's what's happened now to make it better.' *That was kind of the whole point of it. Everybody knows it happened. Look at the Romaine lettuce outbreaks. There's no reason to say it didn't happen because it did and the whole world knows."*

(Lisa Lupo, Personal Communication, 2019)

Coverage of companies' positive changes is important to industry journals. At the same time, coverage of topics that reveal the illegal and unethical doings in the industry serve as a warning. Lupo names the PCA outbreak, recall, investigation, trial, and sentencing as an example of this. "The executives from PCA are in prison, and it's very important for the industry to know that there are repercussions. I definitely think the more of those that we can cover, the better for the industry to see" (Lisa Lupo, Personal Communication, 2019).

Topics and industry participation aside, the larger context of changes in journalism gets in the way of communicating all the intended audiences. Barbara VanRenterghem, PhD, is the Editorial Director at *Food Safety Magazine*. She thinks that the shift from print to digital is challenging not only for the industry, but also for readers.

> *"You have pay walls up by some of your major news reporting groups like* The New York Times *and* The Washington Post *that you get so many free articles a month and then you have to pay if you want to know content. And the additional challenge is that the majority of the incorrect, misleading information is free whereas the fact-based content usually has a price tag associated with it .... people are bombarded with a variety of messages ... the first thing that hits them is what usually sticks. So, unless they really want to get to the bottom of something, there's not a whole lot of research that goes on anymore."*
>
> ***(Barbara VanRenterghem, Personal Communication, 2019)***

As a result, VanRenterghem thinks the biggest challenges in the future for food safety are going to be getting good fact-based, science-based information out there in front of people. Another change factor in journalism and how consumers learn more about the food they purchase is the decrease in qualified investigative journalists at a time when news organizations are experiencing significant shifts in the number of outlets, the ownership of the outlets, and in the resources and prioritization they have for food safety coverage.

With over 30 years of experience covering food safety and health topics for various news agencies and companies, JoNel Aleccia, Senior Correspondent at Kaiser Health News, worries about how trends in the world of journalism will impact the future of food safety.

> *"The thing that really worries me is when I was at NBC [2012-2014] and when I was in Seattle [2014-2016], there were maybe five people in the country—at the most—covering food safety as a beat. Health coverage has been decimated ... it's gotten slimmer and slimmer. Doing the kind of the investigative stories about food safety has, especially in this Trump era, really gotten short shrift. If I can't do it and if some of the other people who were covering food safety before are being pulled away on other issues, it's not getting any coverage right now. I think journalism needs people who are able to pay attention to [food safety issues] and hold people accountable."*
>
> ***(JoNel Aleccia, Personal Communication, 2019)***

One example of this type of investigative reporting that Aleccia highlights is a special report "A Game of Chicken," published by *The Oregonian*, written by Lynne Terry (2015). Terry's work chronicled Oregon and Washington public health officials' investigation of *Salmonella* outbreaks in 2004, 2009, and 2012 that they not only tied to Foster Farms chicken, but also then repeatedly reported to the USDA. Terry wrote about the USDA's reactions in "A Game of Chicken":

> *"The USDA did not warn the public about illnesses associated with Foster Farms chicken until the fourth outbreak. Even then, the alert came three months after the CDC told the USDA of the outbreak. The single Foster Farms recall came as illnesses were subsiding. The peak of the outbreak had occurred nearly 10 months earlier in mid-September 2013. [Al] Almanza [then the Deputy Under Secretary of the USDA's Food Safety Inspection Service] said that if the USDA warned consumers every time an item was suspected in an outbreak, 'we'd be issuing public alerts very often.' Between the time of the public health alert and the recall, more than 250 additional people got sick, the CDC said."*
>
> ***(Terry, 2015.)***

For her work on this investigative report, the Association of Health Care Journalists awarded Terry with a 2016 first place award for public health reporting. According to Aleccia, however, "Lynn Terry doesn't work there at *The Oregonian* anymore: she's a fabulous reporter and she did that whole thing on Foster Farms chicken and *Salmonella* ... and they laid her off [due to] budget cuts. Nobody's covering that anymore" (JoNel Aleccia, Personal Communication, 2019).

The impact on the future job of food safety officials is clear: food safety experts and consumers cannot assume that all media sources—print or online, investigative journalism, or social media—convey the same message about a public health concern. The headlines are a key element in communicating critical information that can influence not only consumers' actions, but also those who work in the food industry.

Changes in consumer advocacy

The last change to consider is that of the future of consumer advocacy. "The customer is always right" has its roots in 19th-century retail stores as a motto prioritizing customer satisfaction. Not all restaurants and retail firms buy into this idea today. Unfortunately, even food safety experts encounter pushback when pointing out unsanitary conditions or unsafe practices. This motto would have customers assuming that their complaints should be treated seriously so that they do not feel cheated, deceived, or harmed.

Another, old, yet related phrase is "let the buyer beware" (or "caveat emptor"). In the context of food, this pushes the role of responsibility onto the consumer, giving a pass to those who should bear liability. Consumers read labels on packages of meat and poultry for safe handling instructions and warning messages on menus regarding food allergens. However, many view these labels as legal loopholes or simply as a way of companies dodging full responsibility for their actions or lack thereof.

While consumers have and will always play a role in food safety, this does not diminish the role of industry. To quote Admiral Hyman Rickover (the Father of the Nuclear Navy), "Responsibility is a unique concept … You may share it with others, but your portion is not diminished. You may delegate it, but it is still with you … If responsibility is rightfully yours, no evasion, or ignorance or passing the blame can shift the burden to someone else" (Rickover, quoted in Cantonwine, 2014).

As discussed earlier, we also have laws to protect consumers. The vast majority of food companies do everything in their power to prioritize and invest in compliance and mitigation. They also train their employees regularly on best practices and on "the why" behind food safety. Still, these laws are broken and those who break them are often not held accountable for their actions in the hospitalizations and deaths of consumers. Often, as discussed in Chapter 5, corporate executives in these situations blame their employees. While "human error" does exist, responsibility rests on the shoulders of every worker—even those in the executive offices.

One fact that has not changed over the course of history is that those who work on farms or in food manufacturing plants or in retail/restaurant settings are also consumers. This is not a landscape where an argument for "Us versus Them" can exist. Those who work in the food industry are also susceptible to becoming a victim of failures in food safety. Further, they have families that often include the most vulnerable of populations (the very young, those who are pregnant, those with compromised immune systems, and the elderly).

The wide variety of contaminated foods, different pathogens, ways in which foods became contaminated, and causes for failures in food safety mitigation all leave experts to assume that a "one-size-fits-all" solution will never exist. At a time when food safety regulations are being modernized and industry leaders are embracing food safety culture alongside new technologies, consumers are bombarded with evidence of the seemingly uninterrupted cycle of crisis and reform.

The human toll from foodborne pathogens in our food supply is too high. Ever since the 1993 Jack in the Box *E. coli* outbreak, the CDC has published estimates that 48 million people get sick, 128,000 are hospitalized, and 3,000 die from foodborne diseases each year in the United States. The vast majority of these cases could be prevented.

The incredible progress by much of the food industry to better protect our food supply can no longer suffer from the failures of those who did not learn from history. Though a complete list of these events would fill a set of books, a few milestones discussed earlier in this book reflect key moments that sparked new levels of awareness.

- The 2018 romaine lettuce outbreaks offered an opportunity for consumers—and the food industry—to learn a lesson about how pathogens can contaminate produce.
- The 2015 and 2016 multiple outbreaks at a single fast-food chain offered an opportunity for restaurants to learn a lesson on food safety priorities, investment, and training.
- The 2008–9 *Salmonella* outbreak and associated criminal outcomes for a peanut company offered an opportunity for executives and quality assurance leaders to learn a lesson about corporate responsibility and legal ramifications for criminal behavior.
- The deaths of four young children during the landmark 1993 *E. coli* outbreak shocked consumers, legislators, journalists, and those who work in the food industry.
- Finally, Upton Sinclair's 1906 novel *The Jungle* sickened consumers around the world and sparked a whole new level of government regulation over food safety.

The simple literary review of Sinclair's novel in a 1906 London newspaper ultimately offered one of the most accurate predictions of the food industry:

> *"The things described by Mr. Sinclair happened yesterday, are happening today, and will happen tomorrow and the next day until some Hercules comes to cleanse the filthy stable."*

Hercules is far from any one single person or entity. Hercules can be found in the voices and in the actions of consumers and those who work in the food industry. The future of food safety will continue to require a Herculean effort—an enormous amount of work, strength, and courage—from all participants along the way from farm to the fork.

Consumers often do not care about food safety failures unless impacted directly. History tells us, however, that the most significant changes in food regulations and industry practices came about after the serious illnesses and deaths of young children. Further improvements demand louder voices not solely from victims, but from *all* Americans. We all must insist that "the customer is always right" to demand safe food. Future food safety policies and legal ramifications for crimes that harm consumers must send a message of "let the maker and seller beware"—not just the buyer.

The firsthand accounts included in this book are intended to achieve the goal of benefiting industry and consumers such that the future of food safety will result in few chairs forever empty at family tables.

References

Association for Food and Drug Officials (AFDO). (2012). Regulatory Guidance for Best Practices: Cottage Foods. Association for Food and Drug Officials. Available from: http://www.afdo.org/resources/temp/Cottage_Foods_013.pdf.

Associated Press. (1991). Food Plant Fire Kills 25; Exits Blocked. The Los Angeles Times. Available from: https://www.latimes.com/archives/la-xpm-1991-09-04-mn-1427-story.html.

Atkin, E. (2019). The Promise and Problem of Fake Meat. The New Republic. Available from: https://newrepublic.com/article/153998/promise-problem-fake-meat-beyond-burger-impossible-foods.

Berlow, A. (2019). Conversation: Ruth Faden and Ali Berlow. Edible Vineyard Magazine. Summer, 2019 Edition.

Carroll, A. (1991). The pyramid of corporate social responsibility: toward the moral management of organizational stakeholders. Business Horizons, 34(4), 39–48.

Colgrass, N. (2015). Bumble Bee Forced to Pay $6M for Worker Cooked Alive. USA Today. Available from: https://www.usatoday.com/story/news/nation/2015/08/13/bumble-bee-forced-pay-6m-worker-cooked-alive/31620881/.

DeMers, J. (2016). 59 Percent of You Will Share this Article Without Even Reading It. Available from: https://www.forbes.com/sites/jaysondemers/2016/08/08/59-percent-of-you-will-share-this-article-without-even-reading-it/.

Food and Drug Administration (FDA). (2019a). Statement from Acting FDA Commissioner Ned Sharpless, M.D., and Deputy Commissioner Frank Yiannas on Steps to Usher the U.S. into a New Era of Smarter Food Safety [Press Release]. Available from: https://www.fda.gov/news-events/press-announcements/statement-acting-fda-commissioner-ned-sharpless-md-and-deputy-commissioner-frank-yiannas-steps-usher.

Food and Drug Administration (FDA). (2019b). Food for Thought—Ideas on How to Begin a New Era of Smarter Food Safety, October 21, 2019. Available from: https://www.fda.gov/media/131682/download.

Fiorilla, V. (2019). Boycotting Chick-fil-A? Here Are 243 Other Companies You Might Want to Avoid. Philadelphia Magazine. Available from: https://www.phillymag.com/news/2019/04/01/chick-fil-a-boycott/.

Flynn, D. (2016). Retail-Host Restaurant Trend is Not Without Food Safety Concerns. Food Safety News. Available from: http://www.foodsafetynews.com/2016/04/retail-host-restaurant-trend-is-not-without-food-safety-concerns/#.Vwun_PkrLIV.

Gabielkov, M., Ramachandran, A., Chaintreau, A., & Legout, A. (2016). Social Clicks: What and Who Gets Read on Twitter? ACM SIGMETRICS/IFIP Performance. Available from: https://hal.inria.fr/hal-01281190/document.

Gottlieb, S. (2018). Statement from FDA Commissioner Scott Gottlieb, M.D., on Findings from the Romaine Lettuce *E. coli* O157:H7 Outbreak Investigation and FDA's Efforts to Prevent Future Outbreaks. FDA. Available from: https://www.fda.gov/news-events/press-announcements/statement-fda-commissioner-scott-gottlieb-md-findings-romaine-lettuce-e-coli-o157h7-outbreak?utm_campaign=11012018_Statement_findings+from+the+romaine+lettuce+E.+coli+O157%3AH7&utm_medium=email&utm_source=Eloqua.

Gynn, C. (1995). Beyond Objectivity and Relativism: A View of Journalism from a Rhetorical Perspective. Doctoral dissertation. The Ohio State University, Columbus, OH. Available from: https://etd.ohiolink.edu/!etd.send_file?accession=osu14878634290946 7&disposition=inline.

Harper, M. (2019). Impact of robotics on food manufacturing. Presentation at the 2019 meeting of the International Association for Food Protection. Louisville, KY.

Healy, K. (2018). A Theory of Human Motivation by Abraham H. Maslow (1942): The British Journal of Psychiatry. Available from: https://www.cambridge.org/core/journals/the-british-journal-of-psychiatry/article/a-theory-of-human-motivation-by-abraham-h-maslow-1942/519D1FAFADE96014EC0C3CE52FC1698F.

Holson, L. (2018). Dallas Restaurant That Defied N.R.A. Donates to 'Gun Sense' Group. The New York Times. Available from: https://www.nytimes.com/2018/05/14/us/politics/nra-boycott-ellens-dallas.html.

Jamrisko, M. (2015). Americans' Spending on Dining Out Just Overtook Grocery Sales for the First Time Ever. Bloomberg News. Available from: http://www.bloomberg.com/news/articles/2015-04-14/americans-spending-on-dining-out-just-overtook-grocery-sales-for-the-first-time-ever.

Jenson, I. (2019). Potential for robotic processing of red meat: food safety implications. Presentation at the 2019 meeting of the International Association for Food Protection. Louisville, KY.

Jones, T. F., Pavlin, B. I., & LaFluer, B. J. (2004). Restaurant inspection scores and foodborne disease. Emerging Infectious Diseases, 10(4). Available from: http://wwwnc.cdc.gov/eid/article/10/4/03-0343_article.

Kelso, A. (2019). Food Delivery Via Drones May Be Closer Than You Think. Forbes Magazine. Available from: https://www.forbes.com/sites/aliciakelso/2019/07/12/food-delivery-via-drones-may-be-closer-than-you-think/#4176ff377438.

Kerry, J. (2019). The climate is changing, are we? Presentation. Martha's Vineyard Film Festival Lecture Series, West Tisbury, MA.

Khaleej Times. (2016) You Can Now Have Your PIZZA Delivered by a Drone. Khaleej Times. Available from: https://www.khaleejtimes.com/offbeat/you-can-now-have-your-pizza-delivered-by-a-drone.

Kurutzdec, S. (2012). The Battlefront in the Front Yard. The New York Times. Available from: https://www.nytimes.com/2012/12/20/garden/gardeners-fight-with-neighbors-and-city-hall-over-their-lawns.html.

Leibrock, A. (2018). Believe It or Not, It May be Illegal to Grow Your Own Food. Sustainable America. Available from: https://sustainableamerica.org/blog/believe-it-or-not-it-may-be-illegal-to-grow-your-own-food/.

Lewis, N. (2018). Desert Heat Lights a Fire Under Dubai's Food Delivery Market. CNN. Available from: https://www.cnn.com/travel/article/dubai-food-delivery-apps/index.html.

Macartney, J. (2008). China Baby Milk Scandal Spreads as Sick Toll Rises to 13,000. The Times. London. Available from: https://www.thetimes.co.uk/article/china-baby-milk-scandal-spreads-as-sick-toll-rises-to-13000-jlxdmrsk9qd.

McCarthy, G. (2019). The climate is changing, are we? Presentation. Martha's Vineyard Film Festival Lecture Series, West Tisbury, MA.

McSwane, D. (2019). Conference for food protection. Presentation at the 2019 International Association for Food Protection, Louisville, KY.

Migala, J. (2019). What is the Beyond Burger and is It Good For You? Womens' Health Magazine. Available from: https://www.womenshealthmag.com/food/a21566428/beyond-meat-burger-ingredients/.

Morran, C. (2010). Breastfeeding Moms Protest Johnny Rockets. The Consumerist. Available from: https://consumerist.com/2010/07/some-breastfeeding-moms-boycotting-johnny-rockets.html.

Morrison, O. (2019). Food is 'Getting Cool': Nestlé CTO Stefan Palzer's Top 7 Predictions on the Future of Food. Food Navigator. Available from: https://www.foodnavigator.com/Article/2019/08/30/Food-is-getting-cool-Nestle-CTO-Stefan-Palzer-s-top-7-predictions-on-the-future-of-food#.

National Gardening Association. (2014). Garden to Table: A 5-Year Look at Food Gardening in America. National Gardening Association. Available from: https://garden.org/special/pdf/2014-NGA-Garden-to-Table.pdf.

National Safety Council. (2015). Food Workers Face Higher Injury, Death Rates: Study. Safety and Health Magazine. Available from: https://www.safetyandhealthmagazine.com/articles/12648-food-workers-face-higher-injury-death-rates-study.

O'Leary (2019). Opening remarks at FoodLogiQ Industry Event, Durham, NC.

Papple, D. (2014). Michigan Loses 'Right To Farm' this Week: A Farewell to Backyard Chickens and Beekeepers. Inquisitr. Available from: https://www.inquisitr.com/1235774/michigan-loses-right-to-farm-this-week-a-farewell-to-backyard-chickens-and-beekeepers/#pWBPjHxvMt8IBhuD.99.

Rickover, H., quoted in Cantonwine, P. (2014). Caught in the Leadership Paradox: Insight from Admiral Rickover. American Nuclear Society. Available from: http://ansnuclearcafe.org/2014/07/03/caught-in-the-leadership-paradox/#sthash.4nTwHCYo.dpbs.

Rockström, J. (2016). How Food Connects All the SDGs. Stockholm University Global Resilience Center. Available from: https://www.stockholmresilience.org/research/research-news/2016-06-14-how-food-connects-all-the-sdgs.html.

Rosenstiel, T., et al. (2014). The Personal News Cycle. The Media Insight Project: An initiative of the American Press Institute and the Associated Press-NORC Center for Public Affairs Research. Available from: https://www.americanpressinstitute.org/wp-content/uploads/2014/03/The_Media_Insight_Project_The_Personal_News_Cycle_Final.pdf.

Schwab, K. (2017). The fourth industrial revolution. New York: Crown Business.

Selyukh, A. (2019). Food for Thought: What Gets to Be a 'Burger'? NPR. Available from: https://www.npr.org/sections/thesalt/2019/07/23/744083270/what-gets-to-be-a-burger-states-restrict-labels-on-plant-based-meat.

Smith, S. (2015). 9 Awful Companies Everyone Should Boycott Right Now. The Daily Dot. Available from: https://www.dailydot.com/via/nestle-whole-foods-horrible-companies-boycott/.

Terry, L. (2015). A Game of Chicken: USDA Repeatedly Blinked When Facing Salmonella Outbreaks involving Foster Farms. The Oregonian. Available from: https://www.oregonlive.com/projects/usda-salmonella/.

Tirado, M. C., Clarke, R., Jaykus, L. A., McQuatters-Gollop, A., & Frank, J. M. (2010). Climate change and food safety: a review Food Research International, 43, 1745–1765.

US Cattlemen's Association (USCA). (2019). Petition for the Imposition of Beef and Meat Labeling Requirements: To Exclude Products Not Derived Directly from Animals Raised and Slaughtered from the Definition of "Beef" and "Meat". US Department of Agriculture. Available from: https://www.fsis.usda.gov/wps/wcm/connect/e4749f95-e79a-4ba5-883b-394c8bdc97a3/18-01-Petition-US-Cattlement-Association020918.pdf?MOD=AJPERES.

US Department of Agriculture (USDA). (2019). USDA and FDA Announce a Formal Agreement to Regulate Cell-Cultured Food Products from Cell Lines of Livestock and Poultry. Available from: https://www.usda.gov/media/press-releases/2019/03/07/usda-and-fda-announce-formal-agreement-regulate-cell-cultured-food.

Interviewee biographies

JoNel Aleccia has a career in journalism that spans 35 years. Aleccia is currently Senior Correspondent at Kaiser Health News. In addition to her work as a Health Reporter at *The Seattle Times*, her career includes serving as the Health Reporter and Editor for MSNBC and NBCNews.com. At *The Spokesman-Review*, she covered health and social service issues in two-state area of Eastern Washington and Northern Idaho. Before that, she worked for 21 years as a Reporter, Editor, and Columnist for *The Mail Tribune*, a regional newspaper in Southern Oregon.

Jeff Almer is a Financial Analyst at Best Buy. His work after the death of his mother to *Salmonella* during the Peanut Corporation of America (PCA) outbreak (2008–9) assisted consumer advocacy groups as well as the federal prosecution team in the trial of the PCA executives.

Mitzi Baum is the CEO at Stop Foodborne Illness, a nonprofit consumer advocacy organization. Baum is also an Adjunct Instructor at Michigan State University. Baum's previous positions include Director of Food Safety at Feeding America, a nonprofit domestic hunger-relief organization.

Alan Baumfalk is a Pet Food Safety Specialist and Food Safety Auditor at Eurofins US Foods Division. He has over 3 decades of experience in human food production facilities. Baumfalk received the 2018 SQF Auditor of the Year award.

Doug Beach is the Manager of the East County Office Ventura County, CA, Environmental Health Division (EHD) of inspectors in the Food Protection Program for thousands of food facilities that sell food to the public in Moorpark, Newbury Park, Simi Valley, Thousand Oaks, and Westlake.

Ali Berlow is the Cohost of "The Local Food Report" on WCAI, Cape and Islands NPR Station. She is the Author of "The Food Activist Handbook: Big & Small Things You Can Do to Help Provide Fresh, Healthy Food for Your Community" (2015) and Co-owner, Editor, and Founding Editor of *Edible Vineyard* Magazine. Berlow has worked with the National Sustainable Agriculture Coalition and the Island Grown Initiative. Early in her career, she was the Assistant Curator of Permanent Collections at the Museum of Science in Boston. Berlow recently started as a student at Vermont Law School, working on her Master of Food and Agriculture Law and Policy.

Dennis Bounds is a former broadcast journalist whose career spans nearly 40 years. For 25 of those years, Bounds sat as the News Anchor at the NBC affiliate KING5 News in Seattle, WA. Bounds earned an Emmy award during his career as a News Anchor.

Linda Byron is a lecturer on investigative reporting at the University of Washington. Her career in journalism spans over 30 years and includes such roles as Investigative Reporter, Criminal Justice Reporter, Special Projects Reporter/Producer, and News Anchor at the NBC affiliate KING5 News in Seattle, WA. Byron received an Edward R. Murrow award and is a 12-time Emmy Award winner.

Joe Corby is the Senior Advisor for the Association of Food and Drug Officials (AFDO), and serves on the Education Advisory Board for the Food Safety Summit and on the Board of Directors for the International Food Protection Training Institute and the Partnership for Food Safety Education. He is currently an instructor for the International Food Protection Training Institute, the National Environmental Health Association (NEHA), and the University of Tennessee. From 2008 to 2018, Corby served as the Executive Director for AFDO. He previously worked for 37 years at the New York State Department of Agriculture and Markets, serving as the Director of the Division of Food Safety and prior to his departure. Corby received the NSF International's prestigious Food Safety Leadership Award at the 2019 Food Safety Summit. He is a past recipient of the Harvey W. Wiley Award, AFDO's most prestigious award that honors members for their exceptional service in the enforcement of food and drug law.

Christine Haughney Dare-Bryan is an Investigative Reporter and Spotlight Fellow at *The Boston Globe*. Her career highlights in print journalism include Agriculture Reporter at *POLITICO*, Staff Reporter at *The New York Times*, Staff Reporter at *The Wall Street Journal*, Editorial Aide/Correspondent for *The Washington Post*, and Staff Reporter for *The Washington Business Journal*. Her career highlights in broadcast journalism include Senior Investigations Editor at Zero Point Zero Production, Inc., where she conceived and developed the web series "Food Crimes," and as their Series Investigative Reporter, where she oversaw a team of reporters investigating global food safety issues for the first season of the Netflix original series "Rotten."

Caroline Smith DeWaal, JD, serves as the International Food Safety Policy Manager at the FDA's Center for Food Safety and Applied

Nutrition (CFSAN). Smith DeWaal previously spent over 21 years at the Center for Science in the Public Interest. As CSPI's Director of Food Safety, she directed policy formulation and execution on food safety issues for a nonprofit consumer research and advocacy organization with 750,000 consumer members in the United States and 100,000 in Canada. This work encompassed components at FDA, USDA, EPA, NOAA, relevant Congressional committees, and numerous international agencies; managed work at the international, Congressional, and regulatory level simultaneously and supervised CSPI staff on diverse issues; made numerous appearances before Congressional Committees to deliver testimony, including top-level White House, OMB, and Secretarial-level meetings; and worked collaboratively with FDA, USDA, consumer, industry, public health, and environmental groups. Smith DeWaal has authored numerous chapters and books, including "Is Our Food Safe?: A Consumer's Guide to Protecting Your Health and the Environment" (2002).

Sandra Eskin, JD, is the Project Director for Food Safety at The Pew Charitable Trusts. Eskin's career includes public policy consulting to consumer and public interest organizations, providing strategic and policy advice on a range of consumer protection issues, including food safety, dietary supplement safety, and food and drug labeling and advertising. Eskin was also a federal government staff attorney, legislative representative for the Consumer Federation of America (CFA), Deputy Director of the Produce Safety Project—a Pew initiative at Georgetown University, and served on numerous federal advisory committees.

Adam Friedlander is a Manager of Food Safety and Technical Services at the Food Marketing Institute (FMI) that focused on advancing food safety, food science, and food regulatory practices for food retailers, wholesalers, and product suppliers. He is an active member of the Institute of Food Technologists (IFT), International Association for Food Protection (IAFP), Conference for Food Protection (CFP), and Association of Food and Drug Officials (AFDO). Friedlander earned a Bachelor of Science in Food Science from Cornell University's College of Agriculture and Life Sciences and a Master of Science in Regulatory Affairs of Food and Food Industries from Northeastern University's College of Professional Studies.

Thomas Gremillion, JD, is the Director of Food Policy at Consumer Federation of America. He oversees the research, analysis, advocacy, and media outreach for the group's food policy activities, and monitors food safety activities at USDA, FDA, and in Congress, where he advocates for strong food safety protections for consumers. He also coordinates the Safe Food Coalition, a group of consumer, trade union, and foodborne illness victim organizations dedicated to reducing foodborne illness by improving government food inspection programs. Prior to joining CFA in 2015, Gremillion practiced environmental law at Georgetown University Law Center's Institute for Public Representation, where he represented community groups and advocacy organizations in litigation against polluters and government regulators. He also served as an associate attorney at the Southern Environmental Law Center in Chapel Hill, NC, where he specialized in transportation and land use issues.

Rylee Gustafson is an award-winning Food Safety Advocate and college student. Gustafson became ill from *E. coli* in spinach in 2006. Her work with STOP Foodborne Illness includes taking part in the production of a training video for the California Leafy Green Products Handler Marketing Agreement (LGMA) that has become part of a comprehensive worker training program for the leafy greens industry. Gustafson received STOP's 2013 Youth Volunteer of the Year and their 2014 Food Safety Heroes Award. Her work with The Pew Charitable Trusts included countless hours of meetings and testimony with legislators to support the passage of the 2010 FDA Food Safety Modernization Act (FSMA).

Jorge Hernandez is the VP of Quality at The Wendy's Company. A former health department sanitarian, Hernandez's career includes serving as Chief Food Safety Officer at Wholesome International, Senior Vice President for Food Safety & Quality Assurance at US FOODS, and VP for Food Safety & Risk Management for the National Restaurant Association. Hernandez is a well-respected voice in the food industry and speaks frequently at events across the country. He has published many articles and is a recognized consultant in the areas of food safety, food safety management systems, food safety accreditation, food safety training, and food safety operations.

Michael Hicks is Cofounder and President, as well as a Board Member for Relevant Systems, Inc., developer of FoodCode-Pro, a fully digital, mobile platform for food safety inspections.

Jill Hollingsworth, DVM, has a career in the food industry that spans 4 decades. Currently the Vice President for Food Safety and Regulatory Affairs at CHEMSTAR, she previously served as a Retail Food Safety Consultant for the National Grocers Association, Senior Vice President for Food

Safety Programs at the Food Marketing Association (FMI), and Senior Vice President at SQF Institute. From 1978 to 1996, Hollingsworth served at the USDA, including in the capacity of Assistant Deputy Administrator for the Food Safety Inspection Service (FSIS).

Anna Jesus is the Vice President for Quality and Food Safety at Amy's Kitchen. Her impressive and diverse career in food safety includes work with Superior Foods Companies as their Director of Quality Assurance, Food Safety and Technical Services, Quality Director at ConAgra Foods, Senior Quality Manager at E&J Gallo Winery, Quality Assurance Supervisor at Dole Fresh Vegetables, Inc., and Quality Assurance Chemist at Cargill, Inc.

John Kobayashi, MD, MPH, is a Clinical Associate Professor at University of Washington. He served as the State Epidemiologist for Communicable Diseases at the Washington State Department of Health from 1982 to 2001. He directed large multistate foodborne outbreak investigations and trained over 25 Epidemic Intelligence Service Officers from the Centers for Disease Control. From 1997 to 2001, he was a member of the National Advisory Committee for Microbiological Standards for Foods. From 2001 to 2008, he was a long-term consultant for the Field Epidemiology Training Program at the National Institute for Infectious Diseases in Tokyo, Japan.

Nathan Libbey is a Sales Manager at CERTUS Food Safety. His previous companies include Cintas, Nestlé, and Dreyer's Grand Ice Cream. He earned a Master of Science in Regulatory Affairs of Food and Food Industries from Northeastern University's College of Professional Studies.

Lisa Lupo has more than 25 years' experience in business communications, newspapers, and magazines. She is currently the Editor of *QA Magazine* (Quality Assurance & Food Safety). Her previous capacities include Executive Vice President, Communications for the International Food Authenticity Assurance Organization, Marketing Communications for Ecolab, and Reporter for Suburban News Publications.

Valerie Madamba, JD, is the Senior Counsel, Regulatory Compliance and Government Affairs at Blue Apron. Her career includes teaching as an Adjunct Professor of Food Law at Brooklyn Law School, serving as Legal Counsel at Bayer, and Senior Associate Director for Drug Regulatory Affairs Advertising & Promotion at Novartis. As Assistant Chief Counsel at the FDA, Madamba provided legal counsel to Center for Food Safety and

Applied Nutrition (CFSAN) and agency leadership on developing, interpreting, and applying regulatory requirements related to foods and dietary supplements.

Bill Marler, JD, is the managing partner of Marler Clark, a Seattle, WA, based law firm that specializes in foodborne illness cases. Marler's advocacy for a safer food supply includes petitioning the USDA to better regulate *E. coli*, working with nonprofit food safety and foodborne illness victims' organizations, and helping spur the passage of the 2010–11 FDA Food Safety Modernization Act. His work has led to invitations to address local, national, and international gatherings on food safety, including testimony before the US House of Representatives Committee on Energy and Commerce. He speaks frequently before food industry groups, associations, and public health groups about the litigation of claims resulting from outbreaks of pathogenic bacteria and viruses and the issues surrounding it. He is the publisher of *Food Safety News*, one of the most respected and recognized sources of information in the industry. In 2010, NSF presented Bill their Food Safety Leadership Award for Education.

Gina McCarthy is Professor of the Practice of Public Health in the Department of Environmental Health at Harvard University and the Director of the Center for Climate, Health, and the Global Environment. She served as the Administrator of the EPA under the Obama Administration from 2013 to 2017. Her tenure as EPA Administrator heralded a paradigm shift in national environmental policy, expressly linking it with global public health. McCarthy has been a leading advocate for common-sense strategies to protect public health and the environment for more than 30 years.

Ann Marie McNamara, PhD, is the former Director of Microbiology, USDA, Food Safety and Inspection Service, Office of Public Health and Science during the Jack in the Box outbreak. She has worked in all areas of food safety: in the government, in manufacturing as Vice President of Food Safety and Technology at *Sara Lee Corporation*, in research/consulting as Vice President of Food Safety and Scientific Affairs at *Silliker, Inc.*, in foodservice as Vice President of Food Safety and Regulatory Affairs at *Jack in the Box, Inc.*, in retail as Vice President of Food and Essentials Safety and Quality Assurance at *Target Corp.*, and in Foodservice and Manufacturing as Vice President of Food Safety and Quality Assurance at *US Foods*. For her work in investigating the Jack in the Box outbreak, Dr. McNamara and her team won a Superior Service Award from the Secretary of Agriculture. Among her honors and awards, she was the recipient of five USDA Superior Service awards including recognition as a coauthor of the USDA Pathogen Reduction/HACCP regulation, and most recently accepted the Food Marketing Institute's Food Safety Innovation Award on behalf of target for the development and implementation of a health inspection management program supported by *Hazel Analytics* automated analysis platform. In 2014, Dr. McNamara received the International Association for Food Protection's Distinguished Service Award (sponsored by Food Safety Magazine). In 2018, she delivered the annual John H. Silliker Lecture at the International Association for Food Protection's meeting in Salt Lake City, UT.

Brad McNamara is the CEO and Cofounder of Freight Farms, Inc., an agricultural technology company that creates tools for a more sustainable and connected food system. McNamara previously worked with the New England Clean Energy Council to evaluate and implement project management software. He is also the Cofounder of United Hydroponics, Inc., that focused on effective and innovative solutions in urban rooftop hydroponic food production.

Sean O'Leary is the Chief Executive Officer at FoodLogiQ. O'Leary has 25 years of experience in the technology industry, building and scaling highly efficient, effective, and successful SaaS companies. Prior to his most recent role as CEO of Atlanta-based Synthio, O'Leary served as President and CEO of KnowledgeTree, Inc., President and CEO of StrikeIron, and held senior executive-level positions at Motorola, Good Technology and Cisco Systems.

Stephen Ostroff, MD, served as the FDA's Deputy Commissioner for Foods and Veterinary Medicine from May 2016 until December 2018. Dr. Ostroff served as the acting FDA Commissioner from April 2015 to late February 2016 and again from January to May 2017. Previously, his FDA capacities include Chief Scientist, the Chief Medical Officer in the Center for Food Safety and Applied Nutrition, and Senior Public Health Advisor to FDA's Office of Foods and Veterinary Medicine. Prior to the FDA, Ostroff served as the CDC's Deputy Director of the National Center for Infectious Diseases at the Centers. He retired from the Commissioned Corps of the US Public Health Service at the rank of Rear Admiral (Assistant Surgeon General). Dr. Ostroff was also the Director of the Bureau of Epidemiology and Acting Physician General for the Commonwealth of Pennsylvania.

Kevin Otto is the Senior Director for Community Engagement at GS1 US, where he leads their cross-industry blockchain efforts bringing together stakeholders from various industries. He also manages the Foodservice GS1 US Standards Initiative. His previous roles include Customer Supply Chain Manager and Supply Chain Analyst at Unilever.

Patrick Quade is the Founder and CEO of Dinesafe, where he leads business development initiatives, seeking out companies and organizations to partner with. Quade brings the intelligence generated by the crowdsourced foodborne illness surveillance platform—Iwaspoisoned.com—to wider audiences to help advance public health and industry.

Tanya Roberts, PhD, is the Chair of the Board of Directors at the Center for Foodborne Illness Research and Prevention. She retired from the USDA as a Senior Economist after 33 years of research and publishing. Roberts is the editor of "Food Safety Economics: Incentives for a Safer Food Supply" (2018). Roberts is also the recipient of the International Association for Food Protection's Ewen C.D. Todd Control of Foodborne Illness Award, recognizing an individual for dedicated and exceptional contributions to the reduction of risks of foodborne illness.

Joseph Robertson is the Global Strategy Director for the nonpartisan nonprofit Citizens' Climate Lobby where he supports the coordination of their citizen engagement groups in Africa, Asia, Europe, Latin America, and Oceania, which leads the Citizens' Climate Engagement Network and represents the organization in the Carbon Pricing Leadership Coalition, UNFCCC negotiations, and other UN processes. He is a member of the Executive Board of the NGO Committee on Sustainable Development-NY and of the Policy and Strategy Group for the World We Want. He is also the founder of Geoversiv.net and the Geoversiv Foundation and the lead strategist supporting the high-level climate dialogue series: Accelerating Progress, Advancing Innovation.

Brian Ronholm is the Senior Director of Regulatory Policy at the law firm of Wilson Sonsini Goodrich & Rosati in Washington, DC. From 2011 to 2017, Ronholm served as the USDA's Deputy Under Secretary for Food Safety. His previous positions included Agriculture Appropriations Associate for US House of Representatives—Office of Rep. Rosa L. DeLauro.

Index

C

D

G

Kolibri 360 GmbH
Ferdinand-Jühlke-Straße 7
99095 Erfurt, Deutschland
produktsicherheit@kolibri360.de